ASBESTOS

SELECTED CANCERS

Committee on Asbestos: Selected Health Effects

Board on Population Health and Public Health Practices

INSTITUTE OF MEDICINE

OF THE NATIONAL ACADEMIES

THE NATIONAL ACADEMIES PRESS
Washington, D.C.
www.nap.edu

THE NATIONAL ACADEMIES PRESS 500 Fifth Street, NW Washington, DC 20001

NOTICE: The project that is the subject of this report was approved by the Governing Board of the National Research Council, whose members are drawn from the councils of the National Academy of Sciences, the National Academy of Engineering, and the Institute of Medicine. The members of the committee responsible for the report were chosen for their special competences and with regard for appropriate balance.

This study was supported by Contract N01-OD-4-2139 between the National Academy of Sciences and the National Institutes of Health. Any opinions, findings, conclusions, or recommendations expressed in this publication are those of the author(s) and do not necessarily reflect the view of the organizations or agencies that provided support for this project.

International Standard Book Number 0-309-10169-7 (Book)
International Standard Book Number 0-309-65952-3 (PDF)

Library of Congress Control Number: 2006928950

Additional copies of this report are available from the National Academies Press, 500 Fifth Street, NW, Lockbox 285, Washington, DC 20055; (800) 624-6242 or (202) 334-3313 (in the Washington metropolitan area); Internet, http://www.nap.edu.

For more information about the Institute of Medicine, visit the IOM home page at: **www.iom.edu.**

Printed in the United States of America.

The serpent has been a symbol of long life, healing, and knowledge among almost all cultures and religions since the beginning of recorded history. The serpent adopted as a logotype by the Institute of Medicine is a relief carving from ancient Greece, now held by the Staatliche Museen in Berlin.

"Knowing is not enough; we must apply.
Willing is not enough; we must do."

—Goethe

INSTITUTE OF MEDICINE

OF THE NATIONAL ACADEMIES

Advising the Nation. Improving Health.

THE NATIONAL ACADEMIES

Advisers to the Nation on Science, Engineering, and Medicine

The **National Academy of Sciences** is a private, nonprofit, self-perpetuating society of distinguished scholars engaged in scientific and engineering research, dedicated to the furtherance of science and technology and to their use for the general welfare. Upon the authority of the charter granted to it by the Congress in 1863, the Academy has a mandate that requires it to advise the federal government on scientific and technical matters. Dr. Ralph J. Cicerone is president of the National Academy of Sciences.

The **National Academy of Engineering** was established in 1964, under the charter of the National Academy of Sciences, as a parallel organization of outstanding engineers. It is autonomous in its administration and in the selection of its members, sharing with the National Academy of Sciences the responsibility for advising the federal government. The National Academy of Engineering also sponsors engineering programs aimed at meeting national needs, encourages education and research, and recognizes the superior achievements of engineers. Dr. Wm. A. Wulf is president of the National Academy of Engineering.

The **Institute of Medicine** was established in 1970 by the National Academy of Sciences to secure the services of eminent members of appropriate professions in the examination of policy matters pertaining to the health of the public. The Institute acts under the responsibility given to the National Academy of Sciences by its congressional charter to be an adviser to the federal government and, upon its own initiative, to identify issues of medical care, research, and education. Dr. Harvey V. Fineberg is president of the Institute of Medicine.

The **National Research Council** was organized by the National Academy of Sciences in 1916 to associate the broad community of science and technology with the Academy's purposes of furthering knowledge and advising the federal government. Functioning in accordance with general policies determined by the Academy, the Council has become the principal operating agency of both the National Academy of Sciences and the National Academy of Engineering in providing services to the government, the public, and the scientific and engineering communities. The Council is administered jointly by both Academies and the Institute of Medicine. Dr. Ralph J. Cicerone and Dr. Wm. A. Wulf are chair and vice chair, respectively, of the National Research Council.

www.national-academies.org

COMMITTEE ON ASBESTOS: SELECTED HEALTH EFFECTS

Jonathan M. Samet, M.D., M.S. (*Chair*), Professor and Chairman, Department of Epidemiology, Bloomberg School of Public Health, Johns Hopkins University, Baltimore, Maryland

Lonnie R. Bristow, M.D., Private Practice and Former President of American Medical Association, Walnut Creek, California

Harvey Checkoway, Ph.D., M.P.H., Professor, Department of Environmental and Occupational Health Sciences, University of Washington, Seattle

Paul Demers, Ph.D., M.Sc., Associate Professor, Department of Health Care and Epidemiology, University of British of Columbia, Vancouver

Ellen A. Eisen, M.S., Sc.D., Adjunct Professor, Department of Environmental Health, Harvard School of Public Health, Boston, Massachusetts

George D. Guthrie, Jr., Ph.D., M.A., Geology and Chemistry Group, Los Alamos National Laboratory, Los Alamos, New Mexico

Rogene F. Henderson, Ph.D., D.A.B.T., Senior Scientist, Lovelace Respiratory Research Institute, Albuquerque, New Mexico

Joseph W. Hogan, Sc.D., Associate Professor, Biostatistics Section and Center for Statistical Sciences Department of Community Health, Brown University, Providence, Rhode Island

Agnes B. Kane, M.D., Ph.D., Professor, Department of Pathology and Laboratory Medicine, Brown University, Providence, Rhode Island

Fadlo R. Khuri, M.D., Professor, Winship Cancer Institute, Emory University School of Medicine, Atlanta, Georgia

Roberta B. Ness, M.D., M.P.H., Chair and Professor, Department of Epidemiology, University of Pittsburgh, Pennsylvania

Michael J. Thun, M.D., M.S., Vice President, Epidemiology and Surveillance Research, American Cancer Society, Atlanta, Georgia

Assistants with Graphical Data

Li Su, Graduate Research Assistant in Biostatistics, Department of Community Health, Brown University

Yunxia Sui, Graduate Research Assistant in Biostatistics, Department of Community Health, Brown University

Staff

Mary Burr Paxton, Study Director

Rose Marie Martinez, Director, Board on Population Health and Public Health Practice

Michael Schneider, Senior Program Associate
Tia S. Carter, Senior Program Assistant
Norman Grossblatt, Senior Editor

Reviewers

This report has been reviewed in draft form by persons chosen for their diverse perspectives and technical expertise in accordance with procedures approved by the National Research Council's Report Review Committee. The purpose of this independent review is to provide candid and critical comments that will assist the institution in making its published report as sound as possible and to ensure that the report meets institutional standards of objectivity, evidence, and responsiveness to the study charge. The review comments and draft manuscript remain confidential to protect the integrity of the deliberative process. We wish to thank the following for their review of this report:

John C. Bailar, Professor Emeritus, University of Chicago, Illinois
Peter R. Buseck, Professor, Department of Geological Sciences and Department of Chemistry and Biochemistry, Arizona State University, Phoenix
Robert G. Coleman, Professor Emeritus, Stanford University, Atherton, California
Arthur Frank, Professor and Chair, Department of Environmental and Occupational Health, School of Public Health, Drexel University, Philadelphia, Pennsylvania
Robert F. Herrick, Lecturer, Department of Environmental Health, Harvard School of Public Health, Boston, Massachusetts
Karl T. Kelsey, Professor, Departments of Cancer Cell Biology and Environmental Health, Harvard School of Public Health, Boston, Massachusetts

Alfred I. Neugut, Program Director, Cancer Epidemiology and Control, Division of Epidemiology, Mailman School of Public Health, Columbia University, New York
H. Catherine Skinner, Research Affiliate and Lecturer, Department of Geology and Geophysics, Yale University, New Haven, Connecticut
Mark Utell, Professor, Departments of Medicine and of Environmental Medicine and Critical Care Division, University of Rochester, New York
Gerald van Belle, Professor, Department of Environmental and Occupational Health Sciences, University of Washington, Seattle
David Wegman, Dean, Health and Environment, University of Massachusetts, Lowell
Noel S. Weiss, Professor, Department of Epidemiology, University of Washington, Seattle

Although the reviewers listed above have provided many constructive comments and suggestions, they were not asked to endorse the conclusions or recommendations nor did they see the final draft of the report before its release. The review of this report was overseen by **Paul D. Stolley,** University of Maryland, School of Medicine, Baltimore, and by **Edward B. Perrin,** University of Washington, Seattle. Appointed by the National Research Council and Institute of Medicine, they were responsible for making certain that an independent examination of this report was carried out in accordance with institutional procedures and that all review comments were carefully considered. Responsibility for the final content of this report rests entirely with the authoring committee and the institution.

Contents

APPENDIXES

Summary

INTRODUCTION

The use of asbestos in many products surged during the 20th century, and asbestos exposure continues despite a sharp reduction in production since the 1980s. Asbestos is an established cause of mesothelioma, an uncommon cancer that arises in the mesothelial cells lining the chest and abdominal cavities, and of lung cancer. It also causes nonmalignant respiratory diseases, including asbestosis, a fibrotic disorder of the lung. In addition, the findings of some epidemiologic studies of asbestos-exposed workers have suggested that exposure to asbestos may increase risk of other cancers. This Institute of Medicine committee was charged with evaluating the evidence relevant to the causation of cancers of the pharynx, larynx, esophagus, stomach, colon, and rectum by asbestos and with judging whether the evidence is sufficient to infer a causal association. The specific charge follows:

> The Institute of Medicine's (IOM) Board on Population Health and Public Health Practices will oversee a study that will comprehensively review, evaluate, and summarize the peer-reviewed scientific and medical literature regarding the association between asbestos and colorectal, laryngeal, esophageal, pharyngeal, and stomach cancers. Based on its examination and evaluation of the extant literature and other information it may obtain in the course of the study, the committee will determine if there is a causal association between asbestos and colorectal, laryngeal, esophageal, pharyngeal, or stomach cancers.

The committee's charge was drawn directly from Senate Bill 852, the Fairness in Asbestos Injury Resolution (FAIR) Act.

COMMITTEE APPROACH

To address the charge, a multidisciplinary committee was appointed by IOM that included experts in biostatistics, epidemiology, mineralogy, oncology, toxicology, and cancer biology. The committee interpreted its charge as requiring a comprehensive and systematic review of evidence on the cancer risk posed by asbestos at the specified sites in humans and in experimental animals. The committee also identified a need to review evidence related to the biologic plausibility of a causal association between asbestos and cancer at the designated sites. Relevant issues included the doses of asbestos fibers reaching the organs, persistence of fibers at the sites, potential interactions with target cells, and plausible mechanisms of carcinogenesis by asbestos fibers at the sites.

The committee was aware that fiber type may be a determinant of risk of developing mesothelioma (and possibly lung cancer) following asbestos exposure. The committee considered whether it should evaluate asbestos-associated risk for the designated cancers in terms of exposure to specific fiber types. In light of the almost universally mixed nature of actual occupational exposure, however, there was not sufficient evidence to have carried out such a review for the selected cancer sites. Consequently, the committee's report describes the level of causal inference in relation to asbestos, without specifying the type.

Accordingly, the committee undertook a systematic review of the available human and toxicologic evidence, setting up a uniform approach for reviewing the full body of relevant epidemiological literature and for abstracting and synthesizing study results. The epidemiologic evidence comes from cohort (follow-up) studies of occupationally exposed persons and from case-control studies of the cancers that assessed occupational exposures as risk factors. The cohort studies generally addressed cancer mortality, and the case-control studies mostly considered incident cases. The studies were further classified by the method of exposure assessment. The results of the studies were then abstracted into a database for descriptive analysis and summary with the technique of quantitative meta-analysis. The units of input for the meta-analysis on each selected cancer site were the most comprehensive risk estimates available on discrete study populations, so a single citation might generate more than one datum (such as separate results for men and women), whereas only the final follow-up results would be used for a series of publications on the same occupational cohort. The meta-analysis on each dataset yielded a summary estimate of cancer risk at the anatomical site associated with asbestos exposure with a confidence interval that accounts for sampling variation within each study and for variation in relative risk among studies. The committee also reviewed the toxicologic literature and the extensive experimental literature on carcinogenesis by asbestos fibers. It addressed the mineralogic and chemical characteristics of asbestos for their relevance to carcinogenicity in the organs of interest. The committee consulted experts on those topics through presentations at its meetings.

Because the committee's charge requires a determination of whether asbestos causes cancer at the specific sites, the committee considered various guidelines for causal inference and terminology for classifying the strength of evidence in support of causation. Its review of approaches led to the uniform application of guidelines for causal inference based on the widely applied criteria or guidelines proposed by Austin Bradford Hill and the similar criteria long used in the reports of the US surgeon general on smoking and health. The criteria for causal inference include consistency, strength of association, temporality, and the coherence or plausibility of the association. The committee selected a four-level classification of the strength of evidence for causal inference, classifying the evidence as *sufficient*, *suggestive*, or *inadequate* to infer causality or suggestive of *no causal association*. For the purpose of its charge, designating an association of asbestos with cancers of the designated sites as causal, the committee required the evidence to reach the level of *sufficient*.

The topic of asbestos and cancer has many facets, including the influence of fiber type on risk and the interactions of asbestos with other factors that produce cancer at the same sites, such as tobacco-smoking for cancer of the larynx. The committee did not consider the issue of fiber type, which was not included in its charge; it did consider information on the combined effect of asbestos with other risk factors when such information was available. The committee also did not attempt to quantify the risk of cancers at the selected sites in relation to magnitude of exposure—a potentially extensive effort that was also beyond its charge.

COMMITTEE FINDINGS

The committee reviewed the evidence from epidemiologic studies and from toxicologic investigations, both animal and in vitro, specifically for each cancer site. The reviews of the evidence related to mineralogy of asbestos and to its carcinogenicity were considered to be generally relevant for all sites, particularly in regard to the causal criterion of coherence or biologic plausibility.

There has been ongoing discussion as to whether there is an absolute difference in the toxicity of the major fiber types, serpentine and amphibole, and whether only amphibole fibers have carcinogenic potential, particularly for mesothelioma, the neoplasm for which the evidence is most suggestive of a difference in risk by fiber type. Recent reviews suggest that, rather than having no carcinogenic activity, chrysotile has a generally lesser degree of potency than amphibole fiber and that the various types of amphibole fiber have differing potency in the extent of their biological activity. With regard to fiber characteristics, the committee noted that several physical and chemical factors may contribute to a mineral particle's potential to induce a pathogenic response. These characteristics differ for serpentine (or chrysotile) and amphibole fibers and may be relevant to their relative carcinogenicity. Many of the properties would be expected to influence how a mineral interacts with biologic fluids under the conditions in the various organs under consideration. Although these properties have been investigated in simplified systems and their potential relevance in processes in natural environments is clear, their roles in mineral-induced pathogenesis of cancer or other diseases have not been extensively studied in the integrated context of whole animals. Size and shape are relevant because they determine site of deposition and also influence interactions with cells. Dissolution may also be relevant because it removes the fibers, but introduces the materials in the fibers, such as metals, into the surrounding fluid with the potential for interaction with target cells. Surface-induced oxidation-reduction is another catalytic pathway that may contribute to carcinogenesis. Ion exchange between the surfaces of the fibers and the surrounding liquid may affect neighboring cells. How these factors play out in terms of producing disease in humans under conditions of real occupational exposure, however, has not been fully studied.

Although there has been little systematic investigation of dispersion of asbestos fibers to extrapulmonary tissues, they do reach the organs covered by the charge. Inhaled materials deposit throughout the respiratory tract, which extends from the nose and mouth to the alveoli, the lung's air sacs. The sites of deposition vary by fiber size; inhaled fibers pass through the pharynx and larynx with the possibility of deposition there. Fibers deposited in the lung are cleared by the mucociliary apparatus, and swallowing of asbestos-containing mucus causes it to pass through the gastrointestinal tract and can lead to potential exposure of the esophagus, stomach, colon, and rectum to asbestos fibers. Encapsulated fibers, known as asbestos bodies, are routinely found in the respiratory tissues of asbestos-exposed individuals; although they have not been systematically sought in other organs, there have been some reports of finding asbestos bodies in extrapulmonary tissues, including the portions of the gastrointestinal tract addressed in this report.

The biologic effects of asbestos fibers depend on their physicochemical properties, dimensions, and deposition and persistence at target sites. On the basis of rodent models of lung cancer and malignant mesothelioma, fiber carcinogenicity is correlated with increased cell proliferation, inflammation, and fibrosis in the lungs and pleura. Several mechanisms have been proposed for the biologic activity of asbestos fibers observed in vitro and in animal models. Long asbestos fibers that are incompletely phagocytized stimulate production of reactive oxygen species that induce DNA damage, oxidant stress, and activation of cell-signaling pathways and lead to cell proliferation. Long asbestos fibers have been shown to interfere physically with the mitotic apparatus and produce chromosomal damage, especially deletions. Asbestos fibers may also directly produce physical injury of target cells and tissues that is repaired by compensatory hyperplasia. There is strong epidemiologic and experimental evidence that asbestos fibers and cigarette smoke are cofactors in the development of lung cancer. Other potential cofactors in malignant mesothelioma are chronic inflammation and viruses (such as SV40). The applicability of these direct and indirect mechanisms of asbestos carcinogenesis to cancers that develop at extrapulmonary sites considered in this report is uncertain.

The committee considered animal-bioassay studies in which animals were administered asbestos by inhalation and the occurrence of cancer was measured. Many studies of that general design have been carried out, but they were directed largely at investigating cancer of the lung and mesothelioma, so only those with comprehensive histopathologic examinations were considered relevant. Among the more limited number of studies with oral administration, the committee found several involving exposure of animals to asbestos fibers mixed into their food particularly relevant. However, the utility of these models for the sites of concern is uncertain.

In addressing its charge, the committee considered both general evidence related to carcinogenicity and site-specific epidemiologic evidence. The committee's reviews and conclusions by site are summarized below. In the following, the relative risk (RR) quantifies the risk of cancer among those exposed to asbestos relative to those not exposed. An RR greater than 1.0 indicates that estimated risk was higher among people who have been exposed, and an RR less than 1.0 indicates that estimated risk was lower among those exposed. An RR of 1.0, sometimes referred to as the null value, corresponds to equal risk in the two groups. The confidence interval (CI) at a given "level of significance" provides an indication of statistical uncertainty.

Pharyngeal Cancer

The committee reviewed six case-control studies of pharyngeal cancer, four of which had exposure assessments of high quality or adjusted for confounding, and the findings on 16 cohort populations. Although the information from the case-control studies was very sparse, the aggregated risk estimate for any asbestos exposure was modest and similar to that for the more numerous cohort studies. The available data did not suggest the presence of a dose-response relationship. In considering the plausibility of a causal association between asbestos exposure and pharyngeal cancer, the committee noted that the epithelium of the oropharynx and hypopharynx differs from that of the respiratory epithelium, although squamous-cell cancers predominate among tumors of the pharynx. The combination of asbestos exposure and tobacco-smoking is an established risk factor for lung cancer, but for pharyngeal cancer only a single case-control study has addressed asbestos exposure as a cofactor with tobacco-smoking. No increase in pharyngeal tumors has been observed in animals exposed chronically to asbestos either by inhalation or by oral feeding.

Although several cohort studies and the larger, better-designed case-control studies suggest an association between asbestos exposure and pharyngeal cancer and asbestos, overall the epidemiologic evidence is limited and biological plausibility has some uncertainty for this site. *Consequently, the committee concluded that the evidence is **suggestive but not sufficient** to infer a causal relationship between asbestos exposure and pharyngeal cancer.*

Laryngeal Cancer

The evidence base for asbestos exposure and laryngeal cancer included more case-control studies (18) than were available for other cancer sites considered by the committee, and the number of cohort populations (35) was similar to the number informative for stomach or colorectal cancer. Subjects in the studies had been exposed to asbestos in a wide array of industries and occupations in North America, South America, Europe, and Japan. Many of the case-control studies collected data that permitted confounding by tobacco-smoking and alcohol consumption to be addressed. Several case-control studies examined the association between asbestos exposure and laryngeal cancer, stratifying on tobacco use, which might potentially interact with or modify the association of asbestos exposure with risk of laryngeal cancer. The committee also reviewed four experimental studies in which rodents were exposed over much of their lifetime to high concentrations of asbestos through inhalation.

The committee found consistency of findings among the epidemiologic studies. Asbestos exposure was associated with increased risk of laryngeal cancer in the nine larger cohort studies and in meta-analyses of the cohort and case-control data. Some evidence of a dose-response relationship was seen in both the cohort and case-control studies. There was no consistent evidence of confounding in case-control studies that reported both age- and multivariate-adjusted RR estimates, and the two studies stratified on asbestos exposure and smoking status suggest synergism between the two factors.

The committee found several bases for considering that asbestos could plausibly cause laryngeal cancer. The larynx, like the lung, is anatomically in the direct path of inhaled asbestos fibers. Inflammation or damage to the vocal cords could disrupt laminar airflow and predispose to the deposition and accumulation of asbestos fibers in the larynx. Squamous-cell carcinomas of the lung and larynx exhibit certain histologic and clinical similarities; cancers at both sites arise from the respiratory epithelium in regions of squamous metaplasia and dysplasia. Tobacco-smoking is the most important risk factor for both sites, and asbestos exposure is an established cause of lung cancer. Tobacco-smoking may lead to laryngeal damage and increased potential for asbestos fibers to deposit in the trachea. Alcohol consumption is also a recognized risk factor for laryngeal cancer, with heavy consumption synergizing markedly with smoking. Together with smoking and drinking, accumulation of asbestos fibers could produce chronic irritation or inflammation, accelerating the progression of neoplasia. However, no clinical data document the accumulation and persistence of asbestos fibers in the larynx, and there is a lack of experimental support from animal studies.

Considering all the evidence, the committee placed greater weight on the consistency of the epidemiologic studies and the biologic plausibility of the hypothesis than on the lack of confirmatory evidence from animal studies or documentation of fiber persistence in the larynx. *The committee concluded that the evidence is **sufficient** to infer a causal relationship between asbestos exposure and laryngeal cancer.*

Esophageal Cancer

Both case-control and cohort studies of esophageal cancer were reviewed, but the available body of evidence was limited. Only three case-control studies met the criteria for inclusion, so there were too few for meta-analysis. There were more cohort populations with relevant results, although the number of cases was often small. The mortality studies did not distinguish between histologic subtypes; if there were specific asbestos-subtype associations, the overall grouping of esophageal cancers would tend to obscure them. In assessing biologic plausibility, the histologic type of cancer, potential dose to the target tissues, and possible mechanisms were considered.

The three case-control studies did not have consistent results, and the number of exposed cases was generally small. Two incorporated adjustment for tobacco-smoking and alcohol consumption. One observed a small excess risk but did not find evidence of a dose-response relationship, and the other found no evidence of an excess. A third, older study found an excess, but it was based on a single case, and so was difficult to interpret. Few cohort studies presented data explicitly on esophageal cancer, because of the rarity of the disease, and their statistical precision was often low. The results for the 25 cohort populations with information on esophageal cancer were mixed. The summary RR computed from the cohort studies was 0.99 (95% CI 0.78-1.27). Although some studies did observe excess risks, overall there was little consistency in the epidemiologic data. Six animal-feeding studies did not find an association with esophageal cancer, and there is no other experimental evidence that asbestos fibers act as a direct or indirect carcinogen specifically in the esophagus.

Some studies have found an association between asbestos exposure and esophageal cancer, but the overall results of epidemiologic studies are mixed. In addition, what little evidence there is from animal experiments about asbestos's carcinogenic potential specifically on esophageal tissues does not support biological activity at this site. *The committee concluded that the evidence is* ***inadequate*** *to infer the presence or absence of a causal relationship between asbestos exposure and esophageal cancer.*

Stomach Cancer

In its final dataset, the committee considered 42 occupational cohorts and five population-based case-control studies that provided data on stomach cancer risk. Overall, the occupational cohorts consistently, although not uniformly, suggested risks increased above risks in the general population (RR = 1.17, 95% CI 1.07-1.28). The results of case-control studies were less consistent (RR = 1.11, 95% CI 0.76-1.64), and suggested neither increased nor lower-than-expected risks associated with asbestos. Considering just the cohort studies, the committee noted that observed risk increases were modest. There were also somewhat consistent patterns supportive of dose-response relations, although trends were not especially strong. Six lifetime feeding studies of asbestos in rodents provided no evidence that asbestos fibers act as a direct or indirect carcinogen in the stomach.

The most frequent histologic type of stomach cancer in western countries is adenocarcinoma, which is most commonly associated with *Helicobacter pylori* infection and inflammation. Tobacco-smoking is also a risk factor for stomach adenocarcinoma. The potential role of asbestos fibers as a cofactor with established risk factors has not been investigated experimentally or epidemiologically. Asbestos bodies have been identified in the stomach and in other sites in the gastrointestinal tract and in other organs. The possibility that asbestos fibers could accumulate at sites of mucosal injury and ulceration has not been explored. There is no experimental evidence from animal toxicology studies that asbestos fibers act as a direct or indirect carcinogen in the stomach.

Overall, the epidemiologic studies revealed fairly modest risk increases and somewhat fragmentary evidence of a dose-response relationship. Animal experimentation has not provided supportive evidence of causation, although the potential for asbestos fibers to accumulate at sites of stomach mucosal injury lends some mechanistic support to potential carcinogenesis. *The committee concluded that the evidence is* ***suggestive but not sufficient*** *to infer a causal relationship between asbestos exposure and stomach cancer.*

Colorectal Cancer

The committee evaluated the overall evidence on colorectal cancer because its charge addressed cancers of the colon and rectum together. The evidence thus included studies providing information on the two sites separately and studies reporting on colorectal cancer overall. Case-control studies of colon or rectal cancers included four studies in which the two outcomes were considered in a single category of colorectal cancer, six studies of only colon cancer, and one of only rectal cancer. In addition, 41 occupational cohorts were reviewed, almost all of which had the necessary information to derive a combined risk estimate for colon and rectal cancers.

There was some inconsistency among the 13 RRs reported from the case-control studies (aggregate RR = 1.16, 95% CI 0.90-1.49), and findings from many of the studies were inconclusive. Although most of the estimated RRs were greater than 1, two of the studies had lower estimated risks for those exposed to asbestos. The case-control study with the most detailed assessment and analysis of asbestos exposure did not find an association between exposure to asbestos and the risk of colorectal cancer. In contrast, the occupational-cohort studies more consistently, although not uniformly, suggested increased risks of colorectal cancer in exposed people than in the general population (RR = 1.15, 95% CI 1.01-1.31).

The summary estimate of association from the case-control studies was similar to that from the cohort studies, but the CI was wider, and evidence of a dose-response relationship in the case-control studies was lacking. The overall observed risk estimate from cohort studies was modestly increased, although it had 95% CI that just excluded 1.0 and some evidence of a dose-response relationship.

There was only limited information available relevant to biologic plausibility. Colorectal tumors in humans are most commonly adenocarcinomas that arise in polyps. Multiple risk factors are associated with colon cancer, including familial predisposition, age, obesity, physical inactivity, and inflammatory bowel disease. The potential role of asbestos fibers as a cofactor has not been investigated in epidemiologic or experimental studies. Asbestos bodies and asbestos fibers have been identified in the colon, including for a small cohort of asbestos workers who had colon cancer. Animal models have failed to produce colon or colorectal cancer, even in studies that involved high-dose feeding of asbestos to rodents. However, studies employing high-dose feeding of chrysotile asbestos to rats did produce benign adenomatous colonic polyps, a precursor to the most common form of colon cancer in humans.

The committee concluded that the evidence is ***suggestive but not sufficient*** *to infer a causal relationship between asbestos exposure and colorectal cancer.*

CLOSING COMMENTS

The committee was charged with reviewing evidence on a widely used material that is known to cause respiratory malignancy. Asbestos has been extensively investigated, epidemiologically and experimentally, as a cause of mesothelioma and lung cancer. However, its potential to cause malignancy at other sites that may also receive a substantial dose of asbestos fibers has not been as extensively investigated.

The committee considered the existing evidence from in vitro and animal experimentation to gain an understanding of mechanisms of carcinogenesis that might plausibly apply to the tissues in question and to determine the extent of toxicologic support for the development of cancers at the specified sites following asbestos exposure. Much of the information reviewed by the committee came from cohort studies of workers that focused on investigating respiratory effects and that reported information on risks of other diseases, including the cancers covered by this committee's charge, only incidentally. Other evidence came from case-control studies that were directed at the causes of the cancers of interest but that were not specifically designed to address asbestos exposure, and their exposure assessments were of varied quality.

Table S.1 provides a distillation of the committee's findings about whether asbestos is a causal factor for cancers at the five sites indicated for evaluation in the committee's charge and the FAIR legislation.

TABLE S.1 Causal Association Between Specified Cancer and Asbestos

Cancer	Evidence for Presence or Absence of Causal Relationship to Asbestos
Laryngeal	Sufficient
Pharyngeal	Suggestive but not sufficient
Stomach	Suggestive but not sufficient
Colorectal	Suggestive but not sufficient
Esophageal	Inadequate

The committee's review identified limitations of the available evidence and the resulting uncertainty in its conclusions. Although the committee was not charged with developing a research agenda to address the information gaps, its review indicated many research needs. Studies directed at doses of fibers received by organs other than the lung are needed; mechanistic studies directed at these organs could be a useful complement to work on respiratory carcinogenesis by asbestos fibers. Studies involving animal models with high risk of cancer at the designated sites might also be considered. Consideration should be given to approaches to strengthen the epidemiologic information on asbestos exposure and risk of cancer at the sites in the committee's charge. Information might be gained from further follow-up of some of the cohorts of asbestos-exposed workers; however, the committee is concerned that further study of these cohorts may be impossible because most were initiated decades ago and their records may not have been maintained. Some effort might be made to determine whether key cohorts could be followed up or new studies on potentially informative populations started.

1

Introduction

STATEMENT OF CHARGE

As contracted through the National Institutes of Health, the committee's charge reads:

> The Institute of Medicine (IOM) Board on Population Health and Public Health Practices will oversee a study that will comprehensively review, evaluate, and summarize the peer-reviewed scientific and medical literature regarding the association between asbestos and colorectal, laryngeal, esophageal, pharyngeal, and stomach cancers. Based on its examination and evaluation of the extant literature and other information it may obtain in the course of the study, the committee will determine if there is a causal association between asbestos and colorectal, laryngeal, esophageal, pharyngeal, or stomach cancers.

CURRENT LEGISLATION

The committee's charge to determine whether asbestos may play a causal role in the occurrence of cancer at the five specified sites was drawn directly from Senate Bill 852, the Fairness in Asbestos Injury Resolution (FAIR) Act. The bill would establish an industry-underwritten $140 billion trust fund for orderly compensation of people suffering health consequences of working with asbestos or of living in Libby, Montana. The legislation as reported out of the Senate Committee on the Judiciary (April 19, 2005) defines asbestos to include:

> (A) chrysotile; (B) amosite; (C) crocidolite; (D) tremolite asbestos; (E) winchite asbestos; (F) richterite asbestos; (G) anthophyllite asbestos; (H) actinolite as-

> bestos; (I) asbestiform amphibole minerals; (J) any of the minerals listed under subparagraphs (A) through (I) that has been chemically treated or altered, and any asbestiform variety, type, or component thereof; and (K) asbestos-containing material, such as asbestos-containing products, automotive or industrial parts or components, equipment, improvements to real property, and any other material that contains asbestos in any physical or chemical form.

People who have a diagnosis of asbestosis, lung cancer, or mesothelioma will be eligible to file a claim documenting their asbestos exposure. Eligibility may also be extended to any additional cancers that are found to be causally associated with asbestos by the report of the present IOM expert committee delineated as item (e) under Subtitle C, Section 121—Medical criteria. The IOM report will be binding on the administrator and the physicians' panel that processes claims against the trust fund. The pending legislation was reported out of the Committee on the Judiciary on June 16, 2005, and was expected to be voted on early in 2006.

Asbestos fibers are known to be carcinogenic. The uniqueness and completeness of the carcinogenic activity of asbestos in mesothelial tissues is clear and undisputed. Most cases of mesothelioma are attributable to asbestos exposure. The role of asbestos in producing lung cancer, particularly in smokers, is also clear. Cancers at the sites included in the charge are largely of epithelial origin, so the underlying causal mechanism would be expected to be similar to that of lung cancer. Inasmuch as the determination of asbestos (in its various forms) as a human carcinogen is long established on the basis of findings of epidemiologic investigations and supportive animal and in vitro studies, this committee viewed its charge to be a more focused evaluation of whether asbestos causes cancer in particular organs. "Biologic plausibility" has been shown for asbestos' carcinogenic potential in general, so this committee's criteria for site-specific causality will differ somewhat from the determinations of whether an agent is a generic human carcinogen, as conducted by the International Agency for Research on Cancer and the US Environmental Protection Agency, for example.

OVERVIEW OF PATTERNS OF ASBESTOS USE AND RECOGNITION OF ITS HEALTH CONSEQUENCES

The physical and chemical properties of minerals classified as asbestos (see Chapter 3) have led to widespread applications of these fibrous substances beginning as long as 2,000 years ago. Those properties include heat stability and fire resistance, thermal and electric insulation, resistance to wear and friction, tensile strength and weavability, and resistance to chemical and biologic degradation (HHS 2004). Uses of asbestos burgeoned as the modern industrial era gained momentum in the 1880s, and industrial consumption peaked in the United States in 1973 (Virta 2002). The gradual recognition that this useful substance was associated with the occurrence of serious health consequences led to increasingly strict curtailment of asbestos's industrial use, but the epidemic of asbestos-caused disease is far from over. Because of the sustained period over which millions of workers were exposed to asbestos in mining, production, and construction and the decades-long latent period of development of asbestos-caused diseases, new cases of these debilitating and often fatal consequences of exposure will continue to be diagnosed for many years to come.

A number of adverse health outcomes are now causally associated with exposure to asbestos. An approximate timeline for recognition of the adverse consequences is provided in this section, as drawn from published sources. The first to be recognized was asbestosis, a pneumoconiosis characterized by fibrosis of the lung and reduction of lung function (Table 1.1), first reported as early as 1907 (Hamilton and Hardy 1974, as cited in Becklake 1976). Iron-coated fibers, called asbestos bodies, are typically found in the tissues of affected lungs. Mesothelioma, an uncommon tumor of the pleural and peritoneal mesothelium (tissues lining the thoracic and abdominal cavities and the organs in them), was linked to asbestos in the early 1960s in clinical case reports, and the increased risk was then further shown in cohort studies of asbestos workers. In the 1950s, epidemiologic studies documented the association of lung cancer with asbestos exposure, and the risk was found to be particularly increased in exposed workers who smoked. As worker cohorts were followed and their cancer risks were tracked, concern arose that asbestos might cause other types of cancers. Complementary information on these cancer sites was reported from studies that assessed site-specific cancer risk in relation to occupational exposures in general; asbestos exposure was specifically addressed in many of these case-control studies. The epidemiologic information is further complemented by an extensive toxicologic literature that includes animal bioassays and investigation of mechanisms of disease production. Since the first rec-

TABLE 1.1 Timeframe for Recognition of Various Health Effects Associated with Asbestos Exposure

Health Effect	Suspected	Probable	Established
Asbestosis	~ 1900	~ 1915	~ 1930
Lung cancer	~ 1930	~ 1945	~ 1955
Mesothelioma	~ 1940	~ 1955	~ 1965
Other cancers	~ 1955	~ 1970	?

SOURCE: Becklake (1976), Liddell (1997), Ross and Nolan (2003).

ognition that asbestos can cause cancer in humans, experimental studies have revealed multiple mechanisms that may contribute to asbestos-related diseases.

COMMITTEE'S APPROACH TO ITS CHARGE

The extensive literature related to the carcinogenic potential of asbestos, including a substantial body of epidemiologic studies plus numerous toxicologic and mechanistic studies, had to be considered in defining the portion relevant to the committee's charge. The committee interpreted its charge as requiring a comprehensive and systematic review of existing evidence on asbestos-related cancer risk at the specified sites in humans and in experimental animals. Accordingly, the committee undertook a systematic review of the available evidence, setting up a uniform approach for reviewing the literature and for abstracting and synthesizing study results. Because the committee's charge requires a determination of whether asbestos "causes" cancer at the specific sites, the committee considered various guidelines for causal inference and the terminology for classifying the strength of evidence in support of causation. That review led to the application of guidelines for causal inference based on the widely applied criteria proposed by Hill (1965) and similar criteria used in the reports of the US surgeon general on smoking and health (HEW 1964, HHS 2004). The committee selected a four-level classification of the strength of evidence for causal inference: sufficient, suggestive but not sufficient, inadequate, and suggestive of no relationship. In addition to searching the published literature systematically, the committee invited experts in several relevant fields to make presentations and provide background information, as indicated in the agendas for open sessions presented in Appendix A.

The topic of asbestos and cancer has many facets, including the influence of fiber type on risk and the interactions of asbestos with other factors that produce cancer at the same sites, such as tobacco-smoking as a cause of cancer of the larynx. The committee did not consider the issue of fiber type, which was not included in its charge; it did consider information on the combined effect of asbestos with other risk factors when such information was available. The committee did not attempt to quantify the risk of cancers at the selected sites; that potentially extensive effort was also beyond the charge.

The committee took into account the limitations of the available epidemiologic information, a key component of the evidence reviewed. The epidemiologic characteristics of the cancers to be investigated (pharyngeal, laryngeal, esophageal, stomach, and colorectal) were considered, including incidence and mortality, survival, and risk factors that might potentially confound or modify the associations of asbestos with risks of cancers at these sites. In any systematic review, another concern is publication bias that may arise from potentially slanted decisions, ranging from researchers' choices of what to study and report, to the tendency of the publication process itself to select for positive findings.

REFERENCES

Becklake M. 1976. Asbestos-related diseases of the lung and other organs: Their epidemiology and implications for clinical practice. *American Review of Respiratory Disease* 114(1): 187-227.

Hamilton A, Hardy H. 1974. Industrial toxicology. In: *Asbestos-Related Diseases of the Lung and Other Organs: Their Epidemiology and Implications for Clinical Practice.* 3rd edition. Acton, MA: Publishing Sciences Group, Inc. Pp. 421.

HEW (US Department of Health Education and Welfare). 1964. *Smoking and Health: Report of the Advisory Committee to the Surgeon General.* Washington, DC: US Government Printing Office.

HHS (US Department of Health and Human Services). 2004. Asbestos CAS No. 1332-21-4. In: *11th Report on Carcinogens.* Washington, DC: National Toxicology Program.

Hill A. 1965. The environment and disease: Association or causation? *Proceedings of the Royal Society of Medicine* 58: 295-300.

Liddell F. 1997. Magic, menace, myth and malice. *Annals of Occupational Hygiene* 41(1): 3-12.

Ross M, Nolan R. 2003. History of asbestos discovery and use and asbestos-related disease in context with the occurrence of asbestos within ophiolite complexes. *Geological Society of America Special Paper* 373: 447-470.

Virta RL. 2002. *Asbestos.* Mineral Yearbook. Reston, VA: US Geological Survey.

2

Committee's Approach to Its Charge and Methods Used in Evaluation

GENERAL APPROACH TO EVIDENCE REVIEW

The committee was charged with assessing the evidence concerning the causation of selected cancers, other than lung cancer and mesothelioma, by exposure to asbestos fibers. The charge required that the committee compile and review the available evidence, attempting to identify all relevant epidemiologic studies, and then evaluate whether the evidence was sufficient to infer the existence of a causal relationship. There are now well-established models for meeting the charge, dating as far back as the landmark 1964 report of the US surgeon general on smoking and health (HEW 1964), which reached the conclusion that smoking causes lung cancer and other diseases. That report assembled the full body of relevant scientific evidence and evaluated it according to formal guidelines. Abundant, comprehensive reviews of various other agents have since been conducted to gauge whether the sets of evidence associating them with particular health outcomes warrant causal conclusions.

Established templates for reviewing scientific evidence set out approaches for gathering evidence and assessing its sufficiency to infer causality of association. With regard to obtaining evidence for review, the approach needs to involve clearly specified search criteria that facilitate collection of all potentially relevant studies for evaluation. For some purposes, there may also be an attempt to capture relevant reports in the "gray literature" (non-peer-reviewed or unpublished findings) to obtain the full set of relevant data and to ensure that publication bias does not skew the evidence evaluated, as may occur when datasets are gathered exclusively from peer-reviewed publications. In the case of an as intensively studied agent as asbestos, however, the committee considered that the findings of most studies would be published. It is possible that only statistically significant or particularly notable results on nonrespiratory endpoints would be included in the published reports on the cohort studies, and this could lead to reporting bias for cancers at the designated sites.

Once germane studies have been identified, they may undergo evaluation so that they can be classified according to the quality of the evidence that they provide. They may be evaluated systematically according to a standardized protocol and placed into tiers on the basis of their quality. In a systematic review, results of studies may be qualitatively evaluated and subjected to an overall judgment; additionally, data may be combined to derive a quantitative summary and to explore variation in results among studies. Analyzing aggregated summaries of studies is often referred to as meta-analysis; on occasion, data from studies are obtained at the level of individual participants and jointly analyzed, an approach sometimes referred to as pooled analysis. Statistical approaches for quantitative meta-analysis have been developed (Petitti 2000), as well as methods for detecting publication bias in meta-analyses (Peters et al. 2006).

Guidelines for causal inference have long been used; perhaps the best-known are those offered in the first report of the US surgeon general on smoking and health (HEW 1964):

- The **consistency** of the association.
- The **strength** of the association.
- The **specificity** of the association.
- The **temporal** relationship of the association.
- The **coherence** of the association.

The guidelines provide principles for interpreting epidemiologic evidence in a context set by biologic plausibility and the coherence of different lines of evidence. This committee has used such criteria in meeting its charge.

Specificity refers to a unique exposure-disease relationship, which is characteristic of diseases caused by infectious organisms. The concept has also been applied for investigating the contribution of physical and chemical agents to disease (Weiss 2002). The association of asbestos with mesothelioma constitutes one of the few examples of a high degree of specificity for a toxic agent and cancer risk, but the committee gave minimal weight to the criterion of specificity because the cancer sites under consideration have multiple causes and more will likely be identified.

From the outset, the committee recognized that asbestos fibers are known to be carcinogenic and that its conclusions with regard to the cancers specified in its charge would rest heavily on the epidemiologic evidence. The committee also believed that information on fiber dose to the target organs would be relevant, because the risk of cancer associated with asbestos fibers is known to be dose-dependent. The committee also gathered information on mechanisms by which asbestos fibers are carcinogenic.

That broad array of evidence was reviewed and synthesized by the committee to make its final determination as to the strength of evidence in support of an inference of causality. A variety of descriptors have been used by committees of the Institute of Medicine (IOM), the National Research Council, and other entities in characterizing the strength of evidence (see NRC 2004 for a review). The classification schemes generally include a category for circumstances in which the data are inadequate for making a judgment and a category for evidence of *no* association. Most schemes include several categories of evidence indicative of a possible causal association ranging from uncertain to fully certain; two or three categories generally serve for this purpose. The IOM approach has also distinguished between association and causality.

For this report, the committee selected a classification scheme similar to that used in the 2004 report of the US surgeon general on smoking and health (HHS 2004). That report used two categories in reference to evidence in support of a causal determination: *sufficient* and *suggestive*. Because the legislation mandating this committee's review requested only a determination of whether asbestos played a causal role in inducing these additional types of cancer, it was the committee's judgment that insertion of an additional category for evidence more weakly supportive of causation would unnecessarily generate another, most probably arbitrary distinction in classifying the evidence below the threshold for causal inference. Therefore, the committee adopted the four-category scheme of the recent US surgeon general's report on smoking and health (HHS 2004) as adequate to meet its charge:

- Evidence **sufficient** to infer a causal relationship.
- Evidence **suggestive but not sufficient** to infer a causal relationship.
- Evidence **inadequate** to infer the presence or absence of a causal relationship, which encompasses evidence that is sparse, of poor quality, or conflicting.
- Evidence **suggestive** of **no** causal relationship.

For the purpose of addressing the charge and the designation of "cause," the committee required that the evidence be judged sufficient. The category of suggestive "but not sufficient" potentially comprises a range of evidence and uncertainty that does not rise to the level of certainty needed for the designation of causality.

For the cancer sites specified in its charge, the committee also needed to consider how asbestos fibers could jointly act with other causal agents to affect risk. For cancers of the larynx and esophagus, tobacco and alcohol are well-established carcinogens, and most cases are attributable to their independent and joint actions. Smoking is also a cause of stomach cancer. Various risk factors for cancers of the colon and rectum are under investigation, including diet and physical activity.

Epidemiologists use the terms effect modification and interaction in referring to the joint consequences of several agents in causing disease. Effect modification in a positive direction, called synergism, increases risk in those exposed to two or more risk factors beyond expectation based on their independent effects. Negative effect modification is called antagonism. To assess the presence of effect modification, stratified and multivariate analytic approaches can be used. The presence of synergism implies that those exposed to one risk factor are at heightened risk when exposed to the additional, interacting factors.

Effect modification by tobacco-smoking has been considered in studies of the association between asbestos exposure and lung cancer. For investigating such effect modification, information is needed on both asbestos exposure and smoking; this requirement is met by some studies, most often of a case-control design. A recent evaluation of the evidence concerning effect modification by smoking on the risk of lung cancer associated with asbestos exposure by the International Agency for Research on Cancer (IARC 2004) concluded that there is synergism; the pattern has not been precisely characterized, however, in part because of methodologic issues.

A related issue is whether asbestos fibers alone can cause cancers at the designated sites. Epidemiologists have conceptually classified causal agents as necessary (presence is required), sufficient (presence is not required, but the agent can cause the disease by itself), and neither necessary nor sufficient (Goodman and Samet 2006, Rothman and Greenland 1998). That classification has proved useful in classifying the span of causation from diseases linked to specific agents to diseases with multiple causes, such as coronary heart disease. For example, causal microbial agents are necessary for infectious diseases and tobacco-smoking alone appears sufficient for lung cancer although there may be genetic and other nontoxicologic factors that lead one smoker but not another to develop lung cancer. Similarly, asbestos fibers are considered sufficient for mesothelioma. Goodman and Samet (2006) stress that for multifactorial diseases, such as cancer, most risk factors are to be regarded as being in the neither-necessary-nor-sufficient category. Agents that behave as synergens, amplifying the effect of another carcinogen, whether or not they appear to function as carcinogens by themselves, would be regarded as causal factors. Ultimately, a convincing demonstration that the **presence compared with absence** of asbestos exposure, all else being equal, **would increase the population risk** of cancer at one of the sites under review would establish a **causal role** for asbestos for that type of cancer.

Finally, although it considered the precision of measures of association reported by the researchers when interpreting the weight of evidence provided by various epidemiologic studies, the committee does not regard statistical significance as a rigid basis for determining causality. A full evaluation needs to consider all types of relevant evidence and take into account uncertainties beyond those of a solely statistical nature.

EVIDENCE CONSIDERED

Assembly of Literature Database

The biomedical literature concerning asbestos is vast (about 25,000 citations in the searchable reference databases MEDLINE and EMBASE), but much of it exclusively addresses asbestos's role in causing asbestosis, lung cancer, and mesothelioma. Given the committee's circumscribed task of answering the question of whether this known carcinogen plays a causal role in producing pharyngeal, laryngeal, esophageal, stomach, or colorectal cancer ("selected cancers"), the committee saw no need to revisit the entire body of information on asbestos's biologic activity or even to review the entire epidemiologic literature on asbestos exhaustively. The subset of epidemiologic literature referring to the selected cancer sites, however, did need to be identified comprehensively, retrieved when possibly pertinent to the task, and thoroughly reviewed when found to be relevant.

MEDLINE and EMBASE are biomedical databases of bibliographic citations and abstracts drawn from biomedical journals (more than 4,600 and 6,500, respectively) published in over 70 countries. Their broad international coverage can be regarded as exhaustive for the developed countries. To ensure the necessary completeness of the desired subset of asbestos literature, those databases were searched by using detailed expansions of synonyms and CAS numbers for asbestos in combination with global search terms for the selected cancers. Before secondary documents and repeated publication of the same material in an English journal and a non-English native language publication were culled, these searches retrieved about 450 English citations and about 100 foreign-language citations.

The secondary literature (e.g., ATSDR 2001; Becklake 1979; EPA 1986; IARC 1977, 1987; Kleinfeld 1973; Landrigan et al. 1999; Li et al. 2004; OSHA 1986) was used to identify articles about the cohorts that have served as the basis of conclusions concerning asbestos's involvement in asbestosis, mesothelioma, and lung cancer. In addition, the reference lists of previous reviews and meta-analyses of asbestos's possible role in the etiology of the "selected cancers" were also searched to identify the primary citations considered. Although the committee would not necessarily accept every study given weight in earlier assessments, the members wanted to be aware of all literature that had been considered. Site-specific reviews were screened for citations on digestive system cancers (Hallenbeck and Hesse 1977, Schneiderman 1974), gastrointestinal cancers (Edelman 1988, Frumkin and Berlin 1988, Goldsmith 1982, Goodman et al. 1999, Kanarek 1989, Miller 1978, Morgan et al. 1985), stomach cancer (Smith 1973), colorectal cancer (Homa et al. 1994, Weiss 1995), colon cancer (Gamble 1994), and laryngeal cancer (Browne and Gee 2000; Chan and Gee 1988; Edelman 1989; Goodman et al. 1999; Griffiths and Molony 2003; Guidotti et al. 1975; Kraus et al. 1995; Libshitz et al. 1974; Liddell 1990; Parnes 1996, 1998; Smith et al. 1990). The primary publications identified in this manner consisted largely of site-specific case-control studies.

"Asbestos cohorts" were defined as those having asbestos as a major exposure and as a primary research focus. That excluded studies of cohorts for which asbestos was merely a component of a poorly characterized, complex exposure; was a confounder of the exposure of real interest to the researchers; or was mentioned as a hypothesized explanation of an observed excess risk. We sought to gather a comprehensive set of citations concerning the asbestos cohorts, but to limit procurement of hard copies to articles most relevant to our mission—the most recent or comprehensive publications on a given cohort and articles specifically addressing the five selected cancers, asbestos exposure, or distribution of asbestos fibers to tissues. All citations related to a given study population were grouped on a spreadsheet to characterize the cohort and how it had been researched over the years. For the cohorts that ultimately provided information on the selected cancers, information from this spreadsheet is tabled in Appendix B. That procedure facilitated recognition of whether any additional publications pertained to a pre-existing study cohort and thereby avoided double-counting of evidence. It also aided in identification of which articles should be obtained as hard copies.

Other search operations were performed manually in PubMed to augment the citations downloaded from MEDLINE and EMBASE into ProCite (2003). PubMed, which contains all MEDLINE citations and an additional 5%, mostly from less prominent foreign journals, is readily accessible for on-line queries and for recovery of citations for importation into ProCite.

To capture any other publications related to the cohorts that might contain information about the "selected cancers" (which might have been deemed peripheral to demonstrating the "known health outcomes"), the names of researchers identified in their author lists were manually searched in PubMed for other asbestos-related publications. Special attention was paid to seeking updates of the identified cohorts that superseded those considered for the evaluations of lung cancer and mesothelioma.

Unless it is found to be associated with the cancer in question, an occupational exposure addressed in a case-control study often is not mentioned in the title, abstract, or keyword field scanned during database searches. Therefore, to avoid bias toward positive results and to ensure full retrieval of case-control studies that considered asbestos and that were published through August 2005, PubMed was screened for cancer, occupation, and case-control (and variants) in combination with synonyms for the selected cancer sites without stipulation of an asbestos-related keyword.

The final ProCite database contains about 2,500 citations. For somewhat more than a fourth of them (754), hard copies were obtained and more closely evaluated for pertinence. Ultimately, about 300 publications directly contributed evidence to our evaluation. Results were abstracted from 36 citations on case-control studies and from about 80 citations on the 40 informative cohort populations for the meta-analyses conducted on epidemiologic findings. Nearly 200 citations contributed asbestos-specific information from animal and in vitro studies, exposure investigations, and mineralogic characterizations.

Selection of Studies for Inclusion

The citations identified by the search procedure described in the previous section were screened for further consideration on the basis of their abstracts. Copies of reviews, meta-analyses, and other secondary sources were obtained for use in searching as described above and for background information, but the cancer-site-specific content was not considered by the committee members before they conducted their own evaluation. For its evidentiary database, however, the committee was interested only in reports of primary investigations. A comprehensive dataset on all asbestos's potential health effects was not being sought, but a wide net was cast by retrieving copies of reports involving the selected cancer sites that might address asbestos exposure specifically and of asbestos-exposed cohorts that might present information on the selected sites of this review along with data on the health outcomes that are now accepted to be asbestos related.

The committee limited the epidemiologic results in its evidentiary database to findings of appropriately designed cohort and case-control studies. Cross-sectional studies, ecologic studies, and case series could at most provide supportive evidence. Furthermore, the committee decided that studies of asbestos in drinking water, primarily ecologic in design, did not provide information that was directly pertinent to the charge.

Although the committee wanted to be as comprehensive as possible, constraints of time and accessibility prevented securing original articles for a large portion of the foreign-language citations and arranging for their translation. When English abstracts were available, they usually stated major findings and conclusions, but the committee's consensus was that study methods needed to be addressed in detail if the reliability of a citation's results were to be evaluated. Therefore, all foreign-language articles were set aside. Consideration of available abstracts and tables did not suggest that the findings reported in those documents differed systematically from findings reported in their English-language counterparts.

Articles that were eligible for inclusion in the evidentiary database were evaluated from several perspectives, as set forth below to determine the overall quality of studies and the consequent reliability of estimates of relative risk (RR) derived from them. As discussed in more detail in the following sections, the design of each study was assessed in terms of how the study sample (cohort members or cases) and comparison group were selected, how the health outcome was determined, how exposure was characterized, and how adequately possible biases and confounders had been addressed. For some of the committee's analyses, subgroups of studies were selected on the basis of design characteristics.

CRITERIA FOR EVIDENCE EVALUATION

Fiber Type

The committee recognized that there is evidence suggesting that the risk associated with asbestos exposure for development of mesothelioma (and possibly of lung cancer) may vary by fiber type. Controversy continues (for example, Hessel et al. 2004, Rice and Heineman 2003) as to whether there is an absolute difference in the toxicity of amphibole and serpentine (chrysotile only) forms of asbestos and whether only amphibole fibers have carcinogenic potential, particularly for mesothelioma, the neoplasm for which a difference seems most apparent. Recent reviews suggest that rather than having no carcinogenic activity, chrysotile has a generally lesser degree of potency than amphibole fibers, and that the various types of amphibole fibera differ in the extent of their biological activity (Britton 2002, IPCS 1998, Roggli 2006, Roggli et al. 1997, Suzuki et al. 2005). In its initial assessment of its charge, the committee evaluated whether its report could address whether associations of asbestos exposure with risk for the designated cancers either depended on the presence of specific type of fibers or varied with type of fiber. With the sole exception of the Montreal study (Dumas et al. 2000; Parent et al. 1998, 2000), the case-control studies did not provide information on fiber type, as self-reported work histories were generally the basis for exposure estimation and the resulting exposure estimates were not specific to fiber type. Consequently, the potentially relevant evidence on fiber type came almost exclusively from the cohort studies of asbestos-exposed populations, and specifically from those that have had relatively pure exposures to a specific fiber type, such as the crocidolite mining and milling workers in Western Australia. In considering the body of evidence from cohort studies for the designated cancer sites, the committee found only limited literature that was specific as to fiber type. The committee considered the physical and chemical characteristics that distinguish the major fiber types and the potential relevance of these characteristics to relative carcinogenicity of the fiber types. The implications of these physical and chemical differences among fiber types for human carcinogenesis have not been extensively studied, specifically under circumstances of occupational exposure. Current evaluations favor the hypothesis that carcinogenicity is not limited to asbestos fibers of the amphibole type (Britton 2002, IPCS 1998, Roggli 2006, Roggli et al. 1997, Suzuki et al. 2005). Consequently, the committee's report describes the level of causal inference in relation to asbestos, without specifying the type.

Grouping of Evidence by Cancer Site

The cancers that this committee was asked to consider are a diverse group of tumors that develop from the upper portions of the respiratory and digestive tracts to the colon and rectum. Even cancers that occur in tissues contiguous to the mouth and pharynx, and that are conventionally grouped together as "head and neck" cancers, differ markedly in their risk factors and descriptive epidemiology. In many epidemiologic studies that have examined the association of asbestos with the cancers of interest in this report, sites have been grouped into various categories to allow statistical analyses of rather sparse data, even when cancers at the subsites have very different etiologies. Optimally, one would consider the evidence concerning these cancers in groupings that reflect generally similar etiology, but extracting what information is available from epidemiologic studies conducted over the last half century under circumstances of evolving understanding of biologic mechanisms and epidemiologic analysis make this objective unattainable.

Given the committee's intention of considering the available data in a comprehensive and inclusive fashion, however, results were first abstracted with notations as to exactly which anatomic sites the researchers were reporting on, according to specific International Classification of Disease (ICD) codes for causes of death (ICD-9; although now superseded, version 9 was in effect at the time of most of the deaths recorded in the studies reviewed) or the comparable oncology codes for cancer type (ICD-O-3). Table 2.1 indicates the equivalence between those coding systems for the cancers under consideration, with some of the common phrases used by researchers to report findings on grouped sets of sites, which often are not accompanied by precise designations.

TABLE 2.1 Standard Codes and Nonstandard Groupings Used to Characterize "Accepted" and "Selected" Cancers

	ICD-9 (for mortality)	ICD-O-3 (for incidence)
"Aerodigestive"		
"Head and Neck"		
Lip, oral cavity, and pharynx	(140-149)	(C00-C14)
Pharynx		
Oro-	***146***	***C09.0, C 09.1, C09.8, C09.9, C10.0, C10.1, C10.2, C10.3, C10.4, C10.8, C10.9***
Naso-	***147***	***C11.0-C11.9***
Hypo-	***148***	***C12.9-C13.9***
Ill-defined sites within lip, oral cavity, and pharyx	149	C14.0, C14.1, C14.2, C14.8
Pharynx, unspecified	***149.0***	
Digestive organs and peritoneum	(150-159)	
"Gastrointestinal" (GI)		
Esophagus	***150***	***C15.0-C15.9***
Stomach	***151***	***C16.0-C16.9***
Small intestine, including duodenum	152	C17.0-C17.9
Colorectal		***C18.0-C20.9***
Colon	***153***	***C18.0-C18.9***
Rectum, rectosigmoid junction, and anus	***154***	***C19.9, C20.9, C21.0-C21.8***
"Other digestive"		
Liver and intrahepatic bile ducts	155	
Gall bladder and extrrahepatic bile ducts	156	
Pancreas	157	
Retroperitoneum and peritoneum	158	C48.0-C48.8
Ill-defined	159	
Respiratory and intrathoracic organs	(160-165)	
Nasal cavities, middle ear, and sinuses (often classified with "Head and Neck")	160	C30.0-C30.1, C31.0-C31.9
Larynx	***161***	***C32.0-C32.9***
Glottic	***161.0***	***C32.0***
Supraglottic	***161.1***	***C32.1***
Subglottic	***161.2***	***C32.2***

continues

TABLE 2.1 Continued

	ICD-9 (for mortality)	ICD-O-3 (for incidence)
Trachea, bronchus, and lung	162	C33.9, C34.0-C34.9
Pleura	163	C38.4
Mesothelioma [applies to tissues otherwise coded as 158 or 163]		
Asbestosis	523.2 or 501	

NOTE: "***Selected cancers***" for consideration as specified by legislation (italicized bold face). "Accepted health outcomes" generally regarded as causally related to asbestos exposure (underlined).

The committee did attempt to note whether effects might be associated with more specific classifications that would be more meaningful from an etiologic perspective. The committee also noted that ICD codes do not capture changes in the subsites involved or their histopathologic classification, which was of particular relevance for esophageal and stomach cancers. When the available data were assembled, the committee considered groupings no broader than "pharynx with oral or buccal cavity," "larynx with epilarynx" (larynx plus portions of the oropharynx specified as ICD codes 146.4, 146.5, and 148.2), and "rectum with colon or intestines" to be meaningful.

Because of the committee's requirement for relatively specific groupings of sites, a considerable number of cohorts were judged uninformative for the "selected cancers." Those cohorts may have been studied intensively with repeated follow-up of vital status, but in most cases the researchers' primary interest was respiratory disease, both malignant and nonmalignant, and information on the cancers of concern in this review was not reported or analyzed.

Study Designs

Epidemiologic designs applied in investigations of environmental and occupational risk factors for cancer are primarily of three types: cohort studies of defined groups (such as worker populations), case-control studies, and "ecologic" studies that compare rates in geographic regions defined by exposure characteristics. Epidemiologic studies can also be classified as exposure-based or general-population-based depending on whether the source population is defined as an exposed group (such as workers in a particular industry or residents of a contaminated community) or the population at large.

Occupational and Environmental Cohort Studies

In general, exposure-based cohort and nested case-control studies (in which cases and controls are selected from a well-defined cohort) provide the most direct observational evidence of associations with occupational carcinogens and industry-related chemicals that may reach the general environment. Their primary advantage is the possibility of linking clearly specified exposures to health outcomes. Limitations of most exposure-based studies are the low frequency of some health outcomes (such as site-specific cancers) and the absence or sparseness of data on lifestyle or constitutional disease risk factors (such as tobacco-smoking and diet) that may confound observed associations with risk.

Population-Based Case-Control Studies

In contrast, population-based case-control studies have the distinct advantages, compared with exposure-based studies, of accruing relatively large case groups and providing an opportunity to obtain data on important potential confounding factors. The weakest aspect of most population-based case-control studies is the poor quality of the exposure characterization, which often lacks agent specificity or quantification.

Ecologic Studies

Although ecologic studies may yield etiologic clues, causal inference is constrained because exposures and health outcomes are correlated at an aggregate level (geographic or population) rather than for individual study subjects. They tend to be most suitable for suggesting exposure-disease relations that may lead to more-focused cohort or case-control studies. Consequently, ecologic studies were not included in the database of epidemiologic studies evaluated and integrated by this committee.

The committee does not view either the case-control or cohort design as being intrinsically preferable or stronger than the other, and does not believe one type should be weighted more heavily than the other. Consideration of the results from both types of design permits viewing the real-world outcomes available for observation by epidemiologists from two different perspectives, with studies of samples defined on the basis of exposure (cohort studies) and with studies of samples defined on the basis of health outcome (case-control studies). Having information from both these types of studies, along with the incorporation of findings from controlled experimentation (as discussed in the coherence criterion section of the causal integration for each cancer site), helps to ensure that the vulnerabilities of one type of evidence are countered by the strengths of the other.

Measurement of Exposure and Outcome

Exposure

The accuracy of exposure assessment is a major determinant of the informativeness of a study for causal inference and of the validity and reliability of risk estimates that can be drawn from study data. Inaccurate exposure assignment can bias study findings with the consequences depending on whether it is nondifferential or differential. Generally, although not always, nondifferential or random exposure misclassification will diminish the likelihood of detecting a true association between an exposure and disease. For asbestos, exposure intensity, timing, and duration are the most relevant considerations for exposure assessment. Sources of exposure misclassification include missing or incomplete data on concentrations or work time, erroneous measurements, and poor sources of data (such as statement of usual occupation on death certificates), but the use of crude exposure classifications (such as "ever exposed" vs "never exposed") is often necessitated by the lack of documentation on actual exposure. Self-reporting of exposure in response to lists of agents can also be a source of misclassification in population-based case-control studies. Because exposures that occurred far in the past are relevant to cancer, the absence of quantitative data and even the lack of a basis for assigning qualitative exposure rankings are common limitations in assessing exposures.

The method used to estimate the exposures of study subjects is crucial in determining the quality of case-control studies. In contrast with cohort studies, it is not feasible to assess asbestos exposure quantitatively in case-control studies using actual measurement data. The most useful case-control studies are those that assign a magnitude or probability of exposure (on an ordinal basis) by using a lifetime work history with details of work activities. That technique was pioneered by researchers in Montreal who used it in several publications included in this review (Dumas et al. 2000; Goldberg et al. 2001; Parent et al. 1998, 2000). In some studies, levels of exposure have been assigned on the basis of occupation or industry using a job-exposure matrix (JEM), occasionally even taking the era when exposure occurred into consideration. Studies that assess exposure with direct questions (for example, "Were you ever exposed to asbestos?") are prone to recall bias and may also suffer from widely varied interpretations among participants of what constitutes exposure. Nonetheless, data derived in such a crude fashion may still yield useful information.

This committee's review did not include hypothesis-generating studies that assessed cancer risks only in association with a large number of occupations or industries and then interpreted the results a posteriori on the basis of exposures assumed to occur in the jobs or industrial sectors found to have increased risks. Some studies used the "usual" occupations and industries entered on death certificates as a source of exposure information, but the committee did not consider them to be adequately reliable for inclusion in this review (Andrews and Savitz 1999; Selikoff 1992), even when interpreted with a JEM. Death certificates may be completed by medical personnel who know little about the work histories of the deceased, they list only a single job, and they do not include dates of employment. Although useful for surveillance, death certificates are a crude source of data for etiologic investigations, particularly for manufacturing workers who may have held many jobs.

The metrics of exposure derived across studies were so diverse that a hierarchy by potential quality could not be applied. The committee adopted a pragmatic approach in order to assess whether classifying a given study population along even a crude exposure gradient would yield evidence for a dose-response relationship between asbestos exposure and risk. The committee recognized limitations of the data available for this purpose and was not seeking accurate quantitative estimates. Initially, the committee defined three levels of exposure-assessment method (EAM) quality for each of the two design types and graded the informative studies accordingly. In practice, it turned out for both designs that the two higher quality grades (now subsumed in EAM = 1) corresponded to the capability to do analyses on dose-gradients (although for the selected cancer sites, the needed data were not necessarily presented in the articles). The committee did consider that evidence of a dose-response relationship is a strong supporting element for inferring causality. Given the limitations of the data available, failure to find an indication of a dose-response relationship was not viewed as evidence against a causal relationship.

Outcome

The primary outcomes for cancer etiology studies are typically cancer mortality and cancer incidence (diagnosis). Cancer mortality is usually ascertained from the underlying cause of death indicated on a death certificate. The National Death Index is an electronic nationwide resource for specific causes of death in the United States; some other countries maintain similar data. The validity of a recording of cancer on a death certificate has been examined and found to be fairly reliable for epidemiologic studies for rapidly fatal cancers (such as lung cancer) (D'Amico et al. 1999, Percy et al. 1981, Sathiakumar et al. 1998). Cancers that metastasize, however, may be listed incorrectly on death certificates, and diagnosed cancers that do not result in death may be missed (as is likely to be the case for laryngeal cancer for which the survival rate is relatively high). Selikoff and Seidman (1992) found death certificate information on primary and contributing causes of death to be problematic for asbestos-related diseases in general, while investigations tracking patients known to have oral and oropharyngeal cancers (Leitner et al. 2001) or colorectal cancers (Ederer et al. 1999) found death certificate information did not reflect the earlier diagnosis with any certainty. In addition, information on death certificates often lacks specificity regarding primary site or histology (for example, simply "pharynx," rather than "oropharynx"). There is no reason to expect the frequency of such errors to be linked to asbestos exposure, but they do decrease the sensitivity of results to any real effect.

Cancer incidence is typically ascertained from a cancer registry—corporation-, state-, or county-based in the United States or national in some countries. The validity of a cancer diagnosis from a statewide cancer registry is generally high because state registries require medical-record validation.

The cohort studies considered by the committee were carried out in multiple locations, and their findings were reported from the 1950s on. In most of the studies, cause-specific mortality was the principal outcome measure. Mortality is a useful indicator of disease occurrence (incidence) for diseases with poor survival, such as lung cancer. The validity of mortality as an indicator of cancer incidence also depends on the accuracy of both identification of cause of death and its coding. Undoubtedly, there was some degree of misclassification in the assignment of cause of death in the cohort studies considered. If random, the result would have been a reduction in sensitivity to detect an effect. As clinicians became aware of the associations of asbestos with various diseases, there may have been a bias toward diagnosing diseases such as lung cancer at higher rates among workers in known asbestos-related industries than in the population at large.

All the case-control studies considered in this review reported results in terms of cancer incidence rather than mortality and identified cases from hospital listings or regional government tumor registries, which are population-based. Aside from nested case-control investigations conducted in the asbestos cohorts under consideration, the committee did not consider nested case-control studies of occupational cohorts that did not have asbestos as a major exposure. Case status may have been determined histologically or from death certificate information, but studies that used histologic confirmation were accorded greater weight in the selection process. In most studies, randomly selected population controls were used. In the studies published by Siemiatycki's group in Montreal (Dumas et al. 2000; Goldberg et al. 2001; Parent et al. 1998, 2000), the controls consisted of a mix of population controls and other controls with other types of cancer.

Validity

Thorough and valid ascertainment of exposures and health outcomes is critical if epidemiologic research is to be informative. Validity is determined by the extent to which the investigators can minimize bias that may result from improper selection of index or comparison groups (exposed and nonexposed subjects in a cohort study, cases and controls in a case-control study), misclassification of health outcome or exposure variables, or failure to minimize confounding by disease risk factors that are also related to the exposure under study.

Precision

Precision of exposure estimates reflects the magnitude of measurement error due to the analytic sampling instrument or the number of measurements made (such as air samples of asbestos fibers). Studies with more subjects tend to be more informative than smaller studies, provided that study size is not achieved at the cost of reduced reliability and validity of the exposure-assessment approach. Sample size is reflected in the precision of estimates of effect as measured by the width of the confidence interval (CI) of an observed RR. Although large studies are desirable, relatively small studies with a high degree of validity are preferable to large studies with questionable validity.

Bias

Detailed discussions of consequences and methods to reduce the three forms of bias—confounding, selection, and information—are provided in standard epidemiologic texts (Rothman and Greenland 1998). The healthy-worker effect (and the related healthy-worker survivor effect) is a source of bias that is both peculiar to occupational epidemiology and ubiquitous, so it warrants further elaboration. As described below, the healthy-worker effect can include elements of both confounding bias and selection bias.

Confounding Bias

Many occupational cohort studies compare disease rates between a worker cohort and the general population. Although comparisons of this type give some indication of overall patterns of relative disease occurrence in the worker cohort, they may also be affected by confounding bias. Specifically, workers in a particular trade may differ from the general population in lifestyle characteristics and health status. For example, tobacco-smoking and alcohol-consumption patterns, known risk factors for laryngeal cancer, may be quite different between blue-collar industrial workers who are exposed to asbestos and the general population, which includes people from all socioeconomic classes. Contrasts in laryngeal-cancer incidence between a worker cohort and the general population might thus be confounded if smoking is not taken into account. The committee could only gauge the potential for confounding to have increased risk estimates from the case-control studies. For comparisons within a specific worker cohort, confounding by smoking and alcohol may be less problematic than in studies in more diverse populations (Kriebel et al. 2004).

Health status also commonly differs between worker and general-population groups because healthy people are selectively hired into the workforce and the general population includes people who are too sick to work; workers may also benefit from the health advantages of higher incomes and employee health plans. Differential employment rates by health status leads to what is known as the healthy-worker effect; it often results in mortality risk estimates that spuriously suggest a health-protective effect in association with occupational exposures. The healthier workers also tend to stay employed longer, resulting in a confounding bias when workers with low cumulative exposure are compared with more highly exposed workers. Thus, the healthy-worker survivor effect may cause bias even in a study based on internal comparisons.

The case-control studies considered by the committee varied a great deal with respect to control for confounding. Nearly all controlled for age and sex either by virtue of original matching criteria for control selection, by statistical adjustment, or by simply reporting on men and women separately. They vary, however, in whether they controlled for smoking, alcohol use, birthplace, region, diet, obesity, physical activity, and educational status. Studies that controlled for smoking and alcohol were given greater weight for pharyngeal and laryngeal cancers.

Selection Bias

The healthy-worker effect and the healthy-worker survivor effect can be viewed as a result of selective hiring of healthy people or of keeping less healthy workers away from exposure in the workplace. The healthy-worker survivor effect is most pronounced for cardiovascular and obstructive lung diseases, but it may also bias research findings for various cancers. Case-control studies are subject to selection bias if controls are poorly chosen in a manner related to the probability of exposure.

Information Bias (Misclassification of Exposure or Outcome)

It is possible for differential misclassification, a classification error associated with the value of other variables, to result in bias toward either overestimation or underestimation of an effect. For instance, the tendency of people who have a disease to search for explanations of their condition may make them more likely to report an exposure of interest, so the possibility of recall bias needs to be anticipated in case-control studies. Independent assessments of documented work histories by occupational hygienists are often applied in an effort to remedy some of the error associated with self-reported exposures in population-based case-control studies. The problem also provides a motivation for using hospital- or registry-identified controls.

In most circumstances, nondifferential misclassification of exposure or health outcome will obscure detection of a real effect by producing an estimated risk closer to the null (RR = 1.0). Of necessity, epidemiologic studies incorporate surrogate exposure indicators for the relevant biologic dose. Exposure and dosimetric modeling may be applied to estimate this dose more precisely, but improper modeling assumptions may introduce misclassification. Similarly, the lower sensitivity of cancer-mortality studies, than of cancer-incidence studies, for cancers with high survival could be regarded as the result of misclassifying deceased people if cancer incidence is the investigation's objective, because the presence of an earlier, nonfatal cancer is unlikely to be recognized.

Statistical Analysis

The validity of a study requires application of appropriate methods for statistical analysis of the data.

Precision

The size of the study population will contribute directly to the precision with which the target effect is estimated; precision is reflected in the standard error or CI associated with the estimated effect. For cohort studies, precision of the estimated effects (and therefore power to test hypotheses) is driven primarily by the expected number of events, which is a function of person-years of follow-up and incidence. For example, two studies with equal numbers of person-years of follow-up will have estimated effects with different precision if one deals with a more common cancer than the other. For case-control studies, precision of estimated effects depends primarily on the size of the sample of cases and controls but also can be affected by adjustment for confounders or method of sampling (matched vs unmatched pairs). Precision thus depends on sample size but may be affected by other characteristics of a study design or method of analysis.

Statistical Modeling

RRs adjusted for confounding can be derived by stratification, by matching on confounders, or by including potential confounders in multiple regression models in which the exposure of interest is the primary independent variable. Models are sometimes preferred over stratified contingency tables because data become sparse in stratified analyses when multiple confounders are present. The most common risk models in environmental and occupational epidemiology are logistic regression, Poisson regression, and Cox proportional hazards models. Parameters estimated from these models can be conveniently interpreted as adjusted odds ratios, mortality or incidence-rate ratios, and hazard-rate ratios, respectively. It is important to keep in mind that all the advantages of modeling can be undermined if the underlying assumptions about the distribution of the outcome or form of the exposure-response relationship are mis-specified. These assumptions are generally known to epidemiologists and biostatisticians working in the field, but are rarely laid out and examined in published papers.

Summary

Ultimately, judgments about the role of any environmental agent in the causation of disease must be based on the critical evaluation of observational studies of exposed subjects. Unlike subjects in clinical trials, epidemiologic studies of environmental or occupational causes of disease cannot randomize subjects into exposed and unexposed groups. Thus, results of even the best observational study may be biased. Recognizing that limitation, the challenge is to assess the collective weight of the evidence across multiple studies of each disease endpoint, with particular attention to the validity of exposure ascertainment.

METHODS USED FOR QUANTITATIVE META-ANALYSIS

The units of input for the meta-analysis on each selected cancer site were the most complete risk estimates available on discrete study populations. A single citation could therefore generate more than one datum (such as separate results for men and for women), whereas only the most recent follow-up giving information on one of the selected cancer sites was used from among a series of publications on the same occupational cohort.

For each cancer site, plots were generated depicting all contributing risk estimates with their respective 95% CIs, plus a summary estimated RR with its associated 95% CI. For each cancer site, plots were constructed separately by study type (case-control vs cohort). The summaries were designed to capture an overall characterization of any exposure vs no exposure, and to capture the available evidence of a dose-related effect by summarizing the available information on the effect for the most extreme exposure category vs no exposure.

The committee carefully considered whether to quantitatively summarize the findings from the diverse body of cohort and case-control studies. The studies were carried out in various worker and general-population samples, and their methods differ to varying extents. In this circumstance, the heterogeneity of the evidence can be statistically considered, as was done by the committee in its aggregating approach. The confidence intervals, however, do not fully reflect the range of uncertainty around the pooled estimates, as differences in exposure and outcome ascertainment and different patterns of potential confounding are not taken into account. The plots provide a graphic display of the range of estimates from the cohort and case-control studies.

Given the heterogeneity of the observational evidence considered, the committee gave weight to the consistency of the findings and to the degree of increase in estimated risk, along with whether there was an indication of a dose-response relationship. The committee proceeded despite concerns that the summary estimates generated by its meta-analyses might convey an unfounded degree of precision or certainty. The committee did not consider indicators of statistical significance arising from the meta-analyses as critical determinants in its decision-making. The summary estimates were useful in considering the extent to which methodologic explanations offered an alternative to causation for observed associations.

The first set of plots for each study type summarizes the distribution of estimated RRs associated with any exposure to asbestos (vs none). A second set of plots presents available evidence of a dose-response relationship. In both the case-control and cohort studies, a subset of studies reported RRs across a gradient of exposure; these were used to summarize the effects of "high" exposure to asbestos. Because the definition of high exposure differed by study, we knowingly summarized RRs over an array of definitions.

For case-control studies, we also summarized the distribution of RRs stratified by exposure-assessment method (EAM). For laryngeal and pharyngeal cancers, we stratified the summaries by whether the reported RRs were adjusted for smoking and alcohol use; similar stratification by confounder adjustment was not possible for cancers at other sites because of small numbers of studies in potential strata.

Summary RRs and associated 95% CIs were computed for the set of RRs overall and for each subgroup by EAMs or with and without confounding adjustment. For cohort studies, this was accomplished by using Poisson regression; for case-control studies, the method of DerSimonian and Laird (1986) was applied. Details of how these aggregate estimates were calculated are provided below.

Summary Plots for Cohort Studies

Organization of Summary Plots

Two plots were constructed for each cancer site. The first summarizes the effect of any exposure to asbestos (vs none), and the second summarizes the effect of high exposure vs none. Each summary plot includes the RR and 95% CI for each cohort listed, and a summary RR with an associated 95% CI. The template for summaries of cohort studies of cancer at each site is given in Table 2.2.

Most of the cohort studies reported results for cancer mortality, but some also, or only, reported on cancer incidence. Incidence is a more comprehensive statistic because it considers all people in whom cancer was diagnosed, not just those who ultimately died from it. Therefore, when there was a choice, incidence findings were reported. A study's caption on a plot indicates when a standardized incidence ratio was reported rather than a standardized mortality ratio.

Plot 1 includes every cohort with a reported finding for any exposure vs none without reference to study characteristics (such as exposure quality and confounder adjustment). The committee decided that the reliability of an estimate of risk for a given cancer type from simply being in an occupational cohort in comparison with a standard population (that is, being categorized as having had "any exposure") would not be affected by a study's thoroughness in determining exposure gradients. Therefore, unlike what was done for case-control results, the cohort results for "any exposure" were not stratified on how exposure quality was measured in the overall study (in which detailed exposure characterization was most often derived

TABLE 2.2 Organization of Summary Plots Used for Cohort Studies Informative for Cancer at Each Site

Plot	Type of RR	Studies Included
1	Any vs none	All
2	Most extreme vs none (If more than one gradient reported, aggregates calculated with smallest and with largest reported RRs)	Studies reporting RR on a gradient

for application to respiratory health outcomes). Most cohort studies did not report explicit confounder adjustment, so stratification on this characteristic was not part of the analysis.

Plot 2 presents RRs for the most extreme category of an exposure gradient vs no exposure. We endeavored to capture the estimated effect in the highest reported categories of exposure (vs none) as a means of detecting dose-response relationships; a positive shift of the summary RR on plot 2 relative to plot 1 is viewed as an indicator of a dose-response relationship. One difficulty in capturing a qualitative sense of that phenomenon is the considerable heterogeneity in how "high exposure" was characterized across studies. Several studies reported RRs on multiple exposure gradients (such as cumulative exposure, duration of exposure, and intensity of exposure). To handle the heterogeneity of reporting scales and metrics, we applied the following procedure to generate plot 2 for each selected cancer site:

- Only studies that reported RRs over an exposure gradient were included on plot 2.
- The RR and CI corresponding to the most extreme category of each reported gradient were abstracted. For example, if a study reported RRs across both probability of exposure and duration of exposure, RRs corresponding to those for whom exposure was most probable and to those with the longest exposure were both abstracted.
- For studies reporting RRs across several metrics reflecting an exposure gradient, both the highest and lowest reported RRs were presented on plot 2. A pair of summary RRs and 95% CIs was computed, first by including the lowest RRs and then the highest RRs. We view the resulting summary as being robust to variability in the metrics and scales used to report exposure gradients.

Computational Conventions Used for Plot Summaries of Cohort Studies

The RR for a cohort study is the ratio of observed to expected events (for example, observed deaths divided by expected deaths). Information needed to compute estimated RRs and 95% CIs was abstracted directly from the published papers. In many cases, an estimated RR and its CI were reported directly. In other cases, CIs were omitted and needed to be computed from available information; we used the following conventions:

- In several studies, the authors supplied incomplete information (for example, RR and observed cases but not expected cases). Whenever two pieces of information were supplied, we calculated the third.
- In many other studies, an RR was given but no CI. However, the CI could be readily obtained from observed and expected counts by using

Byar's approximation, which has been shown by Breslow and Day (1987, page 69) to be very accurate.

- In the uncommon situation in which the RR was given with only a p-value (without observed or expected cases and without a CI), we used the following procedures to recover the CI:

  —When only the point estimate and a p-value were given, the CI was computed by inverting the hypothesis test, as follows. Suppose p denotes the p-value from a two-sided hypothesis test. Let $Z_{p/2}$ denote the ordinate that cuts off probability $p/2$ in the right tail of a standard normal distribution. Then se[log(RR)] = log(RR)/$Z_{p/2}$, and the associated 95% CI for the RR can be computed by exponentiation of log(RR) ± 1.96*se[log(RR)].

  —When an upper bound for a p-value was given (such as $p < 0.05$), we made the conservative assumption that the p-value was equal to its upper limit (such as $p = 0.05$) and computed the standard error (se) as above. (The true CI is narrower than the one derived here.)

  —When a lower bound for a p-value was given (such as $p > 0.05$), we plotted the RR but did not calculate a CI.

- In some cases, RR was zero (the number of expected cases was positive, but the number observed was zero). These cases were entered on the plot with an arrow indicating that the lower confidence bound is at negative infinity; confidence limits were not calculated. These cases were included in the summary RR derived via Poisson regression.

Summary Plots for Case-Control Studies

Organization of Summary Plot

Odds ratios (ORs) were abstracted from the case-control studies as the estimate of cancer risk. Given the relative rarity of the cancers under consideration, those estimates of risk may be considered equivalent to RRs (Koepsell and Weiss 2003, Rothman and Greenland 1998), and so a distinction will not be made between ORs and RRs in the remainder of this report.

Two sets of plots were constructed for each cancer site. Table 2.3 summarizes the organization of plots for the case-control studies at each cancer site. As with the cohort studies, for each of the plots described here, a 95% CI for the weighted average of the RRs is given below the individual study values. For plots with stratification, the aggregate RR and CI are included for each stratum. All the case-control studies that met the committee's criteria for inclusion in the quantitative evidentiary database reported findings exclusively for cancer incidence.

The first set of plots characterizes the effects of any exposure vs none.

TABLE 2.3 Organization of Summary Plots for Case-Control Studies Informative for Cancer at Each Site

Plot	Type of RR	Studies Included	Stratification
1a	Any vs none	All	
1b	Any vs none	All	• EAM = 1 • EAM = 2
1c (larynx and pharynx only)	Any vs none	EAM = 1	• Adjusted for alcohol use and smoking • Not adjusted for alcohol use and smoking
2	Most extreme vs none (If more than one gradient reported, aggregates calculated with smallest and with largest reported RRs)	Those reporting RR on an exposure gradient (EAM = 1)	

Plot 1a includes every study, without reference to study characteristics (exposure ascertainment method and confounder adjustment). Plot 1b is stratified by EAM, where "EAM = 1" indicates higher quality exposure assessment as described previously and "EAM = 2" indicates a lesser quality of exposure assessment. For studies of laryngeal and pharyngeal cancers, we included a third plot (1c) stratified on whether adjustment was made for smoking and alcohol consumption. For other sites, the small number of studies did not permit similar stratification.

The second set of plots characterizes extreme exposure vs none with data from those studies that reported exposure effects on a gradient; we used the same approach applied to cohort studies.

Computational Conventions Used for Plot Summaries of Case-Control Studies

For each study population represented in the plots, its estimated RR and its 95% CI or standard error were abstracted as available from the manuscripts. In most cases, the estimated RR and its CI were obtained directly. In cases in which CIs were not presented in the articles, they were computed if possible from available information:

- In the uncommon situation in which the RR was given with only a p-value, we used the procedures described for cohort studies to recover the CI.

• In the small number of cases in which the estimated RR was zero and no CI was given, we used the standard method of adding 0.5 to each cell in the two-by-two table of case status vs exposure status and calculated the CI by using formulas supplied by Agresti (2002).

• A small number of studies reported an adjusted RR, but neither a p-value nor a CI. For those cases, we compared the crude RR (computed from information usually available in a table giving the total number of cases and the number of cases exposed to asbestos) with the adjusted RR. If the crude RR was within 1 standard error of the adjusted RR, we calculated and used the CI for the crude RR.

Computation of Summary RRs

For each plot (and within each stratum for stratified plots), an estimated aggregate or summary RR and its associated 95% CI are given. An outline of the calculation of those values for cohort and case-control studies follows.

Cohort Studies

In a cohort study, the number of observed events (such as observed deaths) can be assumed to follow a Poisson distribution with the mean equal to the expected number of events in the absence of an exposure effect (such as, expected number of deaths), inflated by the true RR (Armitage et al. 2002). This suggests the model:

$$Y_j \sim Poisson[E_j \exp(\theta)],$$

where for study j, Y_j denotes observed number of cases, E_j denotes expected number, and $\exp(\theta)$ is the average RR across studies.

To estimate θ and its confidence interval, we fit the Poisson regression:

$$\log \mu_j = \log E_j + \theta$$

to the observed event counts across studies, treating θ as an offset term. The standard error calculation took into account extra Poisson variation by using the estimated deviance. The resulting summary RR and its CI for each plot are given by:

$$\exp\left[\hat{\theta} \pm 1.96se\left(\hat{\theta}\right)\right].$$

Case-Control Studies

The summary RR and CI for case-control studies was computed with the method of DerSimonian and Laird (1986). That approach assumes that the distribution of true log RRs across studies follows a normal distribution with mean θ and variance σ^2. The average log RR is computed as a weighted average over studies, where the weights are inversely proportional to the standard error for each estimated log RR (therefore, larger studies contribute more information).

Let θ_j represent the estimated log RR reported from study j, and let s_j denote its standard error. The logarithm of the summary RR is computed by using a weighted average:

$$\hat{\theta} = \sum_j W_j \theta_j \Big/ \sum_j W_j .$$

The weights are given by:

$$W_j = \frac{1}{s_j^2 + \hat{\sigma}^2},$$

where $\hat{\sigma}^2$ is an estimator of the between-study variation in the true log RRs across studies. (The DerSimonian and Laird estimator uses a moment-based procedure to compute $\hat{\sigma}^2$.) The standard error of $\hat{\theta}$ is:

$$\left(\sum_j W_j\right)^{-1/2}.$$

Therefore, the lower and upper 95% confidence limits for the summary RR are given by:

$$\exp\left\{\hat{\theta} \pm \frac{1.96}{\sqrt{\sum_j W_j}}\right\}.$$

INTEGRATION OF DATA

Previous evaluations of specific agents or exposures as contributing to an increased risk of cancer have been conducted by expert panels convened by national and international agencies. The expert panels review, evaluate, and integrate the scientific evidence based on three sources of information: epidemiologic studies of cancer in humans, studies of cancer in experimental animals, and biologic mechanistic data. The present committee critically reviewed and summarized the strengths and weaknesses of the scientific evidence of those three types, guided by the newly revised principles and procedures described in the preamble to the IARC monographs (IARC 2006).

Such guidelines for causal inference are not rigid criteria that can be implemented in a formulaic fashion, so the committee endeavored to achieve comparability across the cancer sites in the application of the criteria it had adopted by following a uniform format for the critical, final sections of Chapters 7 through 11. The concluding section for each site documents the extent of the epidemiologic evidence from the comprehensive search that proved informative for that site, the consistency of that evidence, and the strength of association conveyed by it. The epidemiological evidence was integrated with the complementary evidence on dose, mechanisms, and toxicologic research. All conclusions were made in accord with the prespecified classification for causal inference.

Exposure Data and Epidemiologic Evidence

The committee considered the geographic distribution, commercial applications of asbestos fibers, and exposure data from occupational and environmental sources. The quality of exposure data and the demonstration of dose-response relationships in human epidemiologic studies were major considerations in evaluating the studies. Other considerations used to assess quality included bias and confounding, as discussed above. In addition to case-control studies and cohort analyses, the committee considered a small number of human case reports that examined biomarkers of potential adverse effects of asbestos fibers and dose deposited at target organs that may be relevant for development of cancer at the sites under consideration. The strength of the epidemiologic evidence for a casual relationship between asbestos exposure and development of cancer at each site was distilled, as described above.

Studies in Experimental Animals

The committee reviewed all animal studies published in the peer-reviewed literature related to asbestos exposure and development of cancer at the sites under consideration. Those studies were evaluated qualitatively and quantitatively according to the criteria outlined in the preamble to the IARC monographs, as summarized in Table 2.4.

Biologic Mechanistic Data

The committee reviewed the current mechanistic hypotheses regarding asbestos-related diseases of the lung and pleura. From the information on pulmonary diseases, the following properties of asbestos fibers were considered to be most relevant for pathogenicity: fiber length and diameter, surface reactivity, cytotoxicity, genotoxicity, and persistence at the target site, in that they might contribute to chronic inflammation and cell proliferation. The evidence for fiber deposition, persistence, and induction of mor-

TABLE 2.4 Evaluation of Animal Studies

Qualitative considerations:
1. Adequacy of experimental design
2. Exposure information-route, dose, and duration
3. Animal survival, duration of follow-up, and description of pathologic lesions
4. Consistency of published results across species, sexes, and target organs
Quantitative considerations:
1. Dose-response and time relationships
2. Statistical analysis

SOURCE: IARC 2006.

phologic, cellular, or molecular changes relevant to carcinogenicity at the sites under consideration was evaluated.

The committee evaluated the overall strengths and weaknesses of the scientific evidence based on human epidemiologic studies, animal studies, and biologic mechanistic studies. It then integrated all this information before reaching a conclusion regarding the strength of the evidence for a causal association between asbestos exposure and an increased risk of cancer at each site under consideration. Integration of this evidence—reflecting the consensus reached by the committee—is summarized at the end of each site-specific review.

REFERENCES

Agresti A. 2002. *Categorical Data Analysis.* 2nd edition. New York: Wiley.

Andrews KW, Savitz DA. 1999. Accuracy of industry and occupation on death certificates of electric utility workers: Implications for epidemiologic studies of magnetic fields and cancer. *Bioelectromagnetics* 20(8): 512-518.

Armitage P, Berry G, Matthews JNS. 2002. *Statistical Methods in Medical Research.* 4th edition. Oxford, England: Blackwell Science.

ATSDR (Agency for Toxic Substances and Disease Registry). 2001. *Toxicological Profile for Asbestos.* Atlanta, GA: US Department of Health and Human Services.

Becklake MR. 1979. Environmental exposure to asbestos: A factor in the rising rate of cancer in the industrialized world? *Chest* 76(3): 245-247.

Breslow NE, Day NE. 1987. Statistical methods in cancer research: The design and analysis of cohort studies. *IARC Scientific Publications* 82(2): 1-406.

Britton M. 2002. The epidemiology of mesothelioma. *Seminars in Oncology* 29(1): 18-25.

Browne K, Gee JB. 2000. Asbestos exposure and laryngeal cancer. *Annals of Occupational Hygiene* 44(4): 239-250.

Chan CK, Gee JB. 1988. Asbestos exposure and laryngeal cancer: An analysis of the epidemiologic evidence. *Journal of Occupational Medicine* 30(1): 23-27.

D'Amico M, Agozzino E, Biagino A, Simonetti A, Marinelli P. 1999. Ill-defined and multiple causes on death certificates: A study of misclassification in mortality statistics. *European Journal of Epidemiology* 15(2): 141-148.

DerSimonian R, Laird N. 1986. Meta-analysis in clinical trials. *Controlled Clinical Trials* 7(3): 177-188.

Dumas S, Parent ME, Siemiatycki J, Brisson J. 2000. Rectal cancer and occupational risk factors: A hypothesis-generating, exposure-based case-control study. *International Journal of Cancer* 87(6): 874-879.

Edelman DA. 1988. Exposure to asbestos and the risk of gastrointestinal cancer: A reassessment. *British Journal of Industrial Medicine* 45(2): 75-82.

Edelman DA. 1989. Laryngeal cancer and occupational exposure to asbestos. *International Archives of Occupational and Environmental Health* 61(4): 223-227.

Ederer F, Geisser MS, Mongin SJ, Church TR, Mandel JS. 1999. Colorectal cancer deaths as determined by expert committee and from death certificate: A comparison. The Minnesota Study. *Journal of Clinical Epidemiology* 52(5): 447-452.

EPA (US Environmental Protection Agency). 1986. *Airborne Asbestos Health Assessment Update*. Washington, DC: US Environmental Protection Agency, Office of Health and Environmental Assessment. EPA/600/8-84/003f.

Frumkin H, Berlin J. 1988. Asbestos exposure and gastrointestinal malignancy: Review and meta-analysis. *American Journal of Industrial Medicine* 14(1): 79-95.

Gamble JF. 1994. Asbestos and colon cancer: A weight-of-the-evidence review. *Environmental Health Perspectives* 102(12): 1038-1050.

Goldberg MS, Parent ME, Siemiatycki J, Desy M, Nadon L, Richardson L, Lakhani R, Latreille B, Valois MF. 2001. A case-control study of the relationship between the risk of colon cancer in men and exposures to occupational agents. *American Journal of Industrial Medicine* 39(6): 531-546.

Goldsmith JR. 1982. Asbestos as a systemic carcinogen: The evidence from eleven cohorts. *American Journal of Industrial Medicine* 3(3): 341-348.

Goodman M, Morgan RW, Ray R, Malloy CD, Zhao K. 1999. Cancer in asbestos-exposed occupational cohorts: A meta-analysis. *Cancer Causes and Control* 10(5): 453-465.

Goodman S, Samet J. 2006. Cause and cancer epidemiology. In: *Cancer Epidemiology and Prevention*. 3rd edition. New York: Oxford University Press.

Griffiths H, Molony NC. 2003. Does asbestos cause laryngeal cancer? *Clinical Otolaryngology and Allied Sciences* 28(3): 177-182.

Guidotti TL, Abraham JL, DeNee PB. 1975. Letter: Asbestos exposure and cancer of the larynx. *Western Journal of Medicine* 122(1): 75.

Hallenbeck WH, Hesse CS. 1977. A review of the health effects of ingested asbestos. *Reviews in Environmental Health* 2(3): 157-166.

Hessel PA, Teta MJ, Goodman M, Lau E. 2004. Mesothelioma among brake mechanics: An expanded analysis of a case-control study. *Risk Analysis* 24(3): 547-552.

HEW (US Department of Health Education and Welfare). 1964. *Smoking and Health: Report of the Advisory Committee to the Surgeon General*. Washington, DC: US Government Printing Office.

HHS (US Department of Health and Human Services). 2004. *The Health Effects of Active Smoking: A Report of the Surgeon General*. Washington, DC: US Government Printing Office.

Homa DM, Garabrant DH, Gillespie BW. 1994. A meta-analysis of colorectal cancer and asbestos exposure. *American Journal of Epidemiology* 139(12): 1210-1222.

IARC (International Agency for Research on Cancer). 1977. *Asbestos*. IARC Monographs on the Evaluation of Carcinogenic Risks of Chemicals to Man 14:1-106. Lyon, France: World Health Organization.

IARC. 1987. *Overall Evaluations of Carcinogenity: An Updating of IARC Monographs Volumes 1 to 42*. IARC Monographs on the Evaluation of Carcinogenic Risks of Chemicals to Man. Supplement 7. Lyon, France: World Health Organization.

IARC. 2004. *Tobacco Smoke and Involuntary Smoking.* IARC Monographs on the Evaluation of Carcinogenic Risks to Human. Vol. 83. Lyon, France: World Health Organization.

IARC. 2006. *Preamble.* IARC Monographs on the Evaluation of Carcinogenic Risks to Humans. Lyon, France: World Health Organization.

IPCS (International Programme on Chemical Safety). 1998. *Chrysotile Asbestos: Environmental Health Criteria 203.* Geneva: World Health Organization.

Kanarek MS. 1989. Epidemiological studies on ingested mineral fibres: Gastric and other cancers. *IARC Scientific Publications* 90: 428-437.

Kleinfeld M. 1973. Biologic response to kind and amount of asbestos. *Journal of Occupational Medicine* 15(3): 296-300.

Koepsell TD, Weiss NS. 2003. *Epidemiological Methods: Studying the Occurrence of Illness.* New York: Oxford University Press.

Kraus T, Drexler H, Weber A, Raithel HJ. 1995. The association of occupational asbestos dust exposure and laryngeal carcinoma. *Israel Journal of Medical Sciences* 31(9): 540-548.

Kriebel D, Zeka A, Eisen EA, Wegman DH. 2004. Quantitative evaluation of the effects of uncontrolled confounding by alcohol and tobacco in occupational cancer studies. *International Journal of Epidemiology* 33(5): 1040-1045.

Landrigan PJ, Nicholson WJ, Suzuki Y, Ladou J. 1999. The hazards of chrysotile asbestos: A critical review. *Industrial Health* 37(3): 271-280.

Leitner C, Rogers SN, Lowe D, Magennis P. 2001. Death certification in patients whose primary treatment for oral and oropharyngeal carcinoma was operation: 1992-1997. *British Journal of Oral Maxillofacial Surgery* 39(3): 204-209.

Li L, Sun TD, Zhang X, Lai RN, Li XY, Fan XJ, Morinaga K. 2004. Cohort studies on cancer mortality among workers exposed only to chrysotile asbestos: A meta-analysis. *Biomedical and Environmental Sciences* 17(4): 459-468.

Libshitz HI, Wershba MS, Atkinson GW, Southard ME. 1974. Asbestosis and carcinoma of the larynx: A possible association. *Journal of the American Medical Association* 228(12): 1571-1572.

Liddell FD. 1990. Laryngeal cancer and asbestos. *British Journal of Industrial Medicine* 47(5): 289-291.

Miller AB. 1978. Asbestos fibre dust and gastro-intestinal malignancies: Review of literature with regard to a cause/effect relationship. *Journal of Chronic Diseases* 31(1): 23-33.

Morgan RW, Foliart DE, Wong O. 1985. Asbestos and gastrointestinal cancer: A review of the literature. *Western Journal of Medicine* 143(1): 60-65.

NRC (National Research Council). 2004. *Research Priorities for Airborne Particulate Matter: IV. Continuing Research Progress.* Washington, DC: The National Academies Press.

OSHA (Occupational Safety and Health Administration). 1986. Asbestos: Final Rule. *Federal Register* 51: 22612.

Parent ME, Siemiatycki J, Fritschi L. 1998. Occupational exposures and gastric cancer. *Epidemiology* 9(1): 48-55.

Parent ME, Siemiatycki J, Fritschi L. 2000. Workplace exposures and oesophageal cancer. *Occupational and Environmental Medicine* 57(5): 325-334.

Parnes SM. 1996. Effects of asbestos on the larynx. *Current Opinion in Otolaryngology and Head and Neck Surgery* 4(1): 54-58.

Parnes SM. 1998. Update on the effects of asbestos on the larynx. *Current Opinion in Otolaryngology and Head and Neck Surgery* 6(1): 70-74.

Percy C, Stanek E, Gloeckler L. 1981. Accuracy of cancer death certificates and its effects on cancer mortality statistics. *American Journal of Public Health* 71(3): 242-250.

Peters JL, Sutton AJ, Jones DR, Abrams KR, Rushton L. 2006. Comparison of two methods to detect publication bias in meta-analysis. *Journal of the American Medical Association* 295(6): 676-680.

Petitti D. 2000. *Meta-analysis, Decision Analysis, and Cost-Effectiveness: Methods for Quantitative Synthesis in Medicine.* 2nd edition. New York: Oxford University Press.

ProCite (*ProCite for Windows*). 2003. Version 5.0.3. ISI ResearchSoft.

Rice C, Heineman EF. 2003. An asbestos job exposure matrix to characterize fiber type, length, and relative exposure intensity. *Applied Occupational and Environmental Hygiene* 18(7): 506-512.

Roggli VL. 2006. The role of analytical SEM in the determination of causation in malignant mesothelioma. *Ultrastructal Pathology* 30(1): 31-35.

Roggli VL, Oury TD, Moffatt EJ. 1997. Malignant mesothelioma in women. *Anatomic Pathology* 2: 147-163.

Rothman K, Greenland S. 1998. *Modern Epidemiology.* 2nd edition. Philadelphia, PA: Lippincott-Raven Publishers.

Sathiakumar N, Delzell E, Abdalla O. 1998. Using the National Death Index to obtain underlying cause of death codes. *Journal of Occupational and Environmental Medicine* 40(9): 808-813.

Schneiderman MA. 1974. Digestive system cancer among persons subjected to occupational inhalation of asbestos particles: A literature review with emphasis on dose response. *Environmental Health Perspectives* 9: 307-311.

Selikoff IJ. 1992. Death certificates in epidemiological studies, including occupational hazards: Inaccuracies in occupational categories. *American Journal of Industrial Medicine* 22(4): 493-504.

Selikoff IJ, Seidman H. 1992. Use of death certificates in epidemiological studies, including occupational hazards: Variations in discordance of different asbestos-associated diseases on best evidence ascertainment. *American Journal of Industrial Medicine* 22(4): 481-492.

Smith AH, Handley MA, Wood R. 1990. Epidemiological evidence indicates asbestos causes laryngeal cancer. *Journal of Occupational Medicine* 32(6): 499-507.

Smith WE. 1973. Asbestos, talc and nitrites in relation to gastric cancer. *American Industrial Hygiene Association Journal* 34(5): 227-228.

Suzuki Y, Yuen SR, Ashley R. 2005. Short, thin asbestos fibers contribute to the development of human malignant mesothelioma: Pathological evidence. *International Journal of Hygiene and Environmental Health* 208(3): 201-210.

Weiss NS. 2002. Can the "specificity" of an association be rehabilitated as a basis for supporting a causal hypothesis? *Epidemiology* 13: 6-8.

Weiss W. 1995. The lack of causality between asbestos and colorectal cancer. *Journal of Occupational and Environmental Medicine* 37(12): 1364-1373.

3

Background Information on Asbestos

INTRODUCTION

Asbestos is a term applied to several mineral species when they occur in a fibrous form (asbestiform). When the mineral species are asbestiform, they have the physical characteristics associated with asbestos, such as large aspect ratio of fibers, flexibility, separability and weavability of fibers, and chemical and physical durability. However, in addition to those common properties, each asbestos mineral species has unique chemical and physical properties that make it distinct from the others. Details about the nature and limitations of techniques used to identify and characterize asbestos fibers will not be discussed here, but can be found in reference sources such as Spurny (1994) and Roggli et al. (1992).

This chapter provides an overview of asbestos mineralogy, focusing on characteristics of asbestos fibers that are potentially relevant to carcinogenicity. In particular, the various asbestos mineral species are described, with an emphasis on the characteristics and properties related to their unique biologic properties. Minerals are known to interact dynamically with their environment particularly when they are in contact with a fluid. Such interactions often occur at the interface between the mineral and its environment, in other words, at the mineral's surface. These interactions are critically important in many natural environments and include such phenomena as dissolution and precipitation (which alter the fluid's composition), oxidation and reduction of species in the fluid, sorption, and ion exchange. Each of those phenomena has a potential role in mineral-induced pathogenesis, including carcinogenesis and fibrosis, although understanding of the relationship between mineralogic properties and pathogenesis remains incomplete.

The concept of *mineral species* is fundamental to mineralogy. A mineral species is a crystalline solid with a specific atomic structure and a specific chemical composition (or compositional range). The specific crystal structure and chemical composition of each mineral species imparts a unique set of properties, including how the species interacts physically and chemically with its environment. In a system paralleling that for the plant and animal kingdoms, mineral species are classified hierarchically. A mineral group is roughly equivalent to the *family* classification and consists of minerals with similar compositions or structures. Minerals may also exhibit variability within a species with respect to a particular property. For example, some mineral species may occur with an asbestiform habit (physical form) or a non-asbestiform habit. Those are typically not given distinct mineral-species names but instead are referred to as varieties of the same species; sometimes, they are given varietal names, as in the case of crocidolite, which is the asbestiform variety of the mineral species riebeckite.

Other mineral groups may have species with occasional asbestiform varieties, but the primary mineral groups for asbestos are *amphibole* and *serpentine*. Each species of these groups has a distinct crystal structure, but chemical compositions vary between species within the group. The principal mineral species constituting asbestos are detailed below; they include asbestiform serpentine (chrysotile) and asbestiform varieties of amphibole, such as tremolite, actinolite, anthophyllite, grunerite, riebeckite (also known as crocidolite), winchite, and richterite. Table 3.1 lists the mineral species, varietal names, and mineral groups associated with the common asbestos minerals. Although the three chrysotile mineral species all have the same ideal chemical formula, these polymorphs (or polytypes) differ in the nature of the stacking relationship between successive layers, with clinochrysotile being the most abundant type (Gaines et al. 1997).

"FIBROUS" AND "ASBESTIFORM"

Many minerals may occur as small particles, including particles in the respirable size range, which is less than about 10 μm in aerodynamic diameter. Of these, some may include particles with aspect ratios (length: diameter) of 5:1 or more, usually reflecting a characteristic of the underlying crystal structure. For example, asbestiform amphiboles have fibers that are elongate parallel to the underlying silicate chains in the structure.

Fibrous is a term applied to minerals that consist of fibers, that is, exhibit a large aspect ratio. Although the minimal aspect ratio of a mineral fiber may be debated, for the purpose of definition observed aspect ratios in general are very large (for example, over 5:1 and sometimes over 100:1).

TABLE 3.1 Asbestos Minerals

Mineral Group	Mineral Species	Asbestiform Variety	Ideal Chemical Formula[a]
Serpentine	Clinochrysotile	Chrysotile	$Mg_3Si_2O_5(OH)_4$
Serpentine	Orthochrysotile	Chrysotile	$Mg_3Si_2O_5(OH)_4$
Serpentine	Parachrysotile	Chrysotile	$Mg_3Si_2O_5(OH)_4$
Amphibole	Riebeckite	Crocidolite	$Na_2Fe_5Si_8O_{22}(OH)_2$
Amphibole	Grunerite	Amosite	$(FeMg)_7Si_8O_{22}(OH)_2$
Amphibole	Cummingtonite	Amosite	$(MgFe)_7Si_8O_{22}(OH)_2$
Amphibole	Gedrite	Amosite	$(MgFe)_5Al_2(Si_6Al_2)O_{22}(OH)_2$
Amphibole	Anthophyllite	Asbestiform anthophyllite	$(MgFe)_7(Si)_8O_{22}(OH)_2$
Amphibole	Tremolite	Asbestiform tremolite	$Ca_2Mg_5Si_8O_{22}(OH)_2$
Amphibole	Actinolite	Asbestiform actinolite	$Ca_2(MgFe)_5Si_8O_{22}(OH)_2$
Amphibole	Richterite	Asbestiform richterite	$Na_2Ca(MgFe)_5Si_8O_{22}(OH)_2$
Amphibole	(Alumino)winchite	Asbestiform winchite	$CaNa(MgFe)_4AlSi_8O_{22}(OH)_2$
Amphibole	Ferriwinchite	Asbestiform winchite	$CaNa(FeMg)_4Fe^{3+}Si_8O_{22}(OH)_2$

[a]Simplified representation of the overall stoichiometry of a mineral species. Mineral species typically have chemical modifications, such as substitutions of similar cations and sometimes anions (common examples are Mg^{2+}<->Fe^{2+} and Si^{4+}<->Al^{3+}). Substitutions may cause substantiated deviations from the ideal chemical formula. Limits of chemical variation are defined for each mineral species in Table 3.2.

SOURCE: Gaines et al. (1997).

Asbestiform refers to a subset of fibrous minerals. Among fibrous minerals, some exhibit the additional qualities of flexibility and separability (which contribute to weavability). Such minerals are referred to as asbestiform. Typically, asbestiform minerals also have relatively small fiber diameters (usually under 1 μm) and large fiber lengths (such as 5-10 μm). The asbestiform characteristics are related to properties of the underlying crystal structures, with the specific relationship according to the mineral group. For example, it has been suggested that flexibility is related to defects in the crystal structure of the asbestiform varieties of amphibole (Veblen and Wylie 1993), whereas flexibility in asbestiform serpentine (the various forms of chrysotile) may be related to the hydrogen bonding between concentric sheets of 1:1 layers, as described below.

Some mineral species have both asbestiform and non-asbestiform varieties, and these varieties may have properties beyond just their flexibility that differ. For example, consider the grain boundaries in asbestiform amphibole. Asbestos fibers typically occur as parallel bundles of fibrils (filaments consisting of individual crystals) that are bound together along grain boundaries. The material along the grain boundaries typically is not amphibole but rather a layer silicate, such as talc or mica. When the material is processed, fibers are produced by the breaking apart of packets of fibrils by separation along the structurally weaker grain boundaries, which allows the layer-silicate material to become the surface of the fiber. It is this crystalline material that interacts with the biologic system after inhalation or ingestion. In contrast, the surface of a non-asbestiform variety of amphibole (either an acicular crystal or a cleavage fragment) is often amphibole (and not layer silicate) because the particles are formed either by growth of the original amphibole crystal in the case of acicular fibers or by fracture along weaker atomic planes in the amphibole structure. Hence, asbestiform amphibole is likely to have a different surface structure and composition from non-asbestiform amphibole. Those differences in surface material result in different surface properties between asbestiform and non-asbestiform minerals of the same species, which may in turn result in different biologic responses.

Some fibrous but non-asbestiform minerals also pose potential concern with respect to human exposure. For example, the fibrous zeolite erionite has been associated with human cases of mesothelioma after environmental exposure (Baris et al. 1987).

SERPENTINE ASBESTOS (CHRYSOTILE) MINERALOGY

Chrysotile—sometimes called white asbestos—is the most common type of asbestos to be used commercially, accounting for about 85% of world asbestos production in 1977 (Liddell 1997, Schreier 1989). At present, chrysotile is the only type of asbestos used in manufacturing in the United States (ATSDR 2001). In addition, chrysotile and other serpentine minerals are common naturally, particularly in hydrothermally altered, magnesium-rich rocks, such as altered basalt, peridotite, and dunite. Many such rocks have been almost completely altered to serpentine and are referred to as serpentinites. Although lizardite is the most common form of serpentine in these rocks, chrysotile can also be present, typically having formed as a late-stage mineral filling veins and sometimes replacing the bulk rock. Chrysotile has been commercially exploited in Canada (Quebec and Ontario), the United States (Vermont and California), Zimbabwe, Russia, South Africa, Australia, and elsewhere (Ross 1981), and it has been used in various products, including insulation, friction materials (such as brake pads), and fiber-reinforced composites (such as concrete) (Harrison et al. 1999, Ross and Virta 2001). In addition to synthetic chrysotile-bearing materials, natural deposits are possible sources of exposure to chrysotile, either by direct exposure to chrysotile-bearing rocks and soils or by redistribution of chrysotile fibers from large natural deposits, such as occurs at Coalinga, California (Klein 1993). It has been argued that atmospheric processes have redistributed Coalinga chrysotile over the entire Northern Hemisphere from its occurrence in soils in a 50-mi^2 area (Klein 1993).

Serpentine minerals belong to a family of 1:1 layer silicates, which are composed of a sheet of polymerized SiO_4^{4-} tetrahedra (with silicon at the center of each tetrahedron and oxygen at each apex) that is bonded to a sheet of polymerized $Mg(OH)_6^{4-}$ octahedra (with magnesium at the center of each octahedron and oxygen at each apex) (Figure 3.1). This ratio of tetrahedral to octahedral sheets gives the 1:1 layer silicates their name. The

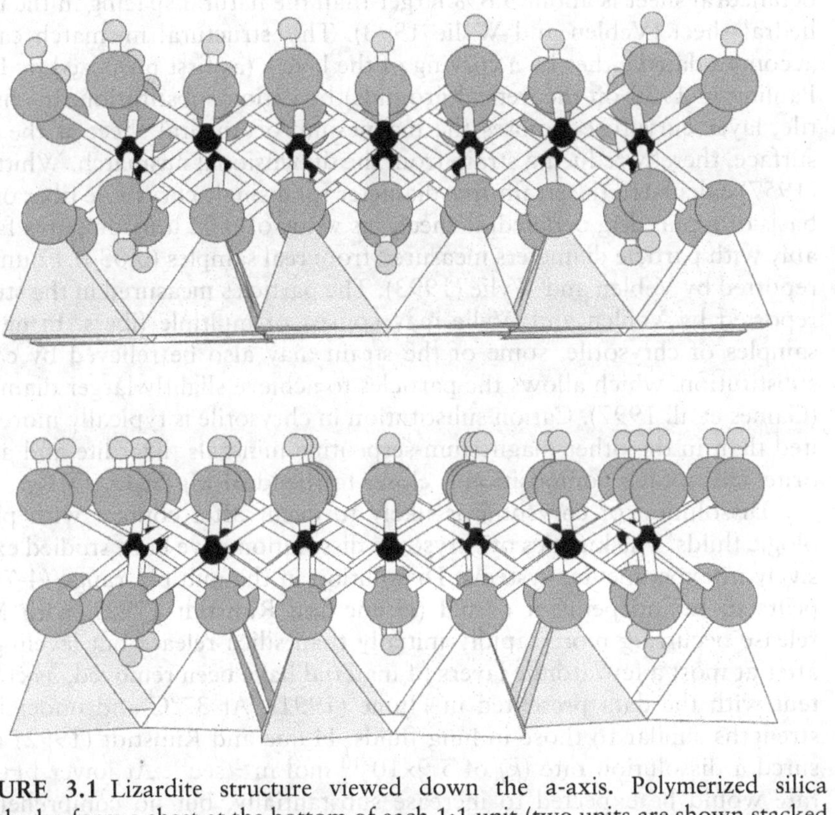

FIGURE 3.1 Lizardite structure viewed down the a-axis. Polymerized silica tetrahedra form a sheet at the bottom of each 1:1 unit (two units are shown stacked vertically), and magnesium hydroxide octahedra form a sheet drawn as ball-and-stick. In chrysotile, the 1:1 units curl with the slightly smaller tetrahedral sheets to the inside, exposing an octahedral sheet to the outside of the particle.
SOURCE: Mellini (1982).

tetrahedral:octahedral (1:1) polymerized layers are stacked one atop another to form the chrysotile structure.

The serpentine group is based on a metal hydroxide sheet containing Mg^{2+} cations, giving rise to a composition of $Mg_3Si_2O_5(OH)_4$.

Chrysotile exhibits a smaller variation in chemical composition than other (non-asbestiform) serpentine minerals, but substitutions do occur. The most common substitutions are $Si^{4+} \rightarrow Al^{3+}$, $Mg^{2+} \rightarrow Fe^{2+}$, and $Mg^{2+} \rightarrow Al^{3+}$; however, these substitutions typically represent much less than 10% of the atomic sites (Veblen and Wylie 1993). Other metal substitutions (such as Ni, Co, Mn, Cr, and Zn) may occur in trace amounts (Ross 1981).

Dimensionally, the octahedral (Mg) sheet is slightly larger than the tetrahedral (Si) sheet. The two sheets are bonded to one another by the sharing of some of their oxygen atoms; the natural spacing of the atoms in the octahedral sheet is about 3.6% larger than the natural spacing in the tetrahedral sheet (Veblen and Wylie 1993). This structural mismatch can be accommodated either by a curving of the layers (as first proposed by Linus Pauling in 1930 on theoretical grounds) by cation substitution. In chrysotile, layer curvature exposes the magnesium octahedral sheet at the fiber surface, thereby reducing strain from the dimensional mismatch. Whittaker (1957) calculated the strain-free diameter for a single chrysotile fiber on the basis of a pure Mg octahedral sheet; his value of 0.02 μm compares favorably with particle diameters measured from real samples (0.03-0.17 μm), as reported by Veblen and Wylie (1993). The particles measured in the studies reported by Veblen and Wylie may consist of multiple fibers. In natural samples of chrysotile, some of the strain may also be relieved by cation substitution, which allows the particles to achieve slightly larger diameters (Gaines et al. 1997). Cation substitution in chrysotile is typically more limited than in the other magnesium-serpentine minerals (lizardite and antigorite; chrysotile's composition is closer to the ideal $Mg_3Si_2O_5(OH)_4$.

Dissolution of chrysotile is likely to occur after contact with physiologic fluids. The kinetics of chrysotile dissolution have been studied extensively in experimental systems. Dissolution in the mid pH range (4-7) appears to be independent of pH (Hume and Rimstidt 1992), with Mg^{2+} release occurring more rapidly initially than silica release but leveling off after at most a few atomic layers of material have been removed, as consistent with the data presented in Hume (1991). At 37°C and under ionic strengths similar to those in lung fluids, Hume and Rimstidt (1992) measured a dissolution rate (k) of 5.9×10^{-10} mol m^{-2} sec^{-1}. At lower pH, the rate would be expected to increase substantially, but no comprehensive quantitative study has been done on chrysotile dissolution rate as a function of pH in acidic environments. At the stated rate, a chrysotile particle, even as thick as 1 μm, would be predicted to be removed from the lung by dissolution in less than a year. The process would remove the pathogenic particle, but it would also release into the surrounding environment any trace metals from the particle, which could be toxic in their own right, although probably in a transient fashion.

AMPHIBOLE ASBESTOS MINERALOGY

Amphiboles are common silicate minerals found in many types of rocks. Although most occurrences of amphibole are non-asbestiform, large deposits of some asbestiform amphiboles have been exploited commercially, particularly from deposits in South Africa, Australia, and Finland. Those that have been exploited commercially typically belong to a small subset of amphibole mineral species (riebeckite or crocidolite, grunerite, anthophyllite, actinolite, and tremolite). As discussed below, other amphiboles may also occur with asbestiform habits, including winchite and richterite, which are associated with human exposures in Libby, Montana. In addition, some amphiboles occur with fibrous but non-asbestiform habits, such as byssolite (the stiff-fibered form of actinolite).

Amphibole minerals form a family of double-chain silicates, which are composed of I-beams, as shown in Figure 3.2. Chains of polymerized silica tetrahedra are on both the top and bottom of the I-beam. Between the

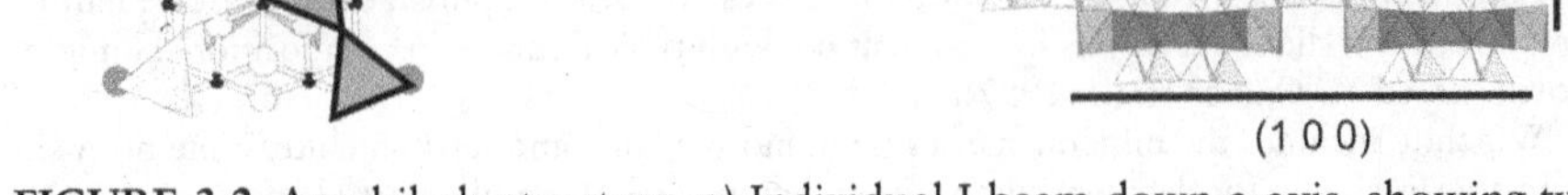

FIGURE 3.2 Amphibole structure. a) Individual I-beam down a-axis, showing two chains of polymerized silica tetrahedra (one darker) overlying strip of metal octahedra (shown as ball-and-stick). A sites are in channels formed by stacked I-beams; B sites appear as larger dark atoms at edges of the octahedral strip; C sites appear as smaller black atoms in middle of octahedral strip; T sites appear as triangles. Larger white atoms are oxygen atoms or hydroxyl groups. b) Individual I-beam down the c-axis, showing two tetrahedral chains on top and bottom of I-beam. c) Amphibole structure down c-axis, showing interconnectivity of I-beams, various cation sites, and common cleavage planes in amphibole that would lead to surfaces found in non-asbestiform amphibole particles.
SOURCE: Papike et al. (1969)

TABLE 3.2 Mineral Names, Varietal Names, and Atomic Site Compositions[a] for Amphiboles That Have Been Commonly Encountered in an Asbestiform Habit

Mineral (variety)	A	B	C	T	Compositional Limits (stoichiometric range)
Riebeckite (crocidolite)		Na_2	$(Fe^{3+}Fe^{2+}Mg)_5$	Si_8	$1.5<Fe^{3+}<2.5$ $Fe^{2+}\geq 2.5$
Grunerite-cummingtonite (amosite)		$(Fe^{2+}Mg)_2$	$(Fe^{2+}Mg)_5$	Si_8	$Mg<4.9$ (total out of B+C)
Gedrite (amosite)	Na_{0-1}	$(MgFe^{2+}Al)_2$	$(MgFe^{2+}Al)_5$	Si_7Al	$0.7<Mg<6.3$ (total out of B+C)
Anthophyllite (asbestiform anthophyllite)		$(MgFe^{2+}Al)_2$	$(MgFe^{2+}Al)_5$	Si_7Al	$0.7<Mg<6.3$ (total out of B+C)
Tremolite (asbestiform tremolite)		Ca_2	Mg_5	Si_8	$4.5\leq Mg$
Actinolite (asbestiform actinolite)		Ca_2	$(Mg,Fe^{2+})_5$	Si_8	$0.5<Fe<2.5$
Winchite[b] (asbestiform winchite)		CaNa	$(MgFe^{2+}AlFe^{3+})_5$	Si_8	(NaK)<0.5 in A site $2.5<Mg$
Richterite (asbestiform richterite)	Na	CaNa	$(MgFe)_5$	Si_8	$2.5<Mg$

[a]Compositions shown for the A, B, C, and T sites are ideal simplified compositions; natural samples exhibit slight variations in composition, with typical ranges in compositional limits as shown, based on Gaines et al. (1997).

[b]Winchite includes the mineral species (alumino)winchite and ferriwinchite. Note no A site occupancy is shown for the ideal composition, but in natural samples partial occupation by Na or K may occur, with a limit of less than 0.5 out of a total of 1 atomic site.

SOURCE: Gaines et al. (1997), Veblen and Wylie (1993).

silica chains lies a sheet of octahedrally coordinated metal ions (specifically, the atomic B sites). At the midpoints along the edges of the I-beam are the eight slightly larger and coordinated C sites. The I-beams—which run the length of the fibers in asbestiform amphibole—are stacked as shown in Figure 3.2c, creating an additional atomic site, the A site.

The complexity of atomic sites in amphiboles is reflected in their chemical complexity. The general formula for amphiboles can be described as $A_{0-1}B_2C_5[T_8O_{22}](OH)_2$, where A sites are coordinated by 12 oxygens and can accommodate large monovalent cations; B sites are coordinated by eight oxygens and can accommodate large monovalent and divalent cations; C sites are coordinated by six oxygens and can accommodate only smaller cations; and T sites are four coordinated tetrahedral sites that can accommodate only very small cations, such as Si^{4+} and Al^{3+}. Table 3.2 lists compositions of amphiboles that have been recognized in association with disease in humans. The compositions shown are idealized chemical formulas, but natural samples often have compositions that differ slightly with respect to both major and trace elements. For example, analysis of the amphibole from Libby, Montana, that has been associated with respiratory disease (Gunter et al. 2003) shows substantial deviation from the ideal chemical formulae for either winchite or richterite because of substitutions of isovalent cations or anions or because of a portion of atomic sites being empty:

$$(K_{0.19}Na_{0.32})(Ca_{1.12}Na_{0.85}Mn_{0.03})(Mg_{4.43}Fe^{3+}{}_{0.34}Fe^{2+}{}_{0.19}Al_{0.02}Mn_{0.01}Ti_{0.01})$$
$$(Si_{7.97}Al_{0.03})O_{22}(OH_{1.63}F_{0.37}).$$

Dimensionally, amphibole asbestos fibers exhibit a range of diameters. As reported in Veblen and Wylie (1993), particle diameters as measured on both bulk and airborne samples fall in the range 0.06-0.70 μm, with riebeckite (crocidolite) particles generally thinner and anthophyllite asbestos particles thicker.

Amphibole dissolution is considerably slower than chrysotile dissolution, as measured experimentally. Although no rates have been reported specifically for dissolution of asbestiform amphibole, experimentally determined rates for amphiboles in general typically fall in the range of 10^{-12}-10^{-10} mol m^{-2} sec^{-1}, that is, orders of magnitude smaller than those for chrysotile. Such dissolution rates imply that a typical amphibole fiber will not dissolve in the lung over the course of a human lifetime. In fact, amphibole fibers often serve as sites of precipitation in the lung, becoming coated with iron-rich material to form an asbestos body. Whether amphiboles would dissolve substantially in lower-pH physiologic fluids, as would be found in the stomach, is not known.

PROPERTIES OF POTENTIALLY HAZARDOUS FIBROUS MINERALS

Several physical and chemical factors may contribute to a mineral particle's pathogenic potential (Table 3.3). Many properties are related to how a mineral interacts with a fluid under various conditions. The impor-

TABLE 3.3 Mineralogic Properties in Relation to Pathogenesis

Mineralogical Property	Potential Relationship to Pathogenesis
Particle size	• Penetration and deposition in lung • Dissolution and chemical reactions between mineral particle and fluid are influenced by surface area per mass of particles • Ability of cells to phagocytize particle
Particle shape	• Particle fate and transport (such as translocation) • Relative proportions of different structural surfaces exposed to fluids and cells • Ability of cells to clear particle by phagocytosis
Dissolution	• Particle removal (chrysotile can dissolve appreciably in human time scales, whereas amphibole cannot) • Change in particle shape or surface structures, leading to alteration in other mineral-fluid interactions • Change in fluid chemistry by release of metals and other mineral components to fluid
Precipitation	• Change in particle shape and/or surface structures, leading to alteration in other mineral-fluid interactions
Sorption	• Mineral surfaces can serve as catalysts for reactions between fluid constituents by changing their effective concentration or by changing their physical orientation to one another (latter is relevant only for molecules)
Ion exchange	• Buffering of activity for aqueous species, such as Na^+, K^+, and Ca^{2+}
Acid-base catalysis	• Mineral surfaces can transfer protons with fluid constituents
Oxidation-reduction	• Mineral surfaces can transfer electrons with fluid constituents

tance of those properties in natural environments is well recognized, but they have not been studied in the context of the pathogenesis of cancer or other diseases by minerals. They are discussed here to provide a context for the potential roles of minerals in biologic processes that lead to disease. Their potential role in pathogenesis will be discussed below. Crystal structure and composition determine a mineral's properties, so each of the different mineral species discussed above will behave somewhat differently as it interacts with body fluids.

Particle size and shape are widely recognized to be important in determining the deposition and translocation of a particle, particularly in the context of respirable particles (e.g., Lehnert 1993). In general, the smaller the particle, the further it can be transported before settling because of gravitational forces. The net effect is that particles with aerodynamic diameters less than about 5 μm are more likely to reach the lower airways, whereas larger particles are usually deposited higher in the respiratory tract and perhaps cleared via the mucociliary escalator. Consequently, the distribution of particle sizes and shapes to which a particular potential target organ or site is exposed may differ from the distribution of the dose to which another site is exposed (Quinn et al. 1997). Different particle size-shape populations may, in turn, have of different physical or chemical characteristics. Two important factors are directly associated with particle size: surface area per mass and size relative to cells. The first factor affects surface-controlled reactions, including many of those discussed below; surface-controlled reactions are those that occur between a mineral surface and its environment (for example, a physiologic fluid), such as dissolution, sorption, and oxidation-reduction. The second factor influences how a cell interacts with a particle, which is most important when a particle is roughly cell-sized or smaller. For example, macrophages have been observed to attempt phagocytosis of particles (fibers in particular) that are around 5-10 μm in length or greater; this process can result in the release of inflammatory agents to the local environment. When particles are much smaller than a macrophage (about 1-2 μm), they are readily cleared via phagocytosis.

Mineral dissolution has several potential roles in the biologic response to exposure to asbestos. One role is to remove a particle. Of the minerals discussed here, only chrysotile is expected to dissolve substantially under most physiologic conditions, and the potential for chrysotile fibers to dissolve while amphibole fibers are far more persistent may be relevant to the relative carcinogenicity of the two main fiber types. Hume and Rimstidt (1992) estimated lifetimes of about 9 months for a 1-μm-diameter fiber, and their model predicts that fibers with diameters of 0.1 μm would require only weeks to dissolve completely. As a mineral dissolves, material is removed from its surface, and this can affect structure and composition and therefore surface properties. Hence, mineral dissolution may affect any pathogenic process that is related to surface interactions (such as those discussed below). Another potential role for dissolution in pathogenesis is the release of trace elements from the crystal structure. In particular, some of the minerals discussed contain trace amounts of polyvalent cations that could have a role in mineral-induced pathogenesis. Such a process has been related to the observed high potency of iron-bearing asbestos minerals in some experimental systems. For example, it has been postulated that iron released from some types of asbestos by dissolution serves as an oxidation-reduction catalyst in a Fenton-type reaction to produce free radicals (Aust and Lund 1990).

Mineral precipitation can occur when the concentration of dissolved aqueous species reaches a critical value that depends on the mineral species. Mineral precipitation has been observed to occur on the surface of some asbestos fibers after a period of time, forming particles known as asbestos bodies or ferruginous bodies. Although the details of formation are not fully known, an asbestos body reflects the precipitation of ferric iron hydroxides on a particle's surface, consequently radically changing the surface properties of the particle. The native asbestos surface is no longer exposed, but instead the surface may consist of a quasi-crystalline material with a high sorption capacity and with relatively low solubility (the solubility of ferric iron, Fe^{3+}, is much lower than the solubility of ferrous iron, Fe^{2+}). Ferruginous coatings have also been observed to form on minerals other than asbestos (Roggli et al. 1992).

Sorption is the process by which atoms or molecules in a fluid bind to the surface of a mineral. Sorption has numerous roles in mineral-fluid interactions, including being a component of many of the processes described here (dissolution, precipitation, oxidation-reduction, and acid-base catalysis). It can also affect reactions in a fluid by allowing atoms and molecules to be concentrated at the mineral surface, thereby effectively raising their activities. Furthermore, sorption processes often orient molecules on the basis of the stereochemistry of the surface and the molecules. Those two aspects of sorption can initiate reactions among fluid species that might otherwise proceed slowly or not at all; for example, Ferris and Ertem (1992) found that the clay mineral montmorillonite catalyzes the oligomerization of ribonuleotides from aqueous solution. Finally, sorption of hazardous molecules (perhaps before introduction of a particle to the physiological environment) can allow the particle to function as an effective delivery agent; this has been suggested to be the case for mineral sorption of constituents from cigarette smoke or diesel exhaust.

Ion exchange is the process by which cations (typically monovalent or divalent cations, such as Na^+, K^+, and Ca^{2+}) that are loosely bound to a mineral are able to exchange with a monovalent or divalent cation in solution. The exchange capacity of the mineral is related to the proportion of exchangeable cation sites that are directly accessible by the fluid (the surface sites) or by cations along rapid-diffusion pathways (such as channels greater than about 0.3 nm); hence, a particle has a finite potential for ion exchange. Nevertheless, ion exchange can effectively buffer the activity of a cation at the surface of a particle for some time. Because of their high surface-area-to-mass ratio, small asbestos particles could have a relatively large ion exchange capacity. Particularly for amphibole fibers with ions in the A sites (such as crocidolite), ion activity is important in many cellular signaling pathways, but whether mineral-induced ion exchange can affect these pathways remains to be investigated.

Mineral surfaces may be the site of catalytic functionalities, such as proton or electron donors and acceptors. Proton donor or acceptor sites can function as acid-base catalysts in many reactions. Numerous types of such sites are present on mineral surfaces (Hochella 1993). In freshly fractured silicate minerals (including asbestos), broken bonds result in surface silica sites that are unde saturated with respect to ionic charge. As those sites interact with water and dissipate the surface charge, they generate free radicals in the fluid. Fubini et al. (1990) have shown that the process can be particularly important in silica-induced pathogenesis. Ultimately, the sites become silanol groups (Si-OH) that will protonate or deprotonate in response to pH. Indeed, many surface oxygens will function similarly, and the acidic strength of protons on these sites depends on the local charge distribution in the underlying mineral.

Surface-induced oxidation-reduction is another catalytic pathway for mineral surfaces. Oxidation-reduction involves the exchange of electrons between the mineral surface and a fluid species; it results in the oxidation of the mineral site and reduction of the fluid species, or vice versa. Such processes are observed in natural environments; the mineral surface donates electrons and thereby reduces species in the fluid and commonly forms metal precipitation at structurally determined sites (Ilton et al. 1992). That process can occur in minerals that contain polyvalent cations (such as Fe^{2+} and Fe^{3+}) in sites that are sufficiently close to allow charge transfer (as in the case of the octahedral strips in amphiboles). In fact, under some pH regimes, mineral surfaces are stronger redox catalysts than iron in solution (Hochella 1993); this suggests that the Fenton reaction proposed for free-radical formation by some asbestos may be as likely with iron on the mineral surface as with dissolved iron in the fluid. Although that process has not been investigated directly in relation to mineral-induced pathogenesis, indirect observations support the idea that it is important in physiologic fluids. For example, observations of mineral particles recovered from the lung show micas with precipitation on the edges consistent with a structurally controlled reduction-precipitation process (Roggli et al. 1992).

REFERENCES

ATSDR (Agency for Toxic Substances and Disease Registry). 2001. *Toxicological Profile for Asbestos.* Atlanta, GA: US Department of Health and Human Services.

Aust AE, Lund LG. 1990. The role of iron on asbestos-catalyzed damage to lipids and DNA. In: Reddy CC, Hamilton GA, Madyastha KM, eds. *Biological Oxidation Systems.* Vol. 1-2. San Diego, CA: Academic Press. Pp. 597-606.

Baris I, Simonato L, Artvinli M, Pooley F, Saracci R, Skidmore J, Wagner C. 1987. Epidemiological and environmental evidence of the health effects of exposure to erionite fibres: A four-year study in the Cappadocian region of Turkey. *International Journal of Cancer* 39(1): 10-17.

Ferris JP, Ertem G. 1992. Oligomerization of ribonucleotides on montmorillonite: Reaction of the 5'-phophorimidazolide of adenosine. *Science* 257: 1387-1389.

Fubini B, Giamello E, Volante M, Bolis V. 1990. Chemical functionalitites at the silica surface determine its reactivity when inhaled formation and reactivity of surface radicals. *Toxicology and Industrial Health* 6(6): 571-598.

Gaines RV, Skinner HCW, Ford EE, Mason B, Rosenzweig A. 1997. *Dana's New Mineralogy.* New York: John Wiley and Sons. P. 1810.

Gunter ME, Dyar MD, Twamley B, Foit F, Cornelius S. 2003. Composition, Fe3+/SFe, and crystal structure of non-asbestiform and asbestiform amphiboles from Libby, Montana, USA. *American Mineralogist* 88: 1970-1978.

Harrison PTC, Levy LS, Patrick G, Pigott GH, Smitt LL. 1999. Comparative hazards of chrysotile asbestos and its substitutes: A European perspective. *Environmental Health Perspectives* 107: 607-612.

Hochella MF. 1993. Surface chemistry, structure, and reactivity of hazardous mineral dust. In: Guthrie GD, Mossman BT, eds. *Health Effects of Mineral Dusts.* Reviews in Mineralogy. Vol. 28. Mineralogical Society of America. Pp. 275-308.

Hume LA. 1991. *The Dissolution of Chrysotile.* M.S. thesis. Virginia Polytechnic Institute and State University, Blacksburg, VA. 46 pp.

Hume LA, Rimstidt JD. 1992. The biodurablity of chrysotile asbestos. *American Mineralogist* 77: 1125-1128.

Ilton ES, Earley D, Marozas D, Veblen DR. 1992. Reaction of some trioctahedral micas with copper-sulfate solutions at 25°C and 1 atomsphere: An electron microphobe and transmission electron microscopy investigation. *Economic Geology* 87: 1813-1829.

Klein C. 1993. Rocks, minerals, and a dusty world. *Reviews in Mineralogy* 28: 6-138.

Lehnert BE. 1993. Defense mechanisms against inhaled particles and associated particle-cell interactions. *Reviews in Mineralogy and Geochemistry* 28: 427-469.

Liddell F. 1997. Magic, menace, myth and malice. *Annals of Occupational Hygiene* 41(1): 3-12.

Mellini M. 1982. The crystal structure of lizardite 1T: Hydrogen bonds and polytypism. *American Mineralogist* 67: 587-598.

Papike JJ, Ross M, Clark JR. 1969. Crystal chemical characterization of clinoamphiboles based on five new structure refinements. *Mineralogical Society of America Special Paper* 2: 117-137.

Pauling L. 1930. The structure of the chlorites. *Proceedings of the National Academy of Sciences of the United States of America* 16: 578-582.

Quinn MM, Ellenbecker MJ, Smith TJ, Wegman DH, Eisen EA. 1997. A model to predict deposition of man-made vitreous fibres in the human tracheobronchial region. *Annals of Occupational Hygiene* 41 (Supplement 1): 197-202.

Roggli VL, Pratt PC, Brody AR. 1992. Analysis of tissue mineral fiber content. In: Roggli V, Greenburg S, Pratt P, eds. *Pathology of Asbestos-Associated Diseases.* 1st edition. New York: Lippincott Williams and Wilkins. Pp. 305-354.

Ross M. 1981. The geologic occurrences and health hazards of amphibole and serpentine asbestos. *Reviews in Mineralogy and Geochemistry* 9A: 279-323.

Ross M, Virta R. 2001. Occurrence, production and uses of asbestos. *Canadian Mineralogist* 5: 79-88.

Schreier H. 1989. *Asbestos in the Natural Environment.* New York: Elsevier Science Publication.

Spurny KR. 1994. Sampling, analysis, identification, and monitoring of fibrous dusts and aerosols. *The Analyst* 119: 41-51.

Veblen DR, Wylie AG. 1993. Mineralogy of amphiboles and 1:1 layer silicates. *Reviews in Mineralogy and Geochemistry* 28: 61-138.

Whittaker EJW. 1957. The structure of chrysotile. V. Diffuse reflexions and fibre texture. *ACTA Crystallographica* 10 (Part 3): 149-156.

4

Exposure and Disposition

EXPOSURE

Introduction

Briefly this section reviews the uses of asbestos, how people may be exposed to it, the magnitude of exposure, and how it is measured. For detailed information, the reader is directed to the more comprehensive reviews conducted by the Agency for Toxic Substances and Disease Registry (ATSDR 2001), the International Agency for Research on Cancer (IARC 1977), and the International Program on Chemical Safety (IPCS 1986).

Asbestos has had a very wide array of uses. It has been used extensively for insulation and in textiles and has been mixed and bonded with cement, plastics, and resins. Production of asbestos products in the United States, Canada, and most other industrialized countries increased rapidly in the 20th century, particularly during World War II, and peaked in the early to mid 1970s. In 1973, the US Environmental Protection Agency (EPA) prohibited spraying of asbestos insulation, and further restrictions were later applied. Many other industrialized countries enacted similar regulations or outright bans, and the use and production of asbestos dropped rapidly.

Although many uses have been discontinued, asbestos is still used in some limited applications. In 2003, asbestos was not produced in the United States, although 6,000 metric tons were consumed—80% for specialized roofing products; 8% for gaskets; 4% for friction products, such as vehicles brake pads, clutches, and transmissions; and 8% for other uses (USGS 2004). Some European countries have banned all uses of asbestos. However, exposure occurs in all countries when buildings, ships, and other structures insulated with asbestos are demolished, when asbestos is removed, or during maintenance and repair of asbestos-containing materials.

Consideration needs to be given to the different measurement methods used when interpreting and comparing the reported levels of airborne exposure in various settings. Historically, airborne asbestos in workplaces was measured with a midget impinger to collect the fibers, a standard occupational hygiene method, and concentrations were expressed as millions of particles per cubic foot (mppcf). More recently, airborne fibers have been collected on membrane filters, and concentration has been reported in terms of either mass (such as nanograms per cubic meter, ng/m^3) or number of fibers (such as fibers per milliliter, f/ml). The latter measure is most commonly used. In water, concentrations may be expressed in terms of fibers per liter. In a given measurement system, fibers may qualify for counting on the basis of criteria such as length (for instance, over 5 μm) or aspect (length:diameter) ratio (for instance, over 3:1), characteristics also relevant to their potential to cause health effects.

Fibers may be counted with either phase-contrast microscopy (PCM) or transmission electron microscopy (TEM). Of the two, TEM is the more sensitive and may measure higher concentrations in the same environment than PCM, because PCM may miss very thin fibers. In addition, PCM may fail to distinguish asbestos from other types of fibers. However, workplace exposures are generally measured with PCM, which is less expensive and considered adequate by regulatory agencies. Conversion between different measures of airborne units is problematic because conversion factors vary with the distribution of fiber thickness and length in the environment of interest. The most valid approach to conversion involves obtaining measurements simultaneously under the same conditions using the different methods for which conversion factors are needed. Using that approach, Dement et al. (1983) found factors for converting PCM to TPM data within the same facilities in the textile industry that ranged from 2.5 to 7.5 f/ml :: 1 mppcf.

Occupational Exposure

Asbestos concentrations observed in occupational settings have been orders of magnitude higher than the highest concentrations observed in residential settings, but some in-home activities, such as shaking out work clothes, can produce levels that may rival those found in the workplace. The highest well-documented exposures have been among workers manufacturing asbestos products or employed in mining and milling operations. Table 4.1 provides selected summary statistics for some asbestos-product manufacturing facilities in the United States based on samples

TABLE 4.1 Concentrations of Fibers in Various US Asbestos-Using Industries

Industry	Plants	Years	Range of Means Within Departments (# fibers >5 μm)/ml, PCM
Insulation plants	5 plants	1966-1971	0.01-74.4
Textile plants	8 plants	1964-1971	0.1-29.9
Friction products plants	5 plants	1968-1971	0.1-14.4
Paper, packing, asphalt products	not reported	1966-1970	0.2-13.6
Cement pipe	7 plants	1969-1970	0.2-6.3
Cement shingle, millboard, gasket	3 plants	1966-1970	0.1-4.4

SOURCE: NIOSH (1972).

collected in 1964-1971 (NIOSH 1972). The table indicates that the highest concentrations were observed in the textile and insulation industries but also that levels of exposure varied considerably between and within industries. Thus, exposure cannot be estimated with any certainty on the basis of descriptions of exposure situations.

The report by Dement et al. (1983) provides a useful example of variability of exposures within an industry. In a large US textile-manufacturing facility, exposures were highest in the 1930s and 1940s and generally, although not uniformly, decreased through the 1970s with the introduction of technologic changes. Concentrations varied among departments by as much as an order of magnitude. In the 1930s, mean concentrations in some areas of fiber preparation were up to 78 f/ml and other areas, such as spinning, had means below 10 f/ml. A similar range of exposures has been reported for the textile industry in Italy (Pira et al. 2005) and in England (Peto et al. 1985).

Concentrations in the mining and milling industries have been similiar to those in manufacturing. For example, in the mid 1960s, mean exposures of 20-100 f/ml were reported at the Wittenoom crocidolite mines and mills in Western Australia; they may have been higher in earlier decades (Armstrong et al. 1988, Reid et al. 2004). Exposures in a similar range have been reported in Quebec (Gibbs and LaChance 1974); Libby, Montana (Amandus et al. 1987); and South Africa (Sluis-Cremer et al. 1992).

Exposure levels of end-users of asbestos are less well documented, at least historically, but appear to be lower when considered as time-weighted averages. Insulation workers constitute a group with potentially high exposures. Although Selikoff et al. (1979) anecdotally reported exposures of 4-12 f/ml, the National Institute of Occupational Safety and Health (NIOSH 1972) reported individual exposures of 0 up to 100 f/ml when shorter-term exposures were considered. Insulation workers engaged in ship building and repair, in which mean exposures may have been as high as 30 f/ml (NIOSH 1972), are of particular concern. Other end-users may have had lower exposures. For example, Corn et al. (1994) reported means during various maintenance activities of 0.008-0.061 f/ml, and other studies have observed similar, highly variable levels of exposure (ATSDR 2001). Mean levels of exposure during asbestos abatement have been measured at 0.006 to 0.76 f/ml (TEM) depending on the material being removed (ATSDR 2001). However, it is important to note that short-term exposures could be quite high.

Limits considered acceptable for occupational exposure have dropped over time. The American Conference of Governmental Industrial Hygienists first proposed a Threshold Limit Value (TLV) of 5 mppcf in 1946 (ACGIH 1998). However, historical sampling data show that many industries did not adhere to that guideline (for example, see Amandus et al. 1987, Dement et al. 1983, Hughes et al. 1987). With the wider recognition of the hazards of asbestos and the regulatory response, exposures rapidly decreased in the industrialized countries. Reductions in exposure due to improved technology have been well documented. An example from the US textile industry is presented in Table 4.2; Dement et al. (1983) converted older measures in mppcf to f/ml using paired samples collected at the same facilities. NIOSH (1972) documented decreasing exposure in many industries. Others noted further dramatic reductions of workplace concentrations in the early and mid 1970s in North America and Europe. For example, mean exposures in the Quebec mining industry declined from 16 f/ml in 1973 to less than 2 f/ml by the late 1970s (LeBel 1995).

TABLE 4.2 Estimated Mean Concentrations (# fibers over 5 mm per ml, PCM) in a Chrysotile Textile Plant (1930-1975)

Operation	Before Controls	After Controls
Fiber preparation	26.2-78.0	5.8-17.2
Carding	10.8-22.1	4.3-9.0
Twisting	24.6-36.0	5.4-7.9
Winding	4.1-20.9	4.1-8.4
Spinning	4.8-8.2	4.8-6.7
Weaving	5.3-30.6	1.4-8.2

SOURCE: Dement et al. (1983).

General Population Exposure

Earlier National Academies committees have considered non-occupational exposure to asbestos (NRC 1984, 1993).

Airborne asbestos fibers can be detected and measured in the general, ambient environment even far from industrial sources. The sources include disturbed natural deposits, improper disposal or transportation of asbestos-containing wastes, and uses that result in friable asbestos, such as motor-vehicle brake pads. Although exposure from undisturbed natural sources is possible, it has not been documented. Concentrations measured in outdoor air are highly variable, ranging from below the limit of detection (0.1 ng/m^3, and estimated to be equivalent to about 0.000003 f/ml as measured with PCM) in rural areas to over 100 ng/m^3 (about 0.003 f/ml, PCM) near industrial sources. In rural areas, typical concentrations are about 0.00001 f/ml (PCM), while urban measurements are typically higher (up to about 0.0001 f/ml, PCM) (ATSDR 2001).

Higher concentrations have been documented in communities near asbestos-related industries. Table 4.3 presents concentrations measured near asbestos manufacturing facilities in Taiwan (Chang et al. 1999). Although concentration appears to drop off with distance, the decreases are not dra-

TABLE 4.3 Asbestos Concentrations in Ambient Air Around Taiwanese Factories

			GM (GSD) Asbestos Concentration (f/ml) Distance from Factory[b]		
Factory Type	No. of Factories	Method[a]	200 m	400 m	600 m
Cement	5	TEM	0.006 (1.230)	0.007 (1.487)	0.006 (1.301)
		PCM	0.01 (3.49)	0.01 (2.91)	<0.01
Friction	3	TEM	0.008 (2.441)	0.008 (1.978)	0.002 (2.221)
		PCM	0.01 (3.22)	0.02 (2.88)	<0.01
Textile	2	TEM	0.012 (2.221)	0.020 (1.432)	0.006 (1.765)
		PCM	0.02 (3.21)	0.02 (3.33)	<0.01
Ground tile	2	TEM	0.033 (1.412)	0.021 (1.421)	0.025 (2.321)
		PCM	0.4 (3.21)	<0.01	0.01 (2.21)
Insulation	1	TEM	0.012 (2.321)	0.020 (2.210)	0.006 (2.773)
		PCM	<0.01	<0.01	<0.01
Refractory	1	TEM	<0.0001<0.0001	<0.0001	
		PCM	<0.01	<0.01	<0.01

[a]TEM = transmission electron microscopy; PCM = phase contrast microscopy.
[b]GM = geometric mean; GSD = geometric standard deviation.

SOURCE: Chang et al. (1999).

matic out to at least 600 m, indicating that the fibers remain airborne. Higher concentrations have been measured historically near asbestos-related open-pit mining and milling operations. For example, in towns near open-pit chrysotile mines in the Canadian province of Quebec, concentrations as high as 0.08 f/ml were measured in the early 1970s, although current concentrations are much lower (Case and Sebastien 1987, ICPS 1998). Residential exposure may also occur in communities with asbestos industries from fibers carried home on the clothing or hair of asbestos workers (Anderson et al. 1979, Case and Sebastien 1989).

Asbestos has been measured in the air inside many public and noncommercial buildings (HEI 1991). Sources of fibers released into the indoor air of non-industrial buildings include asbestos insulation, dry wall, ceiling and floor tiles, and materials used primarily for fireproofing. Exposures may occur by disturbance of asbestos-containing materials that are not well encapsulated (HEI 1991). Nicholson (1987) reported concentrations in buildings from about 0.00003 to 0.006 f/ml (PCM). In a survey of 94 public buildings, EPA (1988) reported concentrations ranging from below the limit of detection to about 0.003 f/ml (PCM), with a mean of 0.0004 f/ml (PCM).

Population exposure may also occur through the consumption of asbestos in drinking water. Asbestos may enter drinking water from erosion of natural deposits, mining operations, or asbestos-containing cement pipes (ATSDR 2001). Although most areas have concentrations less than 10^3 f/ml (PCM), much higher concentrations have been observed, some over 10^5 f/ml (EPA 1976, Kanarek et al. 1980, Sigurdson et al. 1981).

DOSIMETRY

Introduction

For inhaled contaminants, such as asbestos fibers, concepts of exposure and dose have been developed for the respiratory system. Asbestos fibers are particulate matter that is distinguished from other particles present in air by having a length substantially greater than their width. Aspect ratio is the term used for the ratio of length to width. The Occupational Safety and Health Administration defines a fiber as having a length of at least 5 mm and an aspect ratio of 3:1, whereas EPA defines a fiber as having an aspect ratio of over 5:1 (ATSDR 2003). Airborne particles are generally characterized by their aerodynamic diameter, which is determined in reference to the behavior of a sphere of unit density; the aerodynamic diameter corresponds to the size of a unit-density sphere with the same aerodynamic characteristics as the particle of interest.

Much has been learned about particle size and the handling of particles by the respiratory system from experimental findings and the use of physical models of the lung. The mechanisms responsible for particle and fiber deposition are impaction, sedimentation, interception, and diffusion (Asgharian and Yu 1988). Aerodynamic diameter is a key determinant of the likelihood of deposition in the respiratory tract and the site of deposition (see Figure 4.1). Particles greater than 10 μm in aerodynamic diameter are generally captured in the upper respiratory tract, the nose and upper airway, whereas smaller particles can penetrate more deeply and reach the airways and alveoli of the lungs. Particles smaller than about 2.5 μm have a greater likelihood of reaching the alveoli and depositing in this region. Ultrafine particles (less than 0.1 μm) also deposit heavily in the nose. These same considerations apply to inhaled fibers, which can have a range of aerodynamic diameters, depending on size and physical characteristics.

In considering the potential risk posed by inhaled pollutants, including fibers, the critical determinant of injury is the amount of material that reaches the target site—a measure generally referred to as the *biologically effective dose*. As depicted in Figure 4.2, *dose*, without qualification, gener-

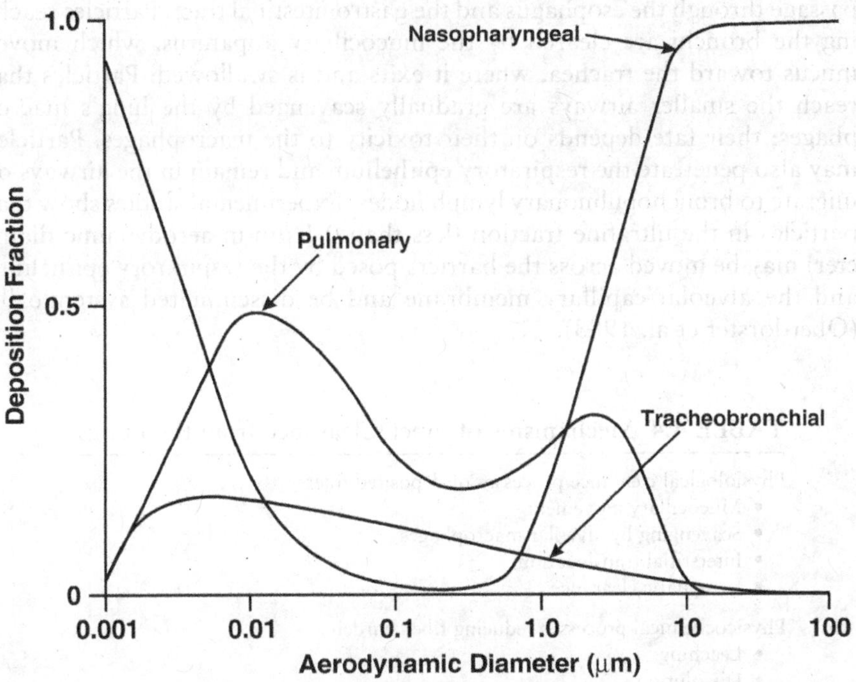

FIGURE 4.1 Effect of aerodynamic diameter on deposition of particles in the respiratory tract.
SOURCE: ICRP (1994).

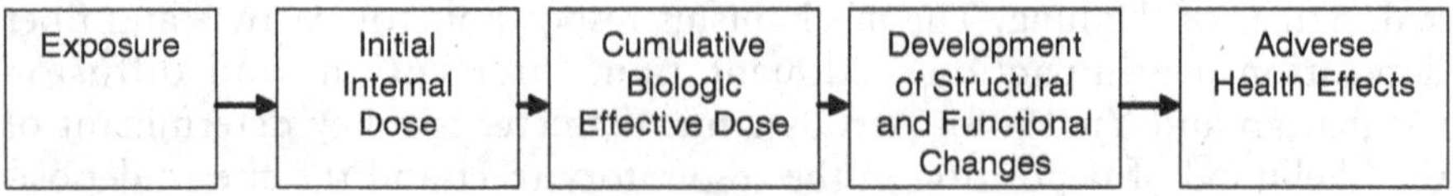

FIGURE 4.2 Exposure and dose-response paradigm in toxicology.
SOURCE: Modified from Lippmann (1992).

ally refers to the amount of material that enters the body; *exposure* refers to the amount of contact with material, with units expressed as concentration multiplied by time. For the respiratory system, models have been developed that relate dose to exposure for inhaled particles (Jarabek et al. 2005); the models are useful in characterizing the chain that begins with the source of an inhaled pollutant and terminates with injury to target tissues.

Various processes remove particles that are deposited in the lung in ways that depend on their size, physicochemical characteristics, and site of deposition (Table 4.4). Particles that reach the upper airways will generally be removed as mucus is swept toward the nostrils or into the pharynx for passage through the esophagus and the gastrointestinal tract. Particles reaching the bronchi are cleared by the mucociliary apparatus, which moves mucus toward the trachea, where it exits and is swallowed. Particles that reach the smaller airways are gradually scavenged by the lung's macrophages; their fate depends on their toxicity to the macrophages. Particles may also penetrate the respiratory epithelium and remain in the airways or migrate to bronchopulmonary lymph nodes. Experimental studies show that particles in the ultrafine fraction (less than 0.1 μm in aerodynamic diameter) may be moved across the barriers posed by the respiratory epithelium and the alveolar-capillary membrane and be disseminated systemically (Oberdörster et al. 1983).

TABLE 4.4 Mechanisms of Fiber Clearance from the Lungs

Physiological clearance processes of deposited fibers
- Mucociliary movement
- Scavenging by alveolar macrophages
- Interstitial translocation
- Lymphatic clearance

Physicochemical processes reducing fiber burden
- Leaching
- Dissolution
- Breakage

SOURCE: Modified from Bernstein et al. (2005).

Fiber dimensions are thought to be important in the pathogenesis of asbestos-related lung diseases (reviewed in Bernstein et al. 2005). Long asbestos fibers are deposited by interception primarily at sites of bifurcations in the conducting airways of the lower respiratory tract (Asgharian and Yu 1988). It is postulated that long asbestos fibers (greater than the diameter of alveolar macrophages about 10-15 μm in rodents and about 14-21 mm in humans) are less likely to be completely phagocytized and are cleared more slowly (reviewed in Bernstein et al. 2005). Fibers that are not removed rapidly by the mucociliary escalator may penetrate into the interstitium of the alveolar walls, be cleared by lymphatic channels, or migrate to the pleura and other extra pulmonary sites. Fibers that are not effectively cleared from the lung may be removed by physicochemical processes, including leaching of ions, dissolution, and breakage (see Chapter 3). Those processes could occur extracellularly in the lung-lining fluid or intracellularly in the phagolysosomal compartment of alveolar and interstitial macrophages. In general, fibers that are long and persistent in the lungs have been shown to be associated with fiber-induced lung disease in animal models (Hesterberg et al. 1996, 1998). The physicochemical properties of asbestos fibers described in Chapter 3 influence the susceptibility of different fiber types to leaching, dissolution, and breakage in the extracellular compartment at neutral pH or in the phagolysosome at acidic pH. In general, amphibole asbestos fibers are more persistent than chrysotile asbestos fibers.

In contrast with studies of fiber deposition in the lower respiratory tract, little is known about fiber deposition and clearance from the upper respiratory tract, particularly the larynx. A recent study by Zhou and Cheng (2005) modeled deposition of carbon fibers with laryngeal casts and predicted that a fraction of inhaled fibers would be deposited in the larynx, especially at the higher ventilation rates associated with moderately heavy work. Gemci et al. (2001) modeled airflow in the larynx by using drug sprays and predicted turbulent flow at the laryngeal constriction. As is seen in the lower airways of cigarette smokers, tobacco-smoking and other causes of chronic laryngeal irritation might impair clearance of fibers from the laryngeal mucosal surfaces.

Considerations for Inhaled Asbestos Fibers

Extension of the general models and definitions to inhaled asbestos fibers provides a framework for considering exposure and the dosimetry of asbestos fibers in the respiratory tract. The exposure measures used in the epidemiologic studies can be considered in the context set by this framework. In the committee's judgment, the most relevant dose measure for cancer is probably the cumulative number of fibers that reach and persist in the target organ, and the biologically effective dose would be related to fibers that interact with target cells. Such measurements are not available, but the epidemiologic studies have not incorporated any attempt to estimate dose, for example, by considering the size distribution of the fibers or the activity of the workers. Instead, a variety of indexes of exposure have been used, ranging from crude indicators of potential for contact to more refined, semi-quantitative measures.

Dose refers to the amount of material potentially available for deposition in the respiratory tract—in this instance, the number of fibers in the air inhaled by the exposed person. Only some fraction of that dose is deposited, and much will be exhaled or cleared. However, studies of lung tissues of asbestos-exposed people show that fibers are retained in the lung and that long, thick fibers are coated with iron, protein, and mucopolysaccharides to form asbestos bodies (ABs) visible with light microscopy (Roggli 2004). ABs have also been documented in other tissues, although their presence may reflect contamination occurring during handling and processing of specimens.

For nonrespiratory organs, concepts of dose are not well developed and related experimental and observational data are limited. For the organs of the gastrointestinal tract (esophagus, stomach, and intestines), fibers cleared from the respiratory tract will move through, with the potential for interaction with target cells in the epithelium. For other abdominal organs (including the liver, pancreas, and kidneys), the routes of movement are uncertain, although fibers have been found in those organs on occasion (Borow et al. 1973, Pooley 1974).

Translocation to the Pleura

After inhalation, asbestos fibers that deposit in the alveolar region of the respiratory tract may be cleared or retained (Figure 4.3). Fibers that persist in the alveolar region may be directly toxic to alveolar epithelial cells or incite a chronic inflammatory response that perpetuates tissue injury followed by episodes of epithelial cell proliferation and fibrosis (Oberdörster 1996). It has been proposed that fibers that penetrate the alveolar lining and enter the interstitium may move to lymphatics and regional lymph nodes. Asbestos fibers that accumulate in subpleural lymphatics may produce diffuse visceral pleural fibrosis and pleural effusions, directly and indirectly (Churg 1988). Asbestos-induced pleural effusions are hypothesized to be caused by cytokines (such as interleukin-8) released from mesothelial cells that trigger inflammation and fluid accumulation in the pleural space (Boylan et al. 1992). Inhaled particles could reach the pleural space after direct transpleural penetration, lymphatic translocation, or indirect transport by the blood (Holt 1981, Lee et al. 1981, Oberdörster et al. 1983). Recent studies in hamsters of inhaled refractory ceramic fibers (mean

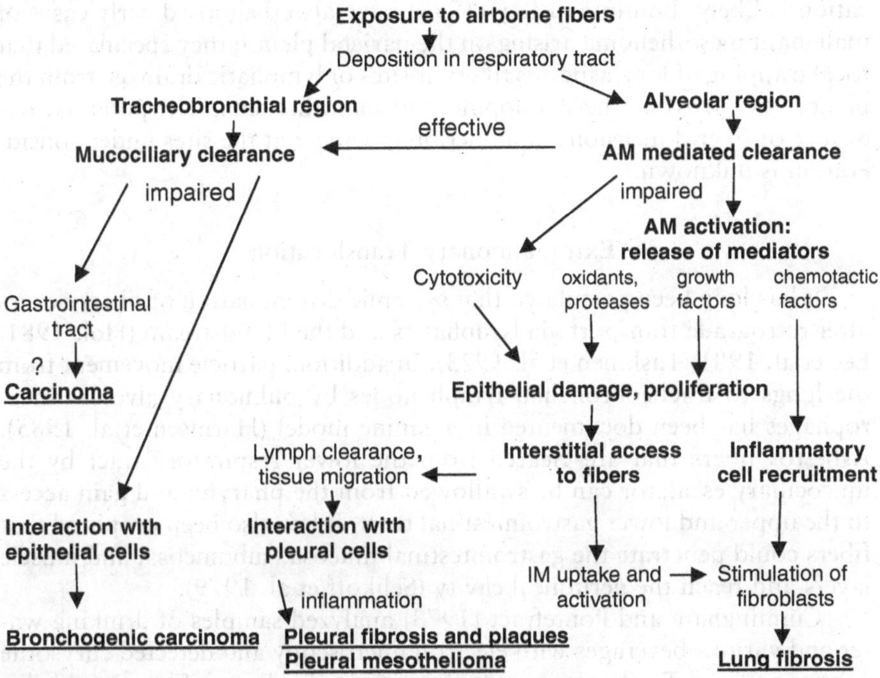

FIGURE 4.3 Translocation of inhaled asbestos fibers and adverse health effects. AM = alveolar macrophage, IM = interstitial macrophage.
SOURCE: Modified from Oberdörster (1996).

length, 20 μm; mean diameter, 1 μm) confirmed rapid translocation of short fibers to the pleural space, followed by inflammation and mesothelial cell proliferation (Gelzleichter et al. 1996a,b).

Few investigators have quantified the mineral-fiber burden in human pleura, but several investigators have found asbestos fibers in the pleural lining of people exposed to asbestos fibers (Dodson et al. 1990, Gibbs et al. 1991, Sebastien et al. 1977, Suzuki and Yuen 2001). Boutin et al. (1996) obtained samples of parietal pleura and lung from workers exposed to asbestos and counted asbestos fibers in dried tissue samples. Anthracotic particles, as well as asbestos fibers, were detected near lymphatic openings on the surface of the parietal pleura. Scanning electron microscopy of these "black spots" revealed focal accumulation of inflammatory cells. The investigators directly visualized black spots with video-assisted fiber-optic thoracoscopy; previous investigators had not been able to identify asbestos fibers in pleural samples, because they sampled tissues at random (Boutin et al. 1996). Identification of particles and fibers at sites of lymphatic drainage on the parietal pleura suggests that local transpleural or lymphatic translocation is likely. Boutin and Rey (1993) have also diagnosed early cases of malignant mesothelioma arising on the parietal pleura; they speculated that focal trapping of long asbestos fibers at sites of lymphatic drainage from the pleura may provoke the development of mesothelioma. The potential relevance of fiber dimensions in induction of cancer at the sites under consideration is unknown.

Extrapulmonary Translocation

It has long been postulated that systemic dissemination of fibers occurs after retrograde transport via lymphatics and the bloodstream (Holt 1981, Lee et al. 1981, Taskinen et al. 1973). In addition, particle movement from the lungs to tracheobronchial lymph nodes by pulmonary alveolar macrophages has been documented in a canine model (Harmsen et al. 1985). Asbestos fibers that are cleared from the lower respiratory tract by the mucociliary escalator can be swallowed from the pharynx and gain access to the upper and lower gastrointestinal tract. It has also been proposed that fibers could penetrate the gastrointestinal mucosa, submucosa, and muscle layers and reach the peritoneal cavity (Selikoff et al. 1979).

Cunningham and Pontefract (1973) analyzed samples of drinking water and various beverages with electron microscopy and detected chrysotile asbestos fibers. To determine whether ingested asbestos fibers could disseminate systemically, they instilled a preparation of short chrysotile asbestos (0.5-2 μm long) in the stomach of rats and sacrificed them after 2-4 days. Using precautions to prevent contamination during necropsy, they sampled blood from the retroorbital plexus, spleen, omentum, heart, brain, and lungs and detected a substantial number of asbestos fibers; the highest concentration was in the omentum (Cunningham and Pontefract 1973). More recent chronic feeding studies conducted by the National Toxicology Program (HHS 1983, 1985, 1988, 1990a, 1990b, 1990c) did not identify any asbestos bodies using light microscopy at the following sites: larynx, lymph nodes, esophagus, stomach, small intestine, colon, cecum, and mesentery (McConnell 2005).

Lee et al. (1981) conducted a subchronic inhalation study with inorganic titanate fibers in hamsters, guinea pigs, and rats and reported fibers and multinucleated giant cells widely disseminated throughout the body, including mediastinal lymph nodes, adipose tissue, spleen, liver, Peyer's patches in the intestine, and the mucosal, submucosal, and muscular layers of the gastrointestinal tract. Tissue responses were minimal except for mild inflammation and fibrosis in the epicardium.

Cook and Olson's (1979) demonstration of asbestos in human urine, which abated when drinking water was filtered, provides substantial evidence that fibers enter into systemic circulation.

Case reports based on human autopsies have noted the presence of asbestos fibers or ABs in abdominal organs, including the spleen, abdominal lymph nodes, liver, omentum, and mesentery (Borow et al. 1973, Dodson et al. 2000, Pooley 1974, Suzuki and Yuen 2001). ABs have also been recovered from sites under consideration by this committee: larynx, esophagus, stomach, and small and large intestines (Roggli 2004). Several caveats must be considered, however, in evaluating reports of asbestos fiber translocation to extrapulmonary sites. A taskforce of the European Respiratory Society (De Vuyst et al. 1998) prepared guidelines for mineral-fiber analyses in biologic samples focusing on the tissues involved in asbestosis, lung cancer, and mesothelioma, but the principles are in large part applicable to techniques that would be used to determine fiber presence in the selected sites considered in this review. First, electron microscopy (EM) is necessary to detect most asbestos fibers, with transmission EM being preferable to scanning EM, but light microscopy is adequate for visualizing ABs; limits of detection should be reported. Second, asbestos fibers and ABs can be identified in lung tissue in most people in the general population, even people who have with no occupational history of asbestos exposure and in the absence of clinical or pathologic evidence of lung disease, meaning that comparison with appropriate controls is essential (De Vuyst et al. 1998). Third, cross-contamination of tissue samples with fibers or particles from surgical gloves, specimen containers, fixatives, scalpel blades, and other organs collected in the surgical or autopsy suite is a serious concern (Cook 1983, De Vuyst et al. 1998; Roggli 2004). Those caveats should be considered in evaluation of the published papers.

In two of five cases, Roggli et al. (1980) found ABs in laryngeal tissues gathered at autopsy from asbestos workers with known pulmonary disease. ABs were not recovered, however, from laryngeal tissue from ten autopsies controls.

Auerbach et al. (1980) used light microscopy to detect ABs in paraffin-embedded tissue samples obtained at autopsy from the lungs and kidneys of a series of 37 cases recorded as having asbestosis, mesothelioma, or pleural plaques. ABs were observed in the lung sections of all but one of these cases and in 38% of the kidney samples. Other organs were available from a subset of these cases. Of the organs for which at least 30 samples were available (heart, liver, spleen, adrenal glands, and pancreas), ABs were detected in 32-62% of cases. Of organs with fewer samples available, stomach, duodenum, and colon were among those in which ABs were found; the others with positive findings were brain, prostate, thyroid, mediastinal lymph nodes, bone, omentum, and spinal cord. The prevalence of ABs in other organs reflected the number of asbestos fibers found in a case's lung sample.

Kobayashi et al. (1987) performed a similar analysis on formalin-fixed tissues from 26 subjects. Esophagus, stomach, and both large and small intestine were among the 13 extrapulmonary organs from which tissues were examined. ABs were detected in some samples from all these organs, and the pattern corresponded with the degree of a given subject's pulmonary burden. The number observed was high for the esophagus. Roggli (2004) noted that the reported results would be consistent with contamination by pulmonary ABs via formalin.

Kambic et al. (1989) examined a cohort of 195 asbestos-cement factory workers and controls in Yugoslavia. Chronic laryngitis was found more frequently in workers than in controls; in 10 workers, biopsies showed changes consistent with hyperplastic chronic laryngitis. Chronic laryngitis was diagnosed clinically in asbestos workers who were nonsmokers or former smokers, as well as in current smokers. Four of the biopsies were examined with scanning EM, and asbestos fibers were observed on the epithelial lining in three.

Ehrlich et al. (1991) determined colonic asbestos burdens with light and electron microscopy in 44 asbestos workers with colon cancer. Chrysotile fibers, amosite fibers, or ABs were identified in the colonic wall in 32% of workers. In contrast, no asbestos fibers or ABs were found in 20 patients who had colon cancer but no history of asbestos exposure.

In addition to technical concerns about reported findings of fibers or ABs in extrapulmonary tissues, there are uncertainties that should be borne in mind when interpreting their biologic meaning. The fact that fibers found in tissues are predominantly amphibole, even when the individual's exposure is documented to have been exclusively to chrysotile with a slight tremolite component, is fully in accord with what is understood about the relative biopersistence of those fiber types (Churg 1994). In the upper respiratory or gastrointestinal tract, are epithelial injury and chronic inflammation (for example, secondary to tobacco-smoking, alcohol use, or persistent bacterial or viral infections) a prerequisite of accumulation of fibers and development of cancer at these sites? Finally, the finding of asbestos fibers or ABs in tissue samples obtained from gastrointestinal tract tumors raises the question of the causal significance of this observation: do the fibers accumulate secondarily at sites of mucosal damage or ulceration associated with a growing tumor?

Few studies have systematically sought evidence of asbestos fibers in the particular extrapulmonary sites of interest in this review, and such investigations are subject to technical difficulties. Nonetheless, there is some documentation that asbestos fibers may disseminate and persist at these selected tissue sites, although not with the regularity that has been established for the lungs, pleura, and lymph nodes.

REFERENCES

ACGIH (American Conference of Governmental Industrial Hygienists). 1998. *Documentation of the Threshold Limit Values and Biological Exposure Indices.* 6th edition. Cincinnati, OH.

Amandus HE, Wheeler R, Jankovic J, Tucker J. 1987. The morbidity and mortality of vermiculite miners and millers exposed to tremolite-actinolite: Part I. Exposure estimates. *American Journal of Industrial Medicine* 11(1): 1-14.

Anderson HA, Lilis R, Daum SM, Selikoff IJ. 1979. Asbestosis among household contacts of asbestos factory workers. *Annals of the New York Academy of Sciences* 330: 387-399.

Armstrong BK, de Klerk NH, Musk AW, Hobbs MS. 1988. Mortality in miners and millers of crocidolite in Western Australia. *British Journal of Industrial Medicine* 45(1): 5-13.

Asgharian B, Yu CP. 1988. Deposition of inhaled fibrous particles in the human lung. *Journal of Aerosol Medicine* 1: 37-50.

ATSDR (Agency for Toxic Substances and Disease Registry). 2001. *Toxicological Profile for Asbestos.* Atlanta, GA: US Department of Health and Human Services.

ATSDR. 2003. *Case Studies in Environmental Medicine.* Atlanta, GA: US Department of Health and Human Services.

Auerbach O, Conston AS, Garfinkel L, Parks VR, Kaslow HD, Hammond EC. 1980. Presence of asbestos bodies in organs other than the lung. *Chest* 77(2): 133-137.

Bernstein D, Castranova V, Donaldson K, Fubini B, Hadley J, Hesterberg T, Kane A, Lai D, McConnell EE, Muhle H, Oberdörster G, Olin S, Warheit DB. 2005. Testing of fibrous particles: Short-term assays and strategies. *Inhalation Toxicology* 17(10): 497-537.

Borow M, Conston A, Livornese L, Schalet N. 1973. Mesothelioma following exposure to asbestos: A review of 72 cases. *Chest* 64(5): 641-646.

Boutin C, Rey F. 1993. Thoracoscopy in pleural malignant mesothelioma: A prospective study of 188 consecutive patients: Part 1. Diagnosis. *Cancer* 72(2): 389-393.

Boutin C, Dumortier P, Rey F, Viallat JR, De Vuyst P. 1996. Black spots concentrate oncogenic asbestos fibers in the parietal pleura: Thoracoscopic and mineralogic study. *American Journal of Respiratory and Critical Care Medicine* 153(1): 444-449.

Boylan AM, Ruegg C, Kim KJ, Hebert CA, Hoeffel JM, Pytela R, Sheppard D, Goldstein IM, Broaddus VC. 1992. Evidence of a role for mesothelial cell-derived interleukin 8 in the pathogenesis of asbestos-induced pleurisy in rabbits. *Journal of Clinical Investigation* 89(4): 1257-1267.

Case BW, Sebastien P. 1987. Environmental and occupational exposures to chrysotile asbestos: A comparative microanalytic study. *Archives of Environmental Health* 42(4): 185-191.

Case BW, Sebastien P. 1989. Fibre levels in lung and correlation with air samples. *IARC Scientific Publications* 90: 207-218.

Chang HY, Chen CR, Wang JD. 1999. Risk assessment of lung cancer and mesothelioma in people living near asbestos-related factories in Taiwan. *Archives of Environmental Health* 54(3): 194-201.

Churg A. 1988. Chrysotile, tremolite, and malignant mesothelioma in man. *Chest* 93(3): 621-628.

Churg A. 1994. Deposition and clearance of chrysotile asbestos. *Annals of Occupational Hygiene* 38(4): 625-633.

Cook PM. 1983. Review of published studies on gut penetration by ingested asbestos fibers. *Environmental Health Perspectives* 53: 121-130.

Cook PM, Olson GF. 1979. Ingested mineral fibers: Elimination in human urine. *Science* 204(4389): 195-198.

Corn M, McArthur B, Dellarco M. 1994. Asbestos exposure of building maintenance personnel. *Applied Occupational Environmental Hygiene* 9(11): 845-852.

Cunningham HM, Pontefract RD. 1973. Asbestos fibers in beverages, drinking water, and tissues: Their passage through the intestinal wall and movement through the body. *Journal—Association of Official Analytical Chemists* 56(4): 976-986.

De Vuyst P, Karjalainen A, Dumortier P, Pairon J, Monso E, Brochard P, Teschler H, Tossavainen A, Gibbs A. 1998. Guidelines for mineral fibre analyses in biological samples: Report of the ERS Working Group. *European Respiratory Journal* 11(6): 1416-1426.

Dement JM, Harris RL Jr, Symons MJ, Shy CM. 1983. Exposures and mortality among chrysotile asbestos workers: Part I. Exposure estimates. *American Journal of Industrial Medicine* 4(3): 399-419.

Dodson RF, Williams MG Jr, Corn CJ, Brollo A, Bianchi C. 1990. Asbestos content of lung tissue, lymph nodes, and pleural plaques from former shipyard workers. *American Review of Respiratory Diseases* 142(4): 843-847.

Dodson R, O'Sullivan M, Huang J, Holiday D, Hammar S. 2000. Asbestos in extrapulmonary sites: Omentum and mesentery. *Chest* 117(2): 486-493.

Ehrlich A, Gordon RE, Dikman SH. 1991. Carcinoma of the colon in asbestos-exposed workers: Analysis of asbestos content in colon tissue. *American Journal of Industrial Medicine* 19(5): 629-636.

EPA (US Environmental Protection Agency). 1976. *Asbestos Fibers in Natural Runoff and Discharges from Sources Manufacturing Asbestos Products: Part II. Non-Point Sources and Point Sources Manufacturing Asbestos Products.* Washington, DC: Office of Toxic Substances.

EPA. 1988. *EPA Study of Asbestos-Containing Materials in Public Buildings: A Report to Congress.* Washington, DC.

Gelzleichter TR, Bermudez E, Mangum JB, Wong BA, Everitt JI, Moss OR. 1996a. Pulmonary and pleural responses in Fischer 344 rats following short-term inhalation of a synthetic vitreous fiber: I. Quantitation of lung and pleural fiber burdens. *Fundamental and Applied Toxicology* 30(1): 31-38.

Gelzleichter TR, Bermudez E, Mangum JB, Wong BA, Moss OR, Everitt JI. 1996b. Pulmonary and pleural responses in Fischer 344 rats following short-term inhalation of a synthetic vitreous fiber: II. Pathobiologic responses. *Fundamental and Applied Toxicology* 30(1): 39-46.

Gemci T, Corcoran TE, Yakut K, Shortall B, Chigier N. 2001. Spray dynamics and deposition of inhaled medications in the throat. *Institute of Liquid Atomization and Spray Systems Europe*: Oral Presentation.

Gibbs AR, Stephens M, Griffiths DM, Blight BJ, Pooley FD. 1991. Fibre distribution in the lungs and pleura of subjects with asbestos related diffuse pleural fibrosis. *British Journal of Industrial Medicine* 48(11): 762-770.

Gibbs G, LaChance M. 1974. Dust-fiber relationships in the Quebec chrysotile industry. *Archives of Environmental Health* 28(2): 69-71.

Harmsen AG, Muggenburg BA, Snipes MB, Bice DE. 1985. The role of macrophages in particle translocation from lungs to lymph nodes. *Science* 230(4731): 1277-1280.

HEI (Health Effects Institute). 1991. *Asbestos in Public and Commercial Buildings: A Literature Review and Synthesis of Current Knowledge: Report of the Asbestos Literature Review Panel.* Cambridge, MA.

Hesterberg TW, Miiller WC, Musselman RP, Kamstrup O, Hamilton RD, Thevenaz P. 1996. Biopersistence of man-made vitreous fibers and crocidolite asbestos in the rat lung following inhalation. *Fundamental and Applied Toxicology* 29(2): 269-279.

Hesterberg TW, Chase G, Axten C, Miller WC, Musselman RP, Kamstrup O, Hadley J, Morscheidt C, Bernstein DM, Thevenaz P. 1998. Biopersistence of synthetic vitreous fibers and amosite asbestos in the rat lung following inhalation. *Toxicology and Applied Pharmacology* 151(2): 262-275.

HHS (US Department of Health and Human Services). 1983. *Lifetime Carcinogenesis Studies of Amosite Asbestos (CAS NO. 12172-73-5) in Syrian Golden Hamsters (Feed Studies)*. NTP TR 249. Research Triangle Park, NC: National Toxicology Program.

HHS. 1985. *Toxicology and Carcinogenesis Studies of Chrysotile Asbestos (CAS No. 12001-29-5) in F344/N Rats (Feed Studies)*. NTP TR 295. Research Triangle Park, NC: National Toxicology Program.

HHS. 1988. *Toxicology and Carcinogenesis Studies of Crocidolite Asbestos (CAS No. 12001-28-4) in F344/N Rats (Feed Studies)*. NTP TR 280. Research Triangle Park, NC: National Toxicology Program.

HHS. 1990a. *Lifetime Carcinogenesis Studies of Chrysotile Asbestos (CAS No. 12001-29-5) in Syrian Golden Hamsters (Feed Studies)*. NTP TR 246. Research Triangle Park, North Carolina: National Toxicology Program.

HHS. 1990b. *Toxicology and Carcinogenesis Studies of Amosite Asbestos (CAS No. 12172-73-5) in F344/N Rats (Feed Studies)*. NTP TR 279. Research Triangle Park, NC: National Toxicology Program.

HHS. 1990c. *Toxicology and Carcinogenesis Studies of Tremolite (CAS No. 14567-73-8) in F344/N Rats (Feed Studies)*. NTP TR 277. Research Triangle Park, NC: National Toxicology Program.

Holt PF. 1981. Transport of inhaled dust to extrapulmonary sites. *Journal of Pathology* 133(2): 123-129.

Hughes JM, Weill H, Hammad YY. 1987. Mortality of workers employed in two asbestos cement manufacturing plants. *British Journal of Industrial Medicine* 44(3): 161-174.

IARC (International Agency for Research on Cancer). 1977. *Asbestos*. IARC Monographs on the Evaluation of Carcinogenic Risks of Chemicals to Man 14: 1-106. Lyon, France: World Health Organization.

ICRP (International Commission on Radiological Protection). 1994. *Human Respiratory Tract Model for Radiolgical Protection*. Oxford: Elsevier.

IPCS (International Programme on Chemical Safety). 1986. *Asbestos and Other Natural Mineral Fibers: Environmental Health Criteria 53*. Geneva: World Health Organization.

IPCS. 1998. *Chrysotile Asbestos: Environmental Health Criteria 203*. Geneva: World Health Organization.

Jarabek AM, Asgharian B, Miller FJ. 2005. Dosimetric adjustments for interspecies extrapolation of inhaled poorly soluble particles (PSP). *Inhalation Toxicology* 17: 317-334.

Kambic V, Radsel Z, Gale N. 1989. Alterations in the laryngeal mucosa after exposure to asbestos. *British Journal of Industrial Medicine* 46(10): 717-723.

Kanarek MS, Conforti PM, Jackson LA, Cooper RC, Murchio JC. 1980. Asbestos in drinking water and cancer incidence in the San Francisco Bay area. *American Journal of Epidemiology* 112(1): 54-72.

Kobayashi H, Ming ZW, Watanabe H, Ohnishi Y. 1987. A quantitative study on the distribution of asbestos bodies in extrapulmonary organs. *ACTA Pathologica Japonica* 37(3): 375-383.

LeBel J. 1995. *Review of Fibre Concentrations in Asbestos Mines and Quebec Asbestos Mining Towns*. Sherbrooke: Quebec Asbestos Mining Association.

Lee KP, Barras CE, Griffith FD, Waritz RS. 1981. Pulmonary response and transmigration of inorganic fibers by inhalation exposure. *American Journal of Pathology* 102(3): 314-323.

Lippmann M. 1992. *Environmental Toxicants: Human Exposures and Their Health Effects*. 1st edition. New York: Wiley.

McConnell EE. 2005 (October 27). *Personal Communication to Mary Paxton for the Committee on Asbestos: Selected Health Effects*. Available in IOM Public Access Files.

Nicholson WJ. 1987. Airborne levels of mineral fibers in the non-occupational environment. *IARC Scientific Publications* 90: 239-261.

NIOSH (National Institute for Occupational Safety and Health). 1972. *Criteria for a Recommended Standard: Occupational Exposure to Asbestos.* Washington, DC.

NRC (National Research Council). 1984. *Asbestiform Fibers: Non-Occupational Health Risks.* Washington, DC: National Academy Press.

NRC. 1993. *Solid-Earth Sciences and Society.* Washington, DC: National Academy Press.

Oberdörster G. 1996. Evaluation and use of animal models to assess mechanisms of fibre carcinogenicity. *IARC Scientific Publications* 140: 107-125.

Oberdörster G, Ferin J, Marcello NL, Meinhold SH. 1983. Effects of intrabronchially instilled amosite on lavagable lung and pleural cells. *Environmental Health Perspectives* 51: 41-48.

Peto J, Doll R, Hermon C, Binns W, Clayton R, Goffe T. 1985. Relationship of mortality to measures of environmental asbestos pollution in an asbestos textile factory. *Annals of Occupational Hygiene* 29(3): 305-355.

Pira E, Pelucchi C, Buffoni L, Palmas A, Turbiglio M, Negri E, Piolatto PG, La Vecchia C. 2005. Cancer mortality in a cohort of asbestos textile workers. *British Journal of Cancer* 92(3): 580-586.

Pooley F. 1974. Locating fibers in the bowel wall. *Environmental Health Perspectives* 9: 235.

Reid A, Ambrosini G, de Klerk N, Fritschi L, Musk B. 2004. Aerodigestive and gastrointestinal tract cancers and exposure to crocidolite (blue asbestos): Incidence and mortality among former crocidolite workers. *International Journal of Cancer* 111(5): 757-761.

Roggli V. 2004. Asbestos bodies and nonasbestos ferruginous bodies. In: Roggli V, Oury T, Sporn T, eds. *Pathology of Asbestos-Associated Diseases.* 2nd edition. New York: Springer. Pp. 34-71.

Roggli VL, Greenberg SD, McLarty JL, Hurst GA, Spivey CG, Heiger LR. 1980. Asbestos body content of the larnyx in asbestos workers: A study of five cases. *Archives of Otolaryngology* 106(9): 533-535.

Sebastien P, Fondimare A, Bignon J, Monchaux G, Desbordes J, Bonnaudi G. 1977. Topographic distribution of asbestos fibers in human lung in relation to occupational and nonoccupational exposure. In: Walton WH, McGovern B, eds. *Inhaled Particles IV.* Oxford: Pergamon Press. Pp. 435-444.

Selikoff IJ, Hammond EC, Seidman H. 1979. Mortality experience of insulation workers in the United States and Canada, 1943-1976. *Annals of the New York Academy of Sciences* 330: 91-116.

Sigurdson EE, Levy BS, Mandel J. 1981. Cancer morbidity investigations: Lessons from the Duluth study of possible effects of asbestos in drinking water. *Environmental Research* 25(1): 50-61.

Sluis-Cremer GK, Liddell FD, Logan WP, Bezuidenhout BN. 1992. The mortality of amphibole miners in South Africa, 1946-80. *British Journal of Industrial Medicine* 49(8): 566-575.

Suzuki Y, Yuen SR. 2001. Asbestos tissue burden study on human malignant mesothelioma. *Industrial Health* 39(2): 150-160.

Taskinen E, Ahlamn K, Wukeri M. 1973. A current hypothesis of the lymphatic transport of inspired dust to the parietal pleura. *Chest* 64(2): 193-196.

USGS (US Geological Survey). 2004. *Mineral Commodity Summaries.* Washington, DC: US Government Printing Office. *http://minerals.usgs.gov/minerals/pubs/mcs/2004/mcs2004.pdf.*

Zhou Y, Cheng YS. 2005. Particle deposition in a cast of human tracheobronchial airways. *Aerosol Science and Technology* 39(6): 492-500.

5

Biological Aspects of Asbestos-Related Diseases

ASBESTOS-RELATED PULMONARY DISEASES AND THEIR MECHANISMS

The causal association between asbestos exposure and nonmalignant and malignant diseases of the lungs and mesothelial linings is well established and supported by epidemiologic, animal, and mechanistic toxicologic studies (IARC 1987). The biologic mechanisms responsible for asbestos-related disease are complex and reflect a chronic, multistep process involving interactions between genetic predisposition and possibly other exposures, including exposure to viruses. Those mechanisms will be discussed in detail after a brief summary of the clinical features and risk factors of lung cancer and malignant mesothelioma.

Asbestos-Related Diseases

The International Agency for Research on Cancer (IARC 1987) has classified various types of asbestos fibers—specifically chrysotile, actinolite, anthophyllite, tremolite, and crocidolite—as known human carcinogens (Group I). Inhalation of asbestos fibers is associated with parenchymal and pleural lung diseases (Table 5.1), all of which have been reproduced in rodent models (reviewed in Bernstein et al. 2005). In chronic rodent inhalation assays, fiber biopersistence and carcinogenicity are associated with persistent inflammation, epithelial cell proliferation, and fibrosis in the lungs (Hesterberg et al. 1993, 1994, 1998). Chronic inflammation and fibrosis are also produced in the lungs and pleural linings of humans exposed to asbestos fibers; these responses are clinically described as asbestosis (or dif-

TABLE 5.1 Pulmonary Diseases Associated with Exposure to Asbestos Fibers

Disease	Humans	Animal Models
Asbestosis (diffuse interstitial fibrosis)	+	+
Carcinoma of the lung	+	+
Nonneoplastic pleural disease:		
Pleural effusion	+	+
Visceral pleural fibrosis	+	+
Parietal pleural plaques	+	+
Malignant mesothelioma of the pleura and peritoneum	+	+

SOURCE: Adapted from Bernstein et al. (2005).

fuse interstitial fibrosis) of the lungs and visceral pleural fibrosis and parietal pleural plaques of the pleural linings (Table 5.1). In the pleura, bilateral and symmetric fibrotic plaques usually reflect environmental or occupational exposure to asbestos fibers, and consequently pleural plaques are considered to be markers of asbestos exposure (Travis et al. 2002). These fibrous scars are not precursors of malignant mesothelioma or lung cancer.

Risk Factors for Lung Cancer and Malignant Mesothelioma

Tobacco-smoking is a major causal risk factor for lung cancer (Table 5.2) and risk of developing lung cancer in current or former smokers is greatly increased by exposure to asbestos fibers. Development of malignant mesothelioma of the pleura or peritoneum has not been found to be associated with tobacco-smoking (Battifora and McCaughey 1995). Exposure to

TABLE 5.2 Risk Factors for Development of Lung Cancer

Certainty	Agent
Established	Cigarette, pipe, or cigar-smoking
	Exposure to environmental tobacco smoke
	Exposure to asbestos fibers
	Exposure to radon
	Occupational exposures (metals and chemicals)
Hypothesized	Air pollution
	Outdoor
	Indoor (cooking fumes)
	HPV (human papilloma virus)

TABLE 5.3 Risk Factors for Development of Malignant Mesothelioma

Certainty	Agent
Established	Exposure to asbestos fibers
	Exposure to erionite fibers
	Exposure to talc or vermiculite contaminated with asbestos fibers
Hypothesized	Radiation therapy
	Chronic inflammation
	SV40 virus

SOURCE: Sporn and Roggli (2004).

environmental erionite fibers has been found to be associated with malignant pleural mesothelioma (Baris et al. 1987, Roushdy-Hammady et al. 2001), while radiation, chronic inflammation, and SV40 virus are also postulated as etiologic factors (Table 5.3).

Genetic Predisposition to Malignant Mesothelioma

Case reports of familial clusters of malignant mesothelioma resulting from occupational or household exposure have been published (Table 5.4). In some of these families, the histological subtype and location were identical, for example, tubulopapillary malignant mesothelioma arising in the peritoneum (Lynch et al. 1994). Recent evidence of an inherited predisposition to malignant mesothelioma after exposure to erionite in two villages in Turkey was published by Roushdy-Hammady et al. (2001).

Malignant mesotheliomas have also been reported in people with inherited cancer-susceptibility syndromes following exposure to asbestos fibers or radiation therapy (Table 5.4). Somatic mutations in the neurofibromatosis type 2 (*Nf2*) gene have been detected in 50% of human malignant

TABLE 5.4 Genetic Predisposition to Malignant Mesothelioma

- Case reports of familial clusters:
  - Genetic predisposition (Roushdy-Hammady et al. 2001)
  - Household exposure (reviewed in Lynch et al. 1994)
- Case report of 40-year-old mechanic with neurofibromatosis type 2 who developed peritoneal malignant mesothelioma (Baser et al. 2002)
- Reports of patients with familial cancer syndromes (Wilms tumor, Li-Fraumeni syndrome) who developed malignant mesothelioma after radiation therapy for primary tumors (Antman 1986, Hisada et al. 1998)
- Report of slightly increased risk of mesothelioma in people exposed to asbestos who have first-degree relatives with Li-Fraumeni syndrome (Heineman et al. 1996)

mesotheliomas (Sekido et al. 1995). Heterozygous *Nf2*-deficient mice show increased susceptibility to induction of peritoneal malignant mesotheliomas after intraperitoneal injection of asbestos fibers (Fleury-Feith et al. 2003), and these mice recapitulate the molecular alterations characteristic of human malignant mesotheliomas (Altomare et al. 2005). Li-Fraumeni syndrome is a rare heritable cancer-susceptibility disorder characterized by carrying a mutant allele of the *p53* gene. Although mutations in the *p53* tumor-suppressor gene are generally rare in human malignant mesotheliomas (Metcalf et al. 1992), individuals with Li-Fraumeni syndrome show increased susceptibility for malignant mesothelioma (Table 5.4). Heterozygous *p53*-deficient mice also show increased susceptibility to and accelerated progression of asbestos-induced mesotheliomas (Marsella et al. 1997, Vaslet et al. 2002). Those murine transgenic models support a role of inactivation of the *Nf2* and *p53* tumor-suppressor gene pathways in the pathogenesis of asbestos-induced malignant mesothelioma.

Properties of Fibers Relevant to Biological Activity

The physical and chemical characteristics related to the carcinogenicity of asbestos fibers include fiber dimensions, chemical composition, biodurability, and surface reactivity (reviewed by Fubini and Oter-Areán 1999). The availability of transition metals, especially iron, to participate in free radical generation (Weitzman and Graceffa 1984) has been hypothesized as playing an important role in asbestos-induced lung diseases (reviewed in Kane 1996). Iron-catalyzed generation of free radicals can cause cell injury, genetic damage, and inflammation in the lungs and pleura (reviewed in Kamp and Weitzman 1999 and in Manning et al. 2002).

Fiber dimensions and biopersistence have been linked mechanistically with persistent inflammation in a variety of toxicologic studies (reviewed in Bernstein et al. 2005). Fiber dimensions influence the extent and rate of fiber deposition and persistence in the lungs, and movement to the pleura (Oberdörster 1996). Long, thin asbestos fibers are trapped at the level of the terminal respiratory bronchioles or deposited in the alveolar spaces. Long fibers are less efficiently phagocytized by alveolar macrophages and stimulate persistent production of proinflammatory mediators, cytokines, and growth factors. Partial phagocytosis impairs macrophage motility and retards fiber clearance. In the absence of effective fiber clearance by the mucociliary escalator, fibers can move to the interstitium of the lung, migrate to the pleura and peritoneum, or even to more distant sites through lymphatics. Fibers that are retained in the walls of the terminal respiratory bronchioles, in the lung interstitium, or on the pleural lining can cause persistent epithelial or mesothelial cell injury, whose repair is accompanied by proliferation. Persistent or chronic macrophage activation can lead to chronic inflammation and fibrosis in the lungs or pleura (summarized in Bernstein et al. 2005).

Mechanisms of Asbestos Carcinogenicity

On the basis of extensive work with in vitro model systems and animal models of asbestosis, lung cancer, and mesothelioma, direct and indirect mechanisms for fiber carcinogenicity have been proposed. The mechanisms may or may not be applicable to tumors that develop at the other sites considered in this report.

Direct mechanisms of asbestos fiber carcinogenesis include genotoxic and nongenotoxic pathways (Table 5.5). It has been hypothesized that long asbestos fibers that are partially phagocytized by macrophages trigger persistent production of reactive oxygen species by the respiratory-burst mechanism. Asbestos fibers contain a high surface content of redox-active iron and generate additional radicals, including the highly reactive hydoxyl radical by Fenton chemistry (Fubini and Oter-Areán 1999, Hardy and Aust 1995). More stable lipid radicals and reactive nitrogen species can be generated secondarily (Goodglick et al. 1989, Park and Aust 1998). Theoretically, those free radicals could be generated in the vicinity of any target cells that are in contact with asbestos fibers. The reactive radicals could damage

TABLE 5.5 Direct Mechanisms of Asbestos-Fiber Carcinogenesis

Mechanism	Experimental Endpoints	References
Genotoxic	Oxidized bases	Chao et al. (1996), Fung et al. (1997)
	DNA breaks	Reviewed in Jaurand (1996)
	Aneuploidy	Reviewed in Jaurand (1996), Jensen et al. (1996)
	Mutations	Park and Aust (1998)
	Deletions	Reviewed in Hei et al. (2000)
Nongenotoxic		
Mitogenic	Target cell proliferation	BéruBé et al. (1996), Goldberg et al. (1997)
	Binding to or activation of surface receptors	Boylan et al. (1995), Pache et al. (1998)
	Growth factor expression	Liu et al. (1996), Brody et al. (1997)
	Activation of signaling pathways	Reviewed in Mossman et al. (1997), Manning et al. (2002)
Cytotoxic	Apoptosis	Broaddus et al. (1996), Goldberg et al. (1997), Levresse et al. (1997)
	Necrosis	Reviewed in Kane (1996)

SOURCE: Bernstein et al. (2005).

DNA or form adducts, such as 8-hydroxydeoxyguanosine (8-OHdG). If the DNA damage is not accurately repaired, mutations or deletions could result (reviewed in Hei et al. 2000). Long asbestos fibers have also been shown to interfere with the mitotic spindle, chromosomal segregation, and cytokinesis in cells in culture (Ault et al. 1995, Hesterberg and Barrett 1985, Jaurand 1996, Jensen et al. 1996). Direct interference with the mitotic apparatus could lead to aneuploidy or polyploidy; these chromosomal alterations have been found in human mesotheliomas (reviewed in Kane 1996, Murthy and Testa 1997).

Several in vivo studies have confirmed the results of these in vitro genotoxicity assays. In the 4 weeks after rats were gavaged with 100 mg/kg chrysotile, Amacher et al. (1974, 1975) found transient increases in DNA synthesis in tissues from the stomachs, small intestines, and colons (but not livers or pancreases), which occurred sooner after treatment in the stomachs than colons. After intratracheal instillation of asbestos fibers in rats, hydroxyl radicals (Schapira et al. 1994) and lipid radicals (Ghio et al. 1997) have been detected. Increased mutation frequencies at the reporter gene locus have been discovered in *lacI* transgenic rats, after inhalation (Rihn et al. 2000) or intraperitoneal injection (Unfried et al. 2002) of crocidolite asbestos fibers.

Both chronic and acute exposure to asbestos fibers increases the proliferation of epithelial and mesothelial cells. Nongenotoxic mechanisms leading to increased cell proliferation include activation of growth factor receptors and intracellular signaling pathways (reviewed in Albrecht et al. 2004). Human and rodent mesotheliomas frequently show constitutive expression and activation of growth-factor pathways, including those of IGF, PDGF, VEGF, and TGF-β (Cacciotti et al. 2005). Alternatively, direct physical damage or free-radical-mediated injury could induce apoptosis or necrosis of target cells that is repaired by compensatory cell proliferation. Repeated episodes of target-cell injury and repair could expand a preneoplastic proliferating cell population during the early stages in the development of lung cancer or malignant mesothelioma (reviewed in Kane 1996).

Epidemiologic studies have established that exposure to asbestos fibers increases the risk of lung cancer, particularly in cigarette smokers (reviewed by Churg 1998). Multiple indirect mechanisms may contribute to a synergistic interaction between smoking and asbestos (IARC 2004). Tobacco-smoking alters mucociliary functions and so may impair clearance of fibers from the bronchi and alveoli (McFadden et al. 1986). In rat tracheal explants and guinea pigs, cigarette smoke enhanced penetration of asbestos fibers into airway epithelium and exacerbated epithelial hyperplasia and small-airway disease (Hobson et al. 1988, Tron et al. 1987). Oxidants in tobacco smoke combined with asbestos-catalyzed generation of reactive oxygen species have been proposed to mediate fiber penetration of airway epithelium (Churg et al. 1989). Inhalation of ozone was also shown to impair clearance and increase retention of asbestos fibers in the lungs of rats (Pinkerton et al. 1989). Because of their large surface area, asbestos fibers may adsorb polycyclic aromatic hydrocarbons (PAHs), transport them into the lungs, and facilitate metabolic activation (Kandaswami and O'Brien 1983, Lakowicz and Bevan 1979). The extent of PAH adsorption on the fiber surface depends on several factors including humidity, phospholipids content of the lung lining fluid, and extent of fiber leaching in the lung. These factors may also influence the kinetics and extent of desorption of PAHs deposited in the tracheobronchial epithelium (Fubini 1993, 1997). PAHs and asbestos fibers were found to be synergistic in inducing squamous metaplasia in tracheal explant cultures (Mossman et al. 1984). Similarly, intratracheal instillation of amosite asbestos fibers plus benzo[a]-pyrene induced a synergistic increase in mutations at the *lacI* reporter gene locus in a rat transgenic model (Loli et al. 2004).

The combined effects of asbestos fibers and tobacco smoke on development of lung cancer may be explained at a molecular level (Table 5.6). *K-ras* and *p53* gene mutations and *FHIT* tumor-suppressor gene deletions have been proposed to be increased by asbestos exposure and related to enhanced chromosomal instability (reviewed in Nelson and Kelsey 2002). Some smokers may be genetically predisposed to lung cancer as a result of mutations in DNA repair pathways (Hartwig 2002, Hu et al. 2002). Alternatively, acquired mutations or deletions in key genes involved in DNA repair may facilitate accumulation of additional genetic mutations induced by tobacco-smoke carcinogens during early stages of development of lung cancer (Hollander et al. 2005). Epigenetic silencing of tumor suppressor genes has been described in human lung cancers (Dammann et al. 2001, Kim et al. 2001) and in human malignant mesotheliomas (Hirao et al. 2002, Toyooka et al. 2001, Wong et al. 2002).

TABLE 5.6 Indirect Mechanisms of Asbestos-Fiber Carcinogenesis

Mechanisms	References
Cofactor with tobacco smoke	Reviewed in Kane (1996), Lee et al. (1998), Nelson and Kelsey (2002)
Epigenetic gene silencing	Reviewed in Esteller (2005)
Persistent inflammation with secondary genotoxicity	Vallyathan and Shi (1997)
Persistent inflammation with release of cytokines and growth factors	Reviewed in Brody et al. (1997)
Cofactor with SV40 virus	Reviewed in Gazdar et al. (2002)

SOURCE: Bernstein et al. (2005).

Persistent inflammation in response to biopersistent asbestos fibers may lead to secondary genotoxicity caused by release of reactive oxygen and nitrogen metabolites from activated macrophages (Vallyathan and Shi 1997). Reactive oxygen metabolites have also been proposed to contribute to altered DNA methylation (Cerda and Weitzman 1997, Govindarajan et al. 2002). Activated macrophages also produce chemokines, cytokines, proteases, and growth factors that perpetuate tissue injury, inflammation, and target-cell proliferation (Robledo et al. 2000). Ultimately, the persistent injury and inflammation can culminate in progressive fibrosis or asbestosis of the lungs. Repair of epithelial injury is achieved by proliferation of type II alveolar cells, which are a potential target for accumulation of additional mutations and development of cancer (reviewed in Brody et al. 1997).

A mechanistic link between chronic inflammation, fibrosis, and cancer has been proposed on the basis of animal models (Coussens and Werb 2002). Although a causal relationship between asbestosis and lung cancer based on epidemiologic studies is controversial, there are plausible biological mechanisms by which fibrosis could mediate an effect. In the lung, chronic inflammation is associated with epithelial cell proliferation and type II hyperplasia (Travis et al. 2002). Mediators derived from activated macrophages or other inflammatory cells may stimulate proliferation of preneoplastic cells. The proliferating population is a target for additional genetic mutations produced by oxidants, viruses, or chemical carcinogens. Activated macrophages and inflammatory cells also release proteases and fibrogenic factors that may increase extracellular matrix turnover and fibrosis. And proteases, in combination with proangiogenic factors, may facilitate invasion and metastasis during later stages of tumor progression (Tlsty 2001).

Polyomaviruses as Possible Cofactors for Cancer

The role of SV40, a polyomavirus, as a cofactor with asbestos fibers in the induction of malignant mesothelioma is controversial (Table 5.7). SV40 viral DNA sequences and oncoproteins have been detected in human pleural malignant mesotheliomas by some investigators (reviewed by Gazdar et al. 2002) but there are technical concerns about these findings (López-Ríos et al. 2004). However, a role for SV40 as a carcinogen or cocarcinogen is biologically plausible on the basis of cellular and animal models (Carbone et al. 2003, Cicala et al. 1993) and the molecular mechanisms of action of these viral oncoproteins (reviewed in Gazdar et al. 2002).

Human JC virus is a member of the polyomavirus family that is closely related to BK virus and SV40 virus. Like SV40 virus, JC virus encodes T and t antigens that function in cell transformation and induction of tumors in experimental animals (reviewed in White et al. 2005). Although JC virus

TABLE 5.7 SV40 Virus and Malignant Mesothelioma

Evidence for a Causal Relationship

1. SV40 viral DNA sequences have been detected in up to 80% of human malignant mesotheliomas in the United States (reviewed in Gazdar et al. 2002).
2. SV40 viral DNA has been detected in tumor cells, not in adjacent stroma or nonneoplastic mesothelial cells (Carbone et al. 1994, 1997; Ranel et al. 1999; Shivapurkar et al. 1999).
3. SV40 T antigen binds to and inactivates p53 and pRb proteins (Carbone et al. 1997, De Luca et al. 1997).
4. SV40 virus preferentially infects and transforms human mesothelial cells (Carbone et al. 2003).
5. Antisense constructs directed against SV40 T antigen induce growth arrest and apoptosis in human mesothelioma cells in vitro (Waheed et al. 1999).
6. SV40 virus induces malignant mesothelioma in hamsters (Cicala et al. 1993).

Evidence Against a Causal Relationship

1. Several studies have failed to detect SV40 viral DNA sequences in human malignant mesotheliomas (López-Ríos et al. 2004, Manfredi et al. 2005).
2. Epidemiologic studies fail to show an increased risk of cancer in individuals likely exposed to SV40 virus in contaminated vaccines (reviewed in IOM 2002).
3. SV40 T antigen is highly immunogenic (reviewed in Butel and Lednicky 1999).
4. Serologic tests for SV40 virus are cross-reactive with JC virus and BK virus which are nearly ubiquitous in humans but do not cause disease in immunocompetent individuals (reviewed in Shah 2004).
5. Distribution of potentially contaminated vaccines coincided with a period of increasing use of asbestos products (reviewed in Gazdar et al. 2002).

is trophic for glial cells of the central nervous system, it can infect tonsillar tissue and is thought to replicate and spread in circulating lymphoid cells. More than 80% of adults have serologic evidence of exposure to JC virus, most likely due to subclinical infection in childhood. JC viral DNA sequences have been detected in the urine, kidney, and gastrointestinal tract of normal people (Bofill-Mas and Girones 2001, Laghi et al. 1999, Ricciardiello et al. 2000). In immunocompromised patients, JC virus can produce a fatal demyelinating disease, progressive multifocal leukoencephalopathy (PML). JC virus has been detected in brain tumors in patients with or without PML (White et al. 2005). It has also been detected in esophageal and colonic tumors (Del Valle et al. 2005, Enam et al. 2002, Laghi et al. 1999). Like the association between SV40 virus and human malignant mesotheliomas, the causal relationship between JC virus and gastrointestinal cancer is disputed (Boland et al. 2004, Newcomb et al. 2004).

SV40 and JC viral T antigens perturb several key cell-signaling and growth-regulatory pathways, both directly by binding to and inactivating pRb and p53 and indirectly by binding to insulin receptor substrate 1 (Fei et al. 1995) and β-catenin (Enam et al. 2002), inducing expression of autocrine and paracrine growth factors (Cacciotti et al. 2001), and altering patterns of gene methylation (Suzuki et al. 2005). In addition, T antigen and agnoprotein encoded by late viral genes may inhibit DNA repair (Digweed et al. 2002) and prevent the cell cycle arrest induced by DNA damage, thereby inducing genetic and karyotypic instability (White et al. 2005). SV40 virus also induces telomerase activity and immortalization of human mesothelial cells (Foddis et al. 2002, Ke et al. 1989). Human mesotheliomas containing SV40 viral sequences show a significantly higher index of gene methylation (Toyooka et al. 2001). One of the most frequently methylated genes, RASSF1A, was shown to be progressively methylated during passage of SV40-infected mesothelial cells in vitro (Toyooka et al. 2002). Thus, SV40 virus may contribute to epigenetic gene silencing during tumor growth and progression.

There is experimental evidence to support the hypothesis that SV40 virus and asbestos fibers can act as cofactors in inducing transformation of human mesothelial cells in culture (Bocchetta et al. 2000) and in hamsters (Krocynska et al. 2005). There are no studies reported on whether asbestos fibers act as a potential cofactor with JC virus in cell transformation in vitro or in tumorigenicity in animal models.

INFORMATION FROM ANIMAL STUDIES

Dosimetry Information

A major consideration in assessing the risk of cancer in the oral cavity, pharynx, larynx, and gut after inhalation exposure to asbestos is the proportion of inhaled fibers that enters those regions and how long the fibers stay there. There is an extensive literature on the deposition and clearance of inhaled particles in animals and humans. Research on the dosimetry of inhaled radionuclides led to the development of extensive models of the deposition and clearance of such inhaled particles because of the ease of detecting the particles in the body. As noted in Chapter 4, the International Commission on Radiological Protection (ICRP 1994) has published its models. A recent dosimetry model for inhaled poorly soluble particles has been published by the Environmental Protection Agency (Jarabek et al. 2005), which allows extrapolation of dosimetry between species.

It is known that poorly soluble particles that deposit in the oropharyngeal, laryngeal, and tracheobronchial region are cleared mainly by coughing or movement up the mucociliary escalator followed by swallowing and passage through the gut. There are fewer studies on deposition and clearance of inhaled fibers. A multiple-path model of fiber deposition in the rat lung developed by Asgharian and Anjilvel (1998) indicated that in oral airways, where deposition is mainly by impaction, the larger the fiber aspect ratio, the lower the deposition by impaction. Modeling by Quinn et al. (1997), however, suggested that greater length would cause fibers to deposit disproportionately higher in the tracheobronchial tree than aerodynamically equivalent spheres. More recently, deposition of fibers in the human respiratory tract was studied by using a cast replica of the tract from the nose to the oral cavity to the fourth bifurcation (Su and Cheng 2005, Zhou and Cheng 2005); the oropharynx was found to be a preferred deposition site, but apparently there was less oral deposition of fibers than of spherical particles. Thus, one might use deposition data for spherical particles as an approximation for fibers.

On the basis of current knowledge, inhalation of asbestos would result in deposition in the oral cavity, pharynx, larynx, and tracheobronchial region—all sites that lead to clearance of fibers through the gut. The toxicology data summarized below suggest that fibers do not persist at the site of deposition or in the gut long enough to induce toxicity in animal models at the cancer sites of concern in this review.

Inhalation Toxicity Studies

The carcinogenicity of asbestos was first noted in humans. Thus, inhalation studies of the toxicity of asbestos in animals have not been directed toward the carcinogenicity of asbestos, but toward more specific issues: mechanisms of fiber-induced toxicity, including neoplasia; deposition and fate of inhaled fibers; and comparison of the toxicity of other fibers with that of asbestos. In that rodents are obligatory nose-breathers, inhalation exposure will not expose the pharynx in a fashion that precisely replicates human exposure. One would, however, expect a large portion of the inhaled fibers ultimately to be ingested because of removal of the fibers from the upper respiratory tract by the mucociliary escalator followed by swallowing.

Inhalation studies have been conducted in F344 rats (Hesterberg et al. 1993, 1994; McConnell et al. 1994a) and Syrian hamsters (McConnell et al. 1994b, 1999) with exposures for 6 hr/day, 5 days/week for up to 24 months. Hesterberg et al. (1993, 1994) exposed F344 rats to chrysotile asbestos fibers at 10 mg/m^3 as a positive control for comparison with responses to glass fibers. At the end of the 2 years of exposure to asbestos, the rats had pulmonary fibrosis, one of 69 rats (1.4%) had mesothelioma, and 13 (19%) had lung tumors (adenomas and carcinomas). No lesions were found in the oropharyngeal region, the gut, or the larynx (McConnell 2005). Using the same species as an animal model, McConnell et al. (1994a) exposed F344 rats to crocidolite asbestos at 10 mg/m^3 in a chronic study to compare the response to asbestos with that to slag wool insulation fibers. The exposure to asbestos fibers was terminated after 10 months because of increased morbidity and mortality, and both mesotheliomas (1%) and lung neoplasms (14%) were observed. No tumors were found in the oropharyngeal region, the gut, or the larynx.

When the Syrian hamster was used as an animal model, mesotheliomas were observed but not lung tumors. In a chronic (24-month) inhalation study of Syrian hamsters exposed to amosite for comparison with glass fibers (McConnell et al. 1999), exposure at 250 fibers/cm^3 for 78 weeks resulted in a mesothelioma incidence of 20%. Again, no lesions of the oropharyngeal region, the gut, or the larynx were observed (McConnell 2005). In another study by McConnell et al. (1994b), Syrian hamsters were exposed to chrysotile asbestos at 10 mg/m^3 for 18 months as a positive control for comparison of responses with those to refractory ceramic fibers. In this case, only pulmonary fibrosis was observed in the exposed hamsters, and there were no neoplasms in the oropharyngeal region, the gut, or the larynx (McConnell 2005).

The above studies indicate that rats are more sensitive to development of pulmonary tumors following asbestos exposure than are Syrian hamsters and that chrysotile is somewhat less potent than the amphiboles. In neither species did chronic asbestos exposures by inhalation lead to tumors in the oropharyngeal region, the gut, or the larynx.

Ingestion Toxicity Studies

One report of the toxicity of ingested asbestos involved F344 rats exposed to asbestos in combination with subcutaneous administration of a known intestinal carcinogen, azoxymethane (AOM) (Ward et al. 1980). The asbestos was administered three times a week for 10 weeks by intragastric bolus dosing (1 mg in 1 ml saline). The first iteration of this experiment included a full complement of control groups and scheduled sacrifice at 34 weeks; neither amosite nor chrysotile appeared to increase the incidence of intestinal tumors above that produced by AOM alone, but they both produced four-to-five-fold increases in metastatic intestinal tumors. A life-span experiment with larger groups, but a more limited design, tested only amosite vs AOM. The lack of untreated vehicle controls made interpretation of the results difficult. Compared to historical controls, there was a nonsignificant increase in neoplastic lesions in the gut of the rats exposed only to asbestos; strictly speaking, one cannot know whether the results observed were associated with the asbestos or with irritation from the procedure, although one would not anticipate that gavage itself would impact the lower portion of the gastrointestinal tract.

The most definitive animal studies of oral exposure to asbestos were a series of studies conducted by the National Toxicology Program (Technical Reports 246, 249, 279, 280, and 295), in which asbestos (chrysotile, crocidolite, and amosite) was administered in the feed of rats and hamsters

(HHS 1983, 1985, 1988, 1990a, 1990b). Nonfibrous tremolite was also tested in rats according to the same protocol (NTP Technical Report 277, HHS 1990c). Animals were exposed to asbestos 1% of the diet, which was estimated by the investigators to be about 70,000 times the greatest possible human exposure in drinking water. The concern at the time of the studies was the potential toxicity of drinking water delivered through asbestos cement pipes, because slightly acidic water was known to leach the cement and release asbestos fibers. Exposure of dams was followed by exposure of the pups by gavage while they were nursing and then in the diet for the remainder of their lives. Examination of the gut was extensive (McConnell 2005). The entire intestinal tract was opened and examined by running it over an "x-ray" view box. Even the smallest inflammatory lesion would have been identified and saved for histopathologic examination. In the gastronintestinal tract, sections of the esophagus, the entire stomach, three levels of small intestine, and the cecum were examined. In addition, the entire colorectum was fixed and then carpet-rolled and sectioned. That allowed histopathologically examination of the entire colorectum (the suspect target tissue). Any crypt lesion should have been identified, if present. The only finding of note in the gastrointestinal tract was a slight increase in the incidence of adenomatous polyps in the large intestine after exposure to the intermediate-length chrysotile (from Quebec) in rats, but preneoplastic changes in the epithelium were not found. No gastrointestinal lesions (inflammatory, preneoplastic, or neoplastic) were found after exposure to the same sample of chrysotile in hamsters, to short chrysotile (from New Idria) in hamsters or rats, to amosite in rats or hamsters, to crocidolite in rats, or to nonfibrous tremolite in rats. The mesentery was examined in detail, as well as mesenteric lymph nodes and sections of the larynx, trachea, and lungs from every animal. No lesions were found in any of those tissues. Asbestos fibers, particularly the amphibole types, are highly tissue-reactive if of the appropriate length and would be hypothesized to produce lesions throughout the gastrointestinal tract if they persisted in sufficient numbers.

Those studies involved extremely high exposures to asbestos in the gut over the lifetime of the animals beginning with nursing pups. The examination of the gut and related tissues was thorough. The studies do not indicate an association between ingested asbestos and neoplasia.

Summary

On the basis of animal studies of asbestos exposure in rats and Syrian hamsters, one would not expect exposure to asbestos fibers at environmental or even occupational concentrations to increase the incidence of tumors in the oropharyngeal region, the larynx, or the gut. Our knowledge of dosimetry suggests that inhalation exposure to asbestos would result in clearance of a large amount of asbestos through the gut, but that the fibers would quickly pass through the gut and be eliminated from the body. The *type* of lesions observed after chronic exposures to asbestos fibers suggests that the fibers were not retained at any site in amounts *needed to cause neoplastic change, although they did produce an increased incidence of (benign) adenomatous polyps in the large intestine of rats at very high exposure levels.*

Although correspondence of tumor sites in humans and experimental animals would constitute intuitively appealing evidence and would likely be mechanistically consistent, *it should be noted, however, that* empirical consideration of epidemiologic and experimental findings for known carcinogens has demonstrated that site-specificity is not necessarily the rule across species (Maronpot et al. 2004). Most of the non-epidemiologic data considered in this chapter do not lend particular credence toward a given extrapulmonary site being the target of carcinogenic action in humans, but serve to establish the precept that asbestos is a human carcinogen.

BIOMARKERS

Role of Biomarkers in Detection of Asbestos-Related Cancer

Biomarkers have not yet been used extensively in the early detection or treatment of cancer. One of the more established biomarkers is the presence of pleural plaques as a marker of pulmonary asbestosis and therefore increased risk of development of pleural mesothelioma. In our review of biomarkers for prediction of the development of laryngeal, pharyngeal, or gastrointestinal tumors, we surveyed the literature for evidence of changes in biomarker expression in animals (primarily rodents) and for serum and radiographic biomarkers in humans. There seems to be no evidence that definitively identifies a biomarker of asbestos exposure that predicts cancers of the larynx, pharynx, esophagus, stomach, colon, or rectum.

Animal Studies

Human malignant mesotheliomas are induced by fibrous dusts, but the nature of the interactions between fibers and target cells, including the molecular mechanisms leading to tumorigenesis, are not fully understood. Several studies in rats monitored mRNA expression patterns at different stages of asbestos-induced carcinogenesis and demonstrated the up-regulation of some proto-oncogenes—including *c-myc*, *fra-1*, and *EGFR* in fiber-induced disease. Several papers point to the possible role of *fra-1* as one of the dimeric proteins generating the immediate early gene (AP-1 transcription factor) family of proteins, and there is some evidence of a dose-dependent increase in expression in mesothelial cells. There is also evidence that asbestos induces mitochondrial DNA damage and dysfunction with dose-related decreases in steady-state mRNA concentrations of cytochrome C oxidases. That result of asbestos exposure led to mRNA expression of pro- and anti-apoptotic genes and increased the numbers of apoptotic cells observed in asbestos-exposed mesothelial cells in murine models. The possible contribution of mitochondrial-derived pathways to asbestos-induced apoptosis was confirmed by its reduction in apoptosis when the cells were pretreated with a caspase-9 inhibitor. Genotoxicity and alterations in DNA synthesis were observed in the livers, and somewhat less consistently in the serum, of rats treated with asbestos.

Human Biomarkers of Asbestos Exposure

Several human studies have attempted to assay biomarkers of asbestos exposure in human serum. Asbestos exposure can lead to early inflammatory responses, such as the release of inflammatory cells that can be collected by non-invasive methods; and several free radicals are involved in the progression of asbestos-related diseases, ultimately leading to cytogenetic changes. Therefore, extensive evaluations have been carried out of antioxidant states and reducing equivalents such as reactive oxygen species. Marczynski et al. (2000a) showed that concentrations of 8-OHdG in DNA of white blood cells of workers highly exposed to asbestos in Germany were significantly increased over those in the control group ($p < 0.001$). The mean concentration for the 496 asbestos-exposed people was 2.61 ± 0.91 8-OHdG/10^5 dG compared to 1.52 ± 0.39 8-OHdG/10^5 dG for the 214 control subjects. Those results indicate that DNA samples from exposed people contain 1.7-2 times the amount of oxidative damage found in controls. The mechanism of action of fiber-induced oxidative damage has been studied with common assays and other procedures. The association between 8-OHdG in the DNA of workers highly exposed to asbestos correlated with a significantly increased risk of cancer compared with non-asbestos-exposed controls, but the risk was not significantly higher ($p > 0.05$) than that in asbestos-exposed patients without tumors of the respiratory tract, gastrointestinal tract, mouth-pharynx-larynx, or urogenital tract. These intriguing data suggest that there is a gradient in the concentrations of 8-OHdG in white blood cells between asbestos-exposed patients with and without cancer and non-asbestos-exposed controls.

There has been extensive work on several DNA-inducible genes as biomarkers of exposure to these agents, including p53 induction of DNA strand breaks, p53 expression, and apoptosis in cell lines, particularly in cultured mesothelial cells. In vitro data show significant biologic effects of asbestos fibers in human blood cells, particularly lymphocytes and neutrophils. There is little evidence to date with regard to asbestos-related biomarkers obtained from human serial sampling other than the aforementioned compelling data in patterns of 8-OHdG descriptions of changes in low-molecular-weight DNA fragmentation in the white cells of workers highly exposed to asbestos (Marczynski et al. 2000b).

Summary

There is evidence of a difference between asbestos-exposed people and non-asbestos-exposed people in modulation of DNA-adduct formation, as demonstrated by a significant elevation in the concentration of 8-OHdG in DNA of white blood cells from asbestos-exposed people. There are no compelling data, however, that can differentiate between the concentrations of these DNA adducts in the lymphocytes of cancer patients exposed to asbestos and of other people exposed to asbestos.

REFERENCES

Albrecht C, Borm PJ, Unfried K. 2004. Signal transduction pathways relevant for neoplastic effects of fibrous and non-fibrous particles. *Mutation Research* 553(1-2): 23-35.

Altomare DA, Vaslet CA, Skele KL, De Rienzo A, Devarajan K, Jhanwar SC, McClatchey AI, Kane AB, Testa JR. 2005. A mouse model recapitulating molecular features of human mesothelioma. *Cancer Research* 65(18): 8090-8095.

Amacher DE, Alarif A, Epstein SS. 1974. Effects of ingested chrysotile on DNA synthesis in the gastrointestinal tract and liver of the rat. *Environmental Health Perspectives* 9: 319-324.

Amacher DE, Alarif A, Epstein SS. 1975. The dose-dependent effects of ingested chrysotile on DNA synthesis in the gastrointestinal tract, liver, and pancreas of the rat. *Environmental Research* 10(2): 208-216.

Antman KH. 1986. Asbestos-related malignancy. *Critical Reviews in Oncology-Hematology* 6(3): 287-309.

Asgharian B, Anjilvel S. 1998. A multiple path model of fiber disposition in the rat lung. *Toxicological Sciences* 44(1): 80-86.

Ault JG, Cole RW, Jensen CG, Jensen LC, Bachert LA, Rieder CL. 1995. Behavior of crocidolite asbestos during mitosis in living vertebrate lung epithelial cells. *Cancer Research* 55(4): 792-798.

Baris I, Simonato L, Artvinli M, Pooley F, Saracci R, Skidmore J, Wagner C. 1987. Epidemiological and environmental evidence of the health effects of exposure to erionite fibres: A four-year study in the Cappadocian region of Turkey. *International Journal of Cancer* 39(1): 10-17.

Baser ME, De Rienzo A, Altomare D, Balsara BR, Hedrick NM, Gutmann DH, Pitts LH, Jackler RK, Testa JR. 2002. Neurofibromatosis 2 and malignant mesothelioma. *Neurology* 59(2): 290-291.

Battifora H, McCaughey WT. 1995. Tumors of the serosal membranes. In: Roasi J, ed. *Atlas of Tumor Pathology*. Third Series. Washington, DC: Armed Forces Institute of Pathology. Pp. 17-27.

Bernstein D, Castranova V, Donaldson K, Fubini B, Hadley J, Hesterberg T, Kane A, Lai D, McConnell EE, Muhle H, Oberdorster G, Olin S, Warheit DB. 2005. Testing of fibrous particles: Short-term assays and strategies. *Inhalation Toxicology* 17(10): 497-537.

BéruBé KA, Quinlan TR, Moulton G, Hemenway D, O'Shaughnessy P, Vacek P, Mossman BT. 1996. Comparative proliferative and histopathologic changes in rat lungs after inhalation of chrysotile or crocidolite asbestos. *Toxicology and Applied Pharmacology* 137(1): 67-74.

Bocchetta M, Di Resta I, Powers A, Fresco R, Tosolini A, Testa JR, Pass HI, Rizzo P, Carbone M. 2000. Human mesothelial cells are unusually susceptible to simian virus 40-mediated transformation and asbestos cocarcinogenicity. *Proceedings of the National Academy of Sciences of the United States of America* 97(18): 10214-10219.

Bofill-Mas S, Girones R. 2001. Excretion and transmission of JCV in human populations. *Journal of Neurovirology* 7(4): 345-349.

Boland CR, Bigler J, Newcomb PA, Lampe JW, Potter JD. 2004. Evidence for an association between JC virus and colorectal neoplasia. *Cancer Epidemiology, Biomarkers and Prevention* 13(12): 2285-2286.

Boylan AM, Sanan DA, Sheppard D, Broaddus VC. 1995. Vitronectin enhances internalization of crocidolite asbestos by rabbit pleural mesothelial cells via the integrin alpha v beta 5. *Journal of Clinical Investigation* 96(4): 1987-2001.

Broaddus VC, Yang L, Scavo LM, Ernst JD, Boylan AM. 1996. Asbestos induces apoptosis of human and rabbit pleural mesothelial cells via reactive oxygen species. *Journal of Clinical Investigation* 98(9): 2050-2059.

Brody AR, Liu JY, Brass D, Corti M. 1997. Analyzing the genes and peptide growth factors expressed in lung cells in vivo consequent to asbestos exposure and in vitro. *Environmental Health Perspectives* 105 (Supplement 5): 1165-1171.

Butel JS, Lednicky JA. 1999. Cell and molecular biology of simian virus 40: Implications for human infections and disease. *Journal of National Cancer Institute* 91(2): 119-134.

Cacciotti P, Libener R, Betta P, Martini F, Porta C, Procopio A, Strizzi L, Penengo L, Tognon M, Mutti L, Gaudino G. 2001. SV40 replication in human mesothelial cells induces HGF/Met receptor activation: A model for viral-related carcinogenesis of human malignant mesothelioma. *Proceedings of the National Academy of Sciences of the United States of America* 98(21): 12032-12037.

Cacciotti P, Mutti L, Gaudino G. 2005. Growth factors and malignant mesothelioma. In: Pass HI, Vogelzang NJ, Carbone M, eds. *Malignant Mesothelioma: Advances in Pathogenesis, Diagnosis, and Translational Therapies.* New York: Springer Science and Business Media. Pp. 112-123.

Carbone M, Pass HI, Rizzo P, Marinetti M, Di Muzio M, Mew DJ, Levine AS, Procopio A. 1994. Simian virus 40-like DNA sequences in human pleural mesothelioma. *Oncogene* 9(6): 1781-1790.

Carbone M, Rizzo P, Grimley PM, Procopio A, Mew DJ, Shridhar V, de Bartolomeis A, Esposito V, Giuliano MT, Steinberg SM, Levine AS, Giordano A, Pass HI. 1997. Simian virus-40 large-T antigen binds p53 in human mesotheliomas. *Nature Medicine* 3(8): 908-912.

Carbone M, Burck C, Rdzanek M, Rudzinski J, Cutrone R, Bocchetta M. 2003. Different susceptibility of human mesothelial cells to polyomavirus infection and malignant transformation. *Cancer Research* 63(19): 6125-6129.

Cerda S, Weitzman SA. 1997. Influence of oxygen radical injury on DNA methylation. *Mutation Research* 386(2): 141-152.

Chao CC, Park SH, Aust AE. 1996. Participation of nitric oxide and iron in the oxidation of DNA in asbestos-treated human lung epithelial cells. *Archives of Biochemistry and Biophysics* 326(1): 152-157.

Churg A. 1998. Neoplastic asbestos-induced disease. In: *Pathology of Occupational Disease.* 2nd edition. Baltimore: Williams and Wilkins. Pp. 339-392.

Churg A, Hobson J, Berean K, Wright J. 1989. Scavengers of active oxygen species prevent cigarette smoke-induced asbestos fiber penetration in rat tracheal explants. *American Journal of Pathology* 135(4): 599-603.

Cicala C, Pompetti F, Carbone M. 1993. SV40 induces mesotheliomas in hamsters. *American Journal of Pathology* 142(5): 1524-1533.

Coussens LM, Werb Z. 2002. Inflammation and cancer. *Nature* 420(6917): 860-867.

Dammann R, Takahashi T, Pfeifer GP. 2001. The CpG island of the novel tumor suppressor gene RASSF1A is intensely methylated in primary small cell lung carcinomas. *Oncogene* 20(27): 3563-3567.

De Luca A, Baldi A, Esposito V, Howard CM, Bagella L, Rizzo P, Caputi M, Pass HI, Giordano GG, Baldi F, Carbone M, Giordano A. 1997. The retinoblastoma gene family pRb/p105, p107, pRb2/p130 and simian virus-40 large T-antigen in human mesotheliomas. *Nature Medicine* 3(8): 913-916.

Del Valle L, White MK, Enam S, Oviedo SP, Bromer MQ, Thomas RM, Parkman HP, Khalili K. 2005. Detection of JC virus DNA sequences and expression of viral T antigen and agnoprotein in esophageal carcinoma. *Cancer* 103(3): 516-527.

Digweed M, Demuth I, Rothe S, Scholz R, Jordan A, Grotzinger C, Schindler D, Grompe M, Sperling K. 2002. SV40 large T-antigen disturbs the formation of nuclear DNA-repair foci containing MRE11. *Oncogene* 21(32): 4873-4878.

Enam S, Del Valle L, Lara C, Gan DD, Ortiz-Hidalgo C, Palazzo JP, Khalili K. 2002. Association of human polyomavirus JCV with colon cancer: Evidence for interaction of viral T-antigen and beta-catenin. *Cancer Research* 62(23): 7093-7101.

Esteller M. 2005. Dormant hypermethylated tumour suppressor genes: Questions and answers. *Journal of Pathology* 205(2): 172-180.

Fei ZL, D'Ambrosio C, Li S, Surmacz E, Baserga R. 1995. Association of insulin receptor substrate 1 with simian virus 40 large T antigen. *Molcular and Cellular Biology* 15(8): 4232-4239.

Fleury-Feith J, Lecomte C, Renier A, Matrat M, Kheuang L, Abramowski V, Levy F, Janin A, Giovannini M, Jaurand MC. 2003. Hemizygosity of *Nf2* is associated with increased susceptibility to asbestos-induced peritoneal tumours. *Oncogene* 22(24): 3799-3805.

Foddis R, De Rienzo A, Broccoli D, Bocchetta M, Stekala E, Rizzo P, Tosolini A, Grobelny JV, Jhanwar SC, Pass HI, Testa JR, Carbone M. 2002. SV40 infection induces telomerase activity in human mesothelial cells. *Oncogene* 21(9): 1434-1442.

Fubini B. 1993. The possible role of surface chemistry in the toxicity of inhaled fibers. In: Warheit D, ed. *Fiber Toxicology*. Newark, DE: Academic Press. Pp. 229-257.

Fubini B. 1997. Surface reactivity in the pathogenic response to particulates. *Environmental Health Perspectives* 105 (Supplement 5): 1013-1020.

Fubini B, Oter-Areán C. 1999. Chemical aspects of the toxicity of inhaled mineral dust. *Chemical Society Review* 28: 373-381.

Fung H, Kow YW, Van Houten B, Mossman BT. 1997. Patterns of 8-hydroxydeoxyguanosine formation in DNA and indications of oxidative stress in rat and human pleural mesothelial cells after exposure to crocidolite asbestos. *Carcinogenesis* 18(4): 825-832.

Gazdar AF, Butel JS, Carbone M. 2002. SV40 and human tumours: Myth, association or causality? *National Reviews of Cancer* 2(12): 957-964.

Ghio AJ, LeFurgey A, Roggli VL. 1997. In vivo accumulation of iron on crocidolite is associated with decrements in oxidant generation by the fiber. *Journal of Toxicology and Environmental Health* 50(2): 125-142.

Goldberg JL, Zanella CL, Janssen YM, Timblin CR, Jimenez LA, Vacek P, Taatjes DJ, Mossman BT. 1997. Novel cell imaging techniques show induction of apoptosis and proliferation in mesothelial cells by asbestos. *American Journal of Respiratory Cellular and Molecular Biology* 17(3): 265-271.

Goodglick LA, Pietras LA, Kane AB. 1989. Evaluation of the causal relationship between crocidolite asbestos-induced lipid peroxidation and toxicity to macrophages. *American Reviews of Respiratory Diseases* 139(5): 1265-1273.

Govindarajan B, Klafter R, Miller MS, Mansur C, Mizesko M, Bai X, LaMontagne K Jr, Arbiser JL. 2002. Reactive oxygen-induced carcinogenesis causes hypermethylation of p16(Ink4a) and activation of MAP kinase. *Molecular Medicine* 8(1): 1-8.

Hardy JA, Aust AE. 1995. The effect of iron binding on the ability of crocidolite asbestos to catalyze DNA single-strand breaks. *Carcinogenesis* 16(2): 319-325.

Hartwig A. 2002. Role of DNA repair in particle- and fiber-induced lung injury. *Inhalation Toxicology* 14(1): 91-100.

Hei TK, Xu A, Louie D, Zhou YL. 2000. Genotoxocity versus carcinogenicity: Implications from fiber toxicity studies. *Inhalation Toxicology* 12(Supplement 3): 141-147.

Heineman EF, Bernstein L, Stark AD, Spirtas R. 1996. Mesothelioma, asbestos, and reported history of cancer in first-degree relatives. *Cancer* 77(3): 549-554.

Hesterberg TW, Barrett JC. 1985. Induction by asbestos fibers of anaphase abnormalities: Mechanism for aneuploidy induction and possibly carcinogenesis. *Carcinogenesis* 6(3): 473-475.

Hesterberg TW, Miller WC, McConnell EE, Chevalier J, Hadley JG, Bernstein DM, Thevenaz P, Anderson R. 1993. Chronic inhalation toxicity of size-separated glass fibers in Fischer 344 rats. *Fundamental and Applied Toxicology* 20(4): 464-476.

Hesterberg TW, Miller WC, Mast R, McConnell EE, Bernstein DM, Anderson R. 1994. Relationship between lung biopersistence and biological effects of man-made vitreous fibers after chronic inhalation in rats. *Environmental Health Perspectives* 102 (Supplement 5): 133-137.

Hesterberg TW, Chase G, Axten C, Miller WC, Musselman RP, Kamstrup O, Hadley J, Morscheidt C, Bernstein DM, Thevenaz P. 1998. Biopersistence of synthetic vitreous fibers and amosite asbestos in the rat lung following inhalation. *Toxicology and Applied Pharmacology* 151(2): 262-275.

HHS (US Department of Health and Human Services). 1983. *Lifetime Carcinogenesis Studies of Amosite Asbestos (CAS NO. 12172-73-5) in Syrian Golden Hamsters (Feed Studies).* NTP TR 249. Research Triangle Park, NC: National Toxicology Program.

HHS. 1985. *Toxicology and Carcinogenesis Studies of Chrysotile Asbestos (CAS No. 12001-29-5) in F344/N Rats (Feed Studies).* NTP TR 295. Research Triangle Park, NC: National Toxicology Program.

HHS. 1988. *Toxicology and Carcinogenesis Studies of Crocidolite Asbestos (CAS No. 12001-28-4) in F344/N Rats (Feed Studies).* NTP TR 280. Research Triangle Park, NC: National Toxicology Program.

HHS. 1990a. *Lifetime Carcinogenesis Studies of Chrysotile Asbestos (CAS No. 12001-29-5) in Syrian Golden Hamsters (Feed Studies).* NTP TR 246. Research Triangle Park, North Carolina: National Toxicology Program.

HHS. 1990b. *Toxicology and Carcinogenesis Studies of Amosite Asbestos (CAS No. 12172-73-5) in F344/N Rats (Feed Studies).* NTP TR 279. Research Triangle Park, NC: National Toxicology Program.

HHS. 1990c. *Toxicology and Carcinogenesis Studies of Tremolite (CAS No. 14567-73-8) in F344/N Rats (Feed Studies).* NTP TR 277. Research Triangle Park, NC: National Toxicology Program.

Hirao T, Bueno R, Chen CJ, Gordon GJ, Heilig E, Kelsey KT. 2002. Alterations of the p16(INK4) locus in human malignant mesothelial tumors. *Carcinogenesis* 23(7): 1127-1130.

Hisada M, Garber JE, Fung CY, Fraumeni JF Jr, Li FP. 1998. Multiple primary cancers in families with Li-Fraumeni syndrome. *Journal of National Cancer Institute* 90(8): 606-611.

Hobson J, Gilks B, Wright J, Churg A. 1988. Direct enhancement by cigarette smoke of asbestos fiber penetration and asbestos-induced epithelial proliferation in rat tracheal explants. *Journal of National Cancer Instiute* 80(7): 518-521.

Hollander MC, Philburn RT, Patterson AD, Velasco-Miguel S, Friedberg EC, Linnoila RI, Fornace AJ Jr. 2005. Deletion of XPC leads to lung tumors in mice and is associated with early events in human lung carcinogenesis. *Proceedings of the National Academy of Sciences of the United States of America* 102(37): 13200-13205.

Hu YC, Sidransky D, Ahrendt SA. 2002. Molecular detection approaches for smoking associated tumors. *Oncogene* 21(48): 7289-7297.

IARC (International Agency for Research on Cancer). 1987. *Overall Evaluations of Carcinogenity: An Updating of IARC Monographs Volumes 1 to 42*. IARC Monographs on the Evaluation of Carcinogenic Risks of Chemicals to Man. Supplement 7. Lyon, France: World Health Organization.

IARC. 2004. *Tobacco Smoke and Involuntary Smoking*. IARC Monographs on the Evaluation of Carcinogenic Risks to Human Vol. 83. Lyon, France: World Health Organization, IARC.

ICRP (International Commission on Radiological Protection). 1994. *Human Respiratory Tract Model for Radiological Protection*. Oxford: Elsevier.

IOM (Institute of Medicine). 2002. *Immunization Safety Review: SV40 Contamination of Polio Vaccine and Cancer*. Washington, DC: National Academy Press.

Jarabek AM, Asgharian B, Miller FJ. 2005. Dosimetric adjustments for interspecies extrapolation of inhaled poorly soluble particles (PSP). *Inhalation Toxicology* 17: 317-334.

Jaurand MC. 1996. Use of in-vitro genotoxicity and cell transformation assays to evaluate the potential carcinogenicity of fibres. *IARC Scientific Publications* 140: 55-72.

Jensen CG, Jensen LCW, Reider CL, Cole RW, Ault JG. 1996. Long crocidolite fibers cause polyploidy by sterically blocking cytokines. *Carcinogenesis* 17: 2013-2021.

Kamp DW, Weitzman SA. 1999. The molecular basis of asbestos induced lung injury. *Thorax* 54(7): 638-652.

Kandaswami C, O'Brien PJ. 1983. Effect of chrysotile asbestos and silica on the microsomal metabolism of benzo(a)pyrene. *Environmental Health Perspectives* 51: 311-314.

Kane AB. 1996. Mechanisms of mineral fibre carcinogenesis. *IARC Scientific Publications* 140: 11-34.

Ke Y, Reddel RR, Gerwin BI, Reddel HK, Somers AN, McMenamin MG, LaVeck MA, Stahel RA, Lechner JF, Harris CC. 1989. Establishment of a human in vitro mesothelial cell model system for investigating mechanisms of asbestos-induced mesothelioma. *American Journal of Pathology* 134(5): 979-991.

Kim DH, Nelson HH, Wiencke JK, Zheng S, Christiani DC, Wain JC, Mark EJ, Kelsey KT. 2001. p16(INK4a) and histology-specific methylation of CpG islands by exposure to tobacco smoke in non-small cell lung cancer. *Cancer Research* 61(8): 3419-3424.

Krocynska B, Cutrone R, Bocchetta M, Yang H, Pass HI, Carbone M. 2005. Asbestos and SV40 are co-carcinogens. *Proceedings of American Association of Cancer Research* 46: 56.

Laghi L, Randolph AE, Chauhan DP, Marra G, Major EO, Neel JV, Boland CR. 1999. JC virus DNA is present in the mucosa of the human colon and in colorectal cancers. *Proceedings of the National Academy of Sciences of the United States of America* 96(13): 7484-7489.

Lakowicz JR, Bevan DR. 1979. Effects of asbetos, iron oxide, silica, and carbon black on the microsomal availability of benzo[a]pyrene. *Biochemistry* 18(23): 5170-5176.

Lee BW, Wain JC, Kelsey KT, Wiencke JK, Christiani DC. 1998. Association between diet and lung cancer location. *American Journal Respiratory and Critical Care Medicine* 158(4): 1197-1203.

Levresse V, Renier A, Fleury-Feith J, Levy F, Moritz S, Vivo C, Pilatte Y, Jaurand MC. 1997. Analysis of cell cycle disruptions in cultures of rat pleural mesothelial cells exposed to asbestos fibers. *American Journal of Respiratory Cell and Molecular Biology* 17(6): 660-671.

Liu JY, Morris GF, Lei WH, Corti M, Brody AR. 1996. Up-regulated expression of transforming growth factor-alpha in the bronchiolar-alveolar duct regions of asbestos-exposed rats. *American Journal of Pathology* 149(1): 205-217.

Loli P, Topinka J, Georgiadis P, Dusinska M, Hurbankova M, Kovacikova Z, Volkovova K, Wolff T, Oesterle D, Kyrtopoulos SA. 2004. Benzo[a]pyrene-enhanced mutagenesis by asbestos in the lung of lambda-lacI transgenic rats. *Mutation Research* 553(1-2): 79-90.

López-Ríos F, Illei PB, Rusch V, Ladanyi M. 2004. Evidence against a role for SV40 infection in human mesotheliomas and high risk of false-positive PCR results owing to presence of SV40 sequences in common laboratory plasmids. *Lancet* 364(9440): 1157-1166.

Lynch HT, Anton-Culver H, Kurosaki T. 1994. Is there a genetic predisposition to malignant mesothelioma? In: Jaurand M, Bignon J, eds. *Mesothelial Cell and Mesothelioma.* New York: Marcel Dekker, Inc. Pp. 47-70.

Manfredi JJ, Dong J, Liu WJ, Resnick-Silverman L, Qiao R, Chahinian P, Saric M, Gibbs AR, Phillips JI, Murray J, Axten CW, Nolan RP, Aaronson SA. 2005. Evidence against a role for SV40 in human mesothelioma. *Cancer Research* 65(7): 2602-2609.

Manning CB, Vallyathan V, Mossman BT. 2002. Diseases caused by asbestos: Mechanisms of injury and disease development. *International Immunopharmacology* 2(2-3): 191-200.

Marczynski B, Kraus T, Rozynek P, Raithel HJ, Baur X. 2000a. Association between 8-hydroxy-2'-deoxyguanosine levels in DNA of workers highly exposed to asbestos and their clinical data, occupational and non-occupational confounding factors, and cancer. *Mutation Research* 468(2): 203-212.

Marczynski B, Rozynek P, Kraus T, Schlosser S, Raithel HJ, Baur X. 2000b. Levels of 8-hydroxy-2'-deoxyguanosine in DNA of white blood cells from workers highly exposed to asbestos in Germany. *Mutation Research* 468(2): 195-202.

Maronpot RR, Flake G, Huff J. 2004. Relevance of animal carcinogenesis findings to human cancer predictions and prevention. *Toxicologic Pathology* 32 (Supplement 1): 40-48.

Marsella JM, Liu BL, Vaslet CA, Kane AB. 1997. Susceptibility of p53-deficient mice to induction of mesothelioma by crocidolite asbestos fibers. *Environmental Health Perspectives* 105 (Supplement 5): 1069-1072.

McConnell EE. 2005 (October 27). *Personal Communication to Mary Paxton for the Committee on Asbestos: Selected Health Effects.* Available in IOM Public Access Files.

McConnell E, Kamstrup O, Musselman R, Hesterberg T, Chevalier J, Miller W, Thevenaz P. 1994a. Chronic inhalation study of size-separated rock and slag wool insulation fibers in Fischer 344/N rats. *Inhalation Toxicology* 6(6): 571-614.

McConnell E, Mast R, Hesterberg T, Chevalier J, Kotin P, Bernstein D, Thevenaz P, Glass L, Anderson R. 1994b. Chronic inhalation toxicity of a kaolin-based refactory ceramic fiber in Syrian golden hamsters. *Inhalation Toxicology* 6(6): 503-532.

McConnell EE, Axten C, Hesterberg TW, Chevalier J, Miller WC, Everitt J, Oberdörster G, Chase GR, Thevenaz P, Kotin P. 1999. Studies on the inhalation toxicology of two fiberglasses and amosite asbestos in the Syrian golden hamster: Part II. Results of chronic exposure. *Inhalation Toxicology* 11(9): 785-835.

McFadden D, Wright JL, Wiggs B, Churg A. 1986. Smoking inhibits asbestos clearance. *American Reviews of Respiratory Diseases* 133(3): 372-374.

Metcalf RA, Welsh JA, Bennett WP, Seddon MB, Lehman TA, Pelin K, Linnainmaa K, Tammilehto L, Mattson K, Gerwin BI. 1992. *p53* and Kirsten-ras mutations in human mesothelioma cell lines. *Cancer Research* 52(9): 2610-2615.

Mossman BT, Eastman A, Bresnick E. 1984. Asbestos and benzo[a]pyrene act synergistically to induce squamous metaplasia and incorporation of [3H]thymidine in hamster tracheal epithelium. *Carcinogenesis* 5(11): 1401-1404.

Mossman BT, Faux S, Janssen Y, Jimenez LA, Timblin C, Zanella C, Goldberg J, Walsh E, Barchowsky A, Driscoll K. 1997. Cell signaling pathways elicited by asbestos. *Environmental Health Perspectives* 105 (Supplement 5): 1121-1125.

Murthy SS, Testa JR. 1997. Asbestos, chromosomal deletions, and tumor suppressor gene alterations in human malignant mesothelioma. *Journal of Cellular Physiology* 180(2): 150-157.

Nelson HH, Kelsey KT. 2002. The molecular epidemiology of asbestos and tobacco in lung cancer. *Oncogene* 21(48): 7284-7288.

Newcomb PA, Bush AC, Stoner GL, Lampe JW, Potter JD, Bigler J. 2004. No evidence of an association of JC virus and colon neoplasia. *Cancer Epidemiology, Biomarkers and Prevention* 13(4): 662-666.

Oberdörster G. 1996. Evaluation and use of animal models to assess mechanisms of fibre carcinogenicity. *IARC Scientific Publications* 140: 107-125.

Pache JC, Janssen YM, Walsh ES, Quinlan TR, Zanella CL, Low RB, Taatjes DJ, Mossman BT. 1998. Increased epidermal growth factor-receptor protein in a human mesothelial cell line in response to long asbestos fibers. *American Journal of Pathology* 152(2): 333-340.

Park SH, Aust AE. 1998. Participation of iron and nitric oxide in the mutagenicity of asbestos in hgprt-, gpt+ Chinese hamster V79 cells. *Cancer Research* 58(6): 1144-1148.

Pinkerton KE, Brody AR, Miller FJ, Crapo JD. 1989. Exposure to low levels of ozone results in enhanced pulmonary retention of inhaled asbestos fibers. *American Review of Respiratory Diseases* 140(4): 1075-1081.

Quinn MM, Ellenbecker MJ, Smith TJ, Wegman DH, Eisen EA. 1997. A model to predict deposition of man-made vitreous fibres in the human tracheobronchial region. *Annals of Occupational Hygiene* 41 (Supplement 1): 197-202.

Ranel M, Nagels J, Heylen H, De Schepper S, Paulussen J, De Maeyer M, Van Haesendonck C. 1999. Detection of SV40 like viral DNA and viral antigens in malignant pleural mesothelioma. *European Respiratory Journal* 14(6): 1381-1386.

Ricciardiello L, Laghi L, Ramamirtham P, Chang CL, Chang DK, Randolph AE, Boland CR. 2000. JC virus DNA sequences are frequently present in the human upper and lower gastrointestinal tract. *Gastroenterology* 119(5): 1228-1235.

Rihn B, Coulais C, Kauffer E, Bottin MC, Martin P , Yvon F, Vigneron JC, Binet S, Monhoven N, Steiblen G, Keith G. 2000. Inhaled crocidolite mutagenicity in lung DNA. *Environmental Health Perspectives* 108(4): 341-346.

Robledo RF, Buder-Hoffmann SA, Cummins AB, Walsh ES, Taatjes DJ, Mossman BT. 2000. Increased phosphorylated extracellular signal-regulated kinase immunoreactivity associated with proliferative and morphologic lung alterations after chrysotile asbestos inhalation in mice. *American Journal of Pathology* 156(4): 1307-1316.

Roushdy-Hammady I, Siegel J, Emri S, Testa JR, Carbone M. 2001. Genetic-susceptibility factor and malignant mesothelioma in the Cappadocian region of Turkey. *Lancet* 357(9254): 444-445.

Schapira RM, Ghio AJ, Effros RM, Morrisey J, Dawson CA, Hacker AD. 1994. Hydroxyl radicals are formed in the rat lung after asbestos instillation in vivo. *American Journal of Respiratory Cell and Molecular Biology* 10(5): 573-579.

Sekido Y, Pass HI, Bader S, Mew DJ, Christman MF, Gazdar AF, Minna JD. 1995. Neurofibromatosis type 2 (NF2) gene is somatically mutated in mesothelioma but not in lung cancer. *Cancer Research* 55(6): 1227-1231.

Shah KV. 2004. Simian virus 40 and human disease. *Journal of Infectious Diseases* 190(12): 2061-2064.

Shivapurkar N, Wiethege T, Wistuba II, Salomon E, Milchgrub S, Muller KM, Churg A, Pass H, Gazdar AF. 1999. Presence of simian virus 40 sequences in malignant mesotheliomas and mesothelial cell proliferations. *Journal of Cellular Biochemistry* 76(2): 181-188.

Sporn T, Roggli V. 2004. Mesothelioma. In: Roggli V, Oury T, Sporn T, eds. *Pathology of Asbestos-Associated Diseases.* 2nd edition. New York: Springer. Pp. 104-168.

Su WC, Cheng YS. 2005. Deposition of fiber in the human nasal airways. *Aerosol Science and Technology* 39(9): 888-901.

Suzuki M, Toyooka S, Shivapurkar N, Shigematsu H, Miyajima K, Takahashi T, Stastny V, Zern AL, Fujisawa T, Pass HI, Carbone M, Gazdar AF. 2005. Aberrant methylation profile of human malignant mesotheliomas and its relationship to SV40 infection. *Oncogene* 24(7): 1302-1308.

Tlsty TD. 2001. Stromal cells can contribute oncogenic signals. *Seminars in Cancer Biology* 11(2): 97-104.

Toyooka S, Pass HI, Shivapurkar N, Fukuyama Y, Maruyama R, Toyooka KO, Gilcrease M, Farinas A, Minna JD, Gazdar AF. 2001. Aberrant methylation and simian virus 40 tag sequences in malignant mesothelioma. *Cancer Research* 61(15): 5727-5730.

Toyooka S, Carbone M, Toyooka KO, Bocchetta M, Shivapurkar N, Minna JD, Gazdar AF. 2002. Progressive aberrant methylation of the RASSF1A gene in simian virus 40 infected human mesothelial cells. *Oncogene* 21(27): 4340-4344.

Travis WD, Colby JV, Koss MN, Rosado-de-Christenson ML, Muller NL, King TE. 2002. Non-neoplastic disorders of the lower respiratory tract. In: Roasi J, ed. *Atlas of Nontumor Pathology.* 1st edition. Washington DC: American Registry of Pathologists and Armed Forces Institute Pathologists. Pp. 814-846.

Tron V, Wright JL, Harrison N, Wiggs B, Churg A. 1987. Cigarette smoke makes airway and early parenchymal asbestos-induced lung disease worse in the guinea pig. *American Review of Respiratory Disease* 136(2): 271-275.

Unfried K, Schurkes C, Abel J. 2002. Distinct spectrum of mutations induced by crocidolite asbestos: Clue for 8-hydroxydeoxyguanosine-dependent mutagenesis in vivo. *Cancer Research* 62(1): 99-104.

Vallyathan V, Shi X. 1997. The role of oxygen free radicals in occupational and environmental lung diseases. *Environmental Health Perspectives* 105 (Supplement 1): 165-177.

Vaslet CA, Messier NJ, Kane AB. 2002. Accelerated progression of asbestos-induced mesotheliomas in heterozygous p53+/- mice. *Toxicological Sciences* 68(2): 331-338.

Waheed I, Guo ZS, Chen GA, Weiser TS, Nguyen DM, Schrump DS. 1999. Antisense to SV40 early gene region induces growth arrest and apoptosis in T-antigen-positive human pleural mesothelioma cells. *Cancer Research* 59(24): 6068-6073.

Ward JM, Frank AL, Wenk M, Devor D, Tarone RE. 1980. Ingested asbestos and intestinal carcinogenesis in F344 rats. *Journal of Environmental Pathology and Toxicology* 3(5-6): 301-312.

Weitzman SA, Graceffa P. 1984. Asbestos catalyzes hydroxyl and superoxide radical generation from hydrogen peroxide. *Archives of Biochemistry and Biophysics* 228(1): 373-376.

White MK, Gordon J, Reiss K, Del Valle L, Croul S, Giordano A, Darbinyan A, Khalili K. 2005. Human polyomaviruses and brain tumors. *Brain Research Reviews* 50(1): 69-85.

Wong L, Zhou J, Anderson D, Kratzke RA. 2002. Inactivation of p16INK4a expression in malignant mesothelioma by methylation. *Lung Cancer* 38(2): 131-136.

Zhou Y, Cheng YS. 2005. Particle deposition in a cast of human tracheobronchial airways. *Aerosol Science and Technology* 39(6): 492-500.

6

Description of Epidemiologic Studies Included in Evidentiary Dataset

COHORT STUDIES

Reports Included in the Evaluation of Cancer Risks

Table 6.1 delineates the 40 main cohort populations that passed the committee's primary eligibility criteria and were found to contain usable information on the risk of cancer at one or more of the sites of interest for this review. Some of the cohorts contained subpopulations (such as men and women) whose results were reported separately. Furthermore, tracking of multiple aspects of the health over decades in many of the cohort populations has resulted in numerous published analyses. Among these, this committee was interested in the most complete, and thus usually the most recent, citation addressing cancer incidence or mortality. Specific citations contributing information to this review are given in the rightmost column. In some instances, different publications provided the most complete information on a given subpopulation or cancer site, so more than one citation may have served as a source of evidence on a single main cohort population. Table B.1 in Appendix B provides more detail about the overall history (such as updates and the nature of asbestos to which the subjects were exposed) of each studied population on a citation-specific basis; boldface indicates particular citations that were the source of evidence abstracted for any of the cancer sites under consideration.

Table 6.2 presents results observed in the informative cohort populations with regard to the recognized asbestos-related health effects: asbestosis, mesothelioma, and lung cancer. Those findings provide a rough indication

TABLE 6.1 Description of Cohorts Informative for Selected Cancers

Cohort Population (location—number, description)	Results for Selected Cancers (ICD range specified; mortality unless otherwise noted)						Source Citation
	Pharynx	Larynx	Esophagus	Stomach	Colon	Rectum	
Patients with Asbestos-Related Disease							
1. Italy—631 women compensated for asbestosis		161		151	153	154	Germani et al. (1999)
2. Finland— a. 1,376 asbestosis patients b. 4,887 patients with pleural disease		161 ?	150 ?	151 ?	153 ?	154 ?	Karjalainen et al. (1999)
3. Poland— a. 907 men with asbestosis b. 490 women with asbestosis		161	150	151	153	154	Szeszenia-Dabrowska et al. (2002)
4. US clinical trial monitoring asbestos-exposed men						153-154 ?	Aliyu et al. (2005)

continues

TABLE 6.1 Continued

Cohort Population (location—number, description)	Results for Selected Cancers (ICD range specified; mortality unless otherwise noted)						Source Citation
	Pharynx	Larynx	Esophagus	Stomach	Colon	Rectum	
Mining							
5. Wittenoom Gorge, Western Australia	140-149, 160 ?	161 ?	150 ?	151 ?		152-154 ?	Armstrong et al. (1988) [mortality to 1980]
	C09.0-C14.8	C32.0-C32.9	C15.0-C15.9	C16.0-C16.9		C18.0-C20.9	Reid et al. (2004) [incidence 1979-2000]
6. Quebec, Canada—Asbestos and Thetford		161	150	151		152-154	McDonald et al. (1993) [through 1976–1988]
Mines		161	#150	151		#152-154	Liddell et al. (1997) [through 1950–1992]
7. Finland—Paakkila and Maljasalmi mines		161 ?	150 ?	151 ?		153-154 ?	Meurman et al. (1994)
8. Balangero, Italy	140-149 ?	161		150-151 ?		152-154 ?	Piolatto et al. (1990)
9. Northern Transvaal, South Africa—North West Cape Blue and Penge Mines	140-149	161	#150	#151	#153	#154	Sluis-Cremer et al. (1992)
10. Libby, MT, US—NIOSH sample				151			Amandus and Wheeler (1987)

Insulation Manufacture/ Insulators (Laggers)							
11. Canada/USA							
a. 632 male insulation workers before 1943 in NY and NJ, US		140-149, 161 ?	150 ?	151 ?		153-154 ?	Selikoff et al. (1979) [through 1976]
b. Paterson, NJ, US—820 men producing amosite asbestos insulation for shipbuilding		140-149, 161 ?	150 ?	151 ?		153-154 ?	Seidman et al. (1986)
c. 17,800 male members of asbestos insulation unions in 1967	146 ?	161	150	151		153-154	Selikoff and Seidman (1991) [through 1986]
12. Uxbridge, UK—Cape [insulation] Boards Plant			150	151	153	154	Acheson et al. (1984)
13. East London, UK—1,400 male laggers (a) (subgroups b and c make up population 32)	140-148	161	150	151	153	154	Berry et al. (2000)
14. Tyler, TX, US—753 white male asbestos pipe-insulation plant workers	140-149	161	150	151	153	154	Levin et al. (1998)

continues

TABLE 6.1 Continued

Cohort Population (location—number, description)	Results for Selected Cancers (ICD range specified; mortality unless otherwise noted)						Source Citation
	Pharynx	Larynx	Esophagus	Stomach	Colon	Rectum	
Asbestos Textile Workers							
15. Italy—889 male and 1,077 female textile workers	140-149	161		151		152-154, 159.0	Pira et al. (2005)
16. Rochdale, Northern England		161 ?	150 ?	151 ?		153-154 ?	Peto et al. (1985)
17. Charleston, SC, US—asbestos-textile workers		161		151			Dement et al. (1994) [through 1990]
Asbestos Cement							
18. Denmark—Danish Eternit Ltd. cement factory	140-148	161		151	153	154	Raffn et al. (1989) [incidence through 1984]
					153	154	Raffn et al. (1996) [incidence through 1990]
19. Emilia Romagna, Italy—10 cement factories	140-149 ?	161					Giaroli et al. (1994)
20. Casale Monferrato, Italy—asbestos-cement production		161 ?		151 ?		153-154 ?	Botta et al. (1991)
21. Lithuainia—Daugeliai and Akmene Factories		161		151		153-154	Smailyte et al. (2004a) [incidence]

22. Southern Sweden—asbestos cement plant				150-152		153-154	Albin et al. (1990) [mortality through 1986]
					153	154	Jakobsson et al. (1994) [incidence through 1989]
23. Tamworth, England, UK—TAC Construction Materials Ltd.		161	150	151	153	154	Gardner et al. (1986)
24. New Orleans, LA, US—workers at two asbestos cement plants	140-149	161	150	151		153-154	Hughes et al. (1987)
Friction Materials							
25. Ontario, Canada—two automotive-parts factories		161					Finkelstein (1989a)
26. Ferodo, UK—friction materials factory		161					Berry (1994)
27. USSR				151 ?			Kogan et al. (1993)
28. New York, US—friction-products manufacture	140-149 ?	161					Parnes (1990)

continues

TABLE 6.1 Continued

Cohort Population (location—number, description)	Results for Selected Cancers (ICD range specified; mortality unless otherwise noted)						Source Citation
	Pharynx	Larynx	Esophagus	Stomach	Colon	Rectum	
Generic "Asbestos Workers"							
29. China—eight asbestos factories		#161 ?	#150 ?	151 ?		#153-154 ?	Zhu and Wang (1993)
30. Qingdao, China—asbestos plant				151 ?			Pang et al. (1997)
31. Federal Republic of Germany—asbestos-related workers in national register				150-151		153-154	Woitowitz et al. (1986)
32. East London, UK—3,000 male (b) and 700 female (c) asbestos factory workers [subgroup a makes up population 13]	140-148	161	150	151	153	154	Berry et al. (2000)
33. Lancashire, UK—gas mask manufacture				151			Acheson et al. (1982)
34. England and Wales, UK—national survey of asbestos workers			150 ?	151 ?	153 ?	154 ?	Hodgson and Jones (1986)
35. US—asbestos industry retirees	140-148	161	150	151	153	154	Enterline et al. (1987)

Other Occupations with Substantial Asbestos Exposure							
36. Ontario, Canada—members of plumbers' and pipefitters' union		161 ?	150 ?	151 ?		153-154 ?	Finkelstein and Verma (2004)
37. Finland—7,775 male shipyard workers		161		151		153-154	Tola et al. (1988) [incidence]
38. Tuscany, Italy—railway-carriage construction and repair	140-149 ?	161 ?		151 ?		152-154 ?	Battista et al. (1999)
39. Genoa, Italy—ship repair, refitting, and construction	140-149	161	150	151		153-154	Puntoni et al. (2001)
40. Gothenburg, Sweden—shipyard workers				151		152-154	Sanden and Jarvholm (1987) [incidence]

NOTES: # = number observed given but no estimated risk; ICD or range = explicit or evident; ICD? or range? = exact sites included in grouping not completely clear.

TABLE 6.2 Rates of Accepted Asbestos-Related Health Outcomes in Cohorts Informative for Selected Cancers

Cohort Population (location—number, description)	Accepted Asbestos-Related Health Outcomes (number observed, RR, 95% CI)			Source Citation
	Asbestosis	Lung Cancer	Mesothelioma	
Patients with Asbestos-Related Disease				
1. Italy—631 women compensated for asbestosis	all	16, 4.8 (2.7-7.8)	14, 64.0 (35.0-107)	Germani et al. (1999)
2. Finland— a. 1,376 asbestosis patients b. 4,887 patients with pleural disease	all	a. 127 M, 6.7 (5.6-7.9); 6 F, 19.80 (7.3-43.1) b. 44 M, 1.3 (1.0-1.8); 0 F	a. 9 M, 31.6 (14.4-60.0); 1 F, 95.7 (2.4-533) b. 4 M, 5.5 (1.5-14.1); 0 F	Karjalainen et al. (1999)
3. Poland— a. 907 men with asbestosis b. 490 women with asbestosis	all all	a. 39, 1.68 (1.22-2.26); b. 13, 6.21 (3.31-10.62)	a. 3, 26.8 (5.5-78.3); b. 3, 72.1 (10.3-146)	Szeszenia-Dabrowska et al. (2002)
4. US clinical trial				Aliyu et al. (2005)
Mining				
5. Wittenoom Gorge, Western Australia—6,505 men		91 M, 1.60 (1.31-1.97)	32	Armstrong et al. (1988) [mortality through 1980]
a. 6,493 men b. 235 women			a. 235 b. 7	Berry et al. (2004) [incidence through 2000]

6. Quebec, Canada—Asbestos and Thetford Mines		646, 1.37	38	Liddell et al. (1997) [1950-1992]
7. Finland—Paakkila and Maljasalmi Mines		76 M, 2.88 (2.27-3.60); 1 F, 2.22 (0.06-12.4)	4 M, 45.6 (12.2-115)	Meurman et al. (1994)
8. Balangero, Italy	16	22, 1.1	2, 6.7	Piolatto et al. (1990)
9. Northern Transvaal, South Africa—North West Cape Blue and Penge Mines	1	63, 1.72 (1.32-2.21)	16	Sluis-Cremer et al. (1992)
10. Libby, MT, US				
a. NIOSH sample		20, 2.23 (1.36-3.45)	Included with lung	Amandus and Wheeler (1987)
b. McGill sample		21	2	McDonald et al. (1986)
Insulation Manufacture/Insulators (Laggers)				
11. Canada/US—17,800 male asbestos insulation unions members in 1967	427	1,168, 4.35, $p<0.001$	458	Selikoff and Seidman (1991)
12. Uxbridge, UK—Cape [insulation] Boards Plant		57, 2.0	5	Acheson et al. (1984)
13. East London, UK—1,400 male laggers (a)		38, 3.67	13	Berry et al. (2000)
14. Tyler, TX, US—753 white male asbestos pipe-insulation plant workers	3	35, 2.77 (1.93-3.85)	4, 28.8 (7.9-73.8)	Levin et al. (1998)

continues

TABLE 6.2 Continued

Cohort Population (location—number, description)	Accepted Asbestos-Related Health Outcomes (number observed, RR, 95% CI)			Source Citation
	Asbestosis	Lung Cancer	Mesothelioma	
Asbestos Textile Workers				
15. Italy—889 male and 1,077 female textile workers	38	76, 2.82 (2.22-3.54)	37, 27.8 (19.6-38.6)	Pira et al. (2005)
16. Rochdale, Northern England	7	132, 1.31, $p<0.01$	11	Peto et al. (1985)
17. Charleston, SC, US—546 black and 1,247 white male and 1,229 white female asbestos textile workers		4, 1.55 (0.53-3.55)	2	Dement et al. (1994)
Asbestos Cement				
18. Denmark—Danish Eternit Ltd. cement factory		162, 1.80 (1.54-2.10)	10, 5.46 (2.62-10.1)	Raffn et al. (1989) [incidence through 1984]
		1.63 (1.26-2.08)		Raffn et al. (1996) [incidence through 1990]
19. Emilia Romagna, Italy—10 cement factories		33, 1.24 (0.91-1.66)	6, 4.11	Giaroli et al. (1994)
20. Casale Monferrato, Italy—asbestos cement production	85 M; 4 F	110 M, 2.71 (2.23-3.27); 7 F, 3.96 (1.59-8.16)		Botta et al. (1991)

21. Lithuainia—Daugeliai and Akmene Factories	29 M, 0.9 (0.7-1.3); 1 F, 0.7 (0.1-4.6)	0 M; 1 F, 20.1 (2.9-142)	Smailyte et al. (2004a)
22. Southern Sweden—asbestos cement plant	35, 1.8 (0.90-3.7)	13, 7.2 (0.97-54)	Albin et al. (1990)
23. Tamworth, England, UK—TAC Construction Materials LTD	34 M, 0.9 (0.6-1.3); 6 F, 1.4 (0.5-3.1)	1 M; 0 F	Gardner et al. (1986)
24. New Orleans, LA, US—workers at two asbestos cement plants	154, 1.34	1	Hughes et al. (1987)
Friction Materials			
25. Ontario, Canada—two automotive parts factories	11, 1.40	Included with lung	Finkelstein (1989a)
26. Ferodo, UK—friction materials factory			Berry (1994)
27. USSR	2, 0.11		Kogan et al. (1993)
28. New York, US—friction products manufacture	15, 0.95		Parnes (1990)

continues

TABLE 6.2 Continued

Cohort Population (location—number, description)	Accepted Asbestos-Related Health Outcomes (number observed, RR, 95% CI)			Source Citation
	Asbestosis	Lung Cancer	Mesothelioma	
Generic "Asbestos Workers"				
29. China—eight asbestos factories		67, 4.2		Zhu and Wang (1993)
30. Qingdao, China—asbestos plant		3 M, 5.1; 6 F, 6.8		Pang et al. (1997)
31. Federal Republic of Germany—asbestos-related workers from national register		a. 26, 1.70 b. 12, 4.62	a. 6 b. 6	Woitowitz et al. (1986)
32. East London, UK—3,000 male (b) and 700 female (c) asbestos factory workers		b. 157, 2.55 c. 37, 7.46	b. 60 c. 25	Berry et al. (2000)
33. Lancashire, UK—gas mask manufacture		22, 2.00	3	Acheson et al. (1982)
34. England and Wales, UK—national survey of asbestos workers	11	157, 1.30	34	Hodgson and Jones (1986)
35. US—asbestos industry retirees	22	77, 2.71	Included with lung	Enterline et al. (1987)

Other Occupations with Substantial Asbestos Exposure				
36. Ontario, Canada—members of plumbers' and pipefitters' union		393, 1.27 (1.13-1.42)	8	Finkelstein and Verma (2004)
37. Finland—7,775 male shipyard workers		227, 1.18 (1.03-1.35) for all 7,775 shipyard workers	1, 1.13—in a machinist, not pipe fitter	Tola et al. (1988) [incidence]
38. Tuscany, Italy—railway carriage construction and repair		26, 1.24 (0.87-1.72) [90%CI]	5, 13.27, (5.23-27.9) [90%CI]	Battista et al. (1999)
39. Genoa, Italy—ship repair, refitting, and construction	18, 46.6 (27.6-73.6)	298, 1.77 (1.57-1.98)	60, 5.24, (4.00-6.74)	Puntoni et al. (2001)
40. Gothenburg, Sweden—shipyard workers		11, 1.12 (0.56-2.0)	4	Sanden and Jarvholm (1987)

of asbestos exposure and of how informative each of the cohorts might be expected to be in contributing evidence to the committee's evaluation of asbestos's role in others cancers.

For the cohorts that provided information on at least one of the selected cancer sites, Figure 6.1 gives a graphic indication of the period when exposure was occurring and of the length of the most recent (most complete) follow-up of the vital status of the cohort members. The figure also includes the percentage of the original cohort members found to have died as an index of a cohort's "maturity," which suggests how much additional information might be garnered if follow-up were extended for the cohort.

Figure 6.2 presents an analogous picture for the roughly six dozen asbestos-exposed cohorts that the committee screened for the selected cancers but found no usable information. The most recent citation related to cancer outcomes is specified. The considerably greater number of cohorts in the uninformative category gives an indication of the extent to which research has focused on reporting respiratory outcomes of asbestos exposure.

The cohort studies retained for the evidentiary dataset addressed defined occupational cohorts in specific asbestos industries (such as mining and milling, cement, textile, and friction products), in less clearly specified industries (such as "asbestos factory"), or employed in certain occupations with documented asbestos exposures (such as insulators). Some of the cohort studies derived qualitative categories of asbestos exposure based on individual work history or clinical factors (such as presence of pleural plaques). Quantitative exposure assessments to enable dose estimation were available only for a small percentage of the studies.

We summarized findings from reports of cohort studies of asbestos-exposed workers in which cancer-risk data were available on at least one of the specific cancers of interest as delineated in Table 6.1. The main cohort populations were made up of workers employed in asbestos mining (6); manufacturing and use of insulation (3), textiles (4), cement (7), friction materials (4), and various other asbestos products, such as gas masks (7); and in other occupations with substantial asbestos exposure (5). The most recent report of a cohort study was selected if there had been repeated follow-ups; this was the case for studies of the London East End factory (Berry et al. 2000), US textile workers (Dement et al. 1994), Quebec miners (Liddell et al. 1997, McDonald et al. 1993), and North American insulation workers (Selikoff and Seidman 1991); see Table B.1 for a listing of the citations that were superseded.

We also included in our review three studies of cohorts of patients with asbestosis or nonmalignant pleural disease who had worked in any of numerous unspecified industries and occupations (Germani et al. 1999, Karjalainen et al. 1999, Szeszenia-Dabrowska et al. 2002) under the assumption that there was a high likelihood of exposure of cohort members

Cohort Population (location – number, description)	1900 * 1920 * 1940 * 1960 * 1980 * 2000 * Time Elapsed to Final Follow-up (+ marks earliest exposure, if known)	Percent Original Cohort Dead
Patients with Asbestos-Related Disease		
1. Italy – 631 women compensated for asbestosis	---------	44%
2. Finland –		
a. 1,376 asbestosis patients	-------------	Inc
b. 4,887 patients with pleural disease	-------------	Inc
3. Poland –		
a. 907 men with asbestosis	----------------	33%
b. 490 women with asbestosis	----------------	25%
4. US clinical trial monitoring 3,897 asbestos-exposed men	----------	Inc
Mining		
5. Wittenoom Gorge, Western Australia – crocidolite mining industry workers	+ ----------	
6. Quebec, Canada - Asbestos and Thetford Mines – 9,708 men	+ ----------------------	82%
7. Finland - Paakkila and Maljasalmi Mines – 736 men, 167 women	--------------------	Inc
8. Balangero, Italy – 1,058 men	--------------------	40%
9. Northern Transvaal, South Africa - North West Cape Blue and Penge Mines – 7,317 white men	-----------------	17%
10. Libby, MT, US - NIOSH sample – 575 men	-----	28%
Insulation Manufacture/Insulators		
11. Canada and US		
a. 632 male insulation workers before 1943 in NY and NJ, US	------------------	76%
b. Paterson, NJ, US – 820 men producing amosite asbestos insulation for shipbuilding	---------------------	72%
c. 17,800 male members in 1967 of asbestos insulation unions	------------	28%
12. Uxbridge, UK - Cape [insulation] Boards Plant – 5,969 men	-----------------	7%
13. East London, UK – 1,400 male laggers	---------------	
14. Tyler, TX, US – 753 white male asbestos pipe-insulation plant workers	+ --------------	30%
	1900 * 1920 * 1940 * 1960 * 1980 * 2000 *	

continues

FIGURE 6.1 Follow-up on informative cohorts.

Cohort Population (location – number, description)	Time Elapsed to Final Follow-up (+ marks earliest exposure, if known) 1900 1920 1940 1960 1980 2000	Percent Original Cohort Dead
Asbestos Textile Workers		
15. Italy – 889 male and 1,077 female textile workers	------------------------	28%
16. Rochdale, Northern England – 3,639 asbestos textile workers	--	35%
17. Charleston, SC, US – 3,022 asbestos textile workers	------------------------	42%
Asbestos Cement		
18. Denmark - Danish Eternit Ltd. cement factory – 8,580 employees	-----------------------------	18%
Colorectal cancer only	--------------------------------	25%
19. Emilia Romagna, Italy – 10 cement factories – 3,341 workers	--------------------	8%
20. Casale Monferrato, Italy – asbestos cement production – 3,367 workers	+ ------------	30%
21. Lithuainia - Daugeliai and Akmene Factories – 1,887 workers	+ ----------	25%
22. Southern Sweden – 1,929 asbestos cement plant workers	-----------------------------	40%
2,507 workers followed for colon cancer	--------------	Inc
23. Tamworth, England, UK – 2,167 TAC Construction Materials Ltd. Employees	----------------------	22%
24. New Orleans, LA, US – 6,931 workers at two asbestos cement plants	---------------------	31%
Friction Materials		
25. Ontario, Canada – 1,657 workers at two automotive parts factories	-------------------	?
26. Ferodo, UK – 13,450 friction materials factory workers	----------------------	19%
27. USSR – 2,990 workers	------------------	?
28. New York, US – 2,057 friction products manufacturers	---------------------	13%
	1900 1920 1940 1960 1980 2000	

continues

FIGURE 6.1 Continued

Cohort Population (location – number, description)	Time Elapsed to Final Follow-up (+ marks earliest exposure, if known) 1900 * 1920 * 1940 * 1960 * 1980 * 2000 *	Percent Original Cohort Dead
Generic "Asbestos Workers"		
29. China – 5,893 workers from eight asbestos factories	-------	8%
30. Qingdao, China – 530 asbestos plant workers	------------	?
31. Federal Republic of Germany – 3,735 asbestos-related workers from national register	---	7%
32. East London, UK – 3,000 male (b) and 700 female (c) asbestos factory workers (subgroup a makes up pop 13)	---------------	~24%
33. Lancashire, UK – 1,327 female gas mask manufacturers	--------------	33%
34. England and Wales, UK – national survey of 31,150 male asbestos workers	------	4%
35. USA – 1,074 white male asbestos industry retirees	-------------------	88%
Other Occupations with Substantial Asbestos Exposure		
36. Ontario, Canada – 25,285 members of plumbers' and pipefitters' union	--------------------	11%
37. Finland – 7,775 male shipyard workers	-------------------	Inc
38. Tuscany, Italy – 734 railway-carriage construction and repair workers	+ --------------	27%
39. Genoa, Italy – 3,959 workers in ship repair, refitting, and construction	------------	60%
40. Gothenburg, Sweden – 3,787 shipyard workers	---	Inc
	1900 * 1920 * 1940 * 1960 * 1980 * 2000 *	

FIGURE 6.1 Continued

to asbestos. Additionally, we included a cohort of asbestos-exposed people who had been monitored in a clinical trial (Aliyu et al. 2005).

We reviewed but did not include cancer-risk data from studies of cohorts of workers in several industries in which modest asbestos exposure occurred in conjunction with major exposure to other toxic agents, such as a refinery and petrochemical plant (Tsai et al. 1996), rubber industry (Straif et al. 1999), and a nitric acid factory (Hilt et al. 1991).

Health Outcome Data

In most of the cohort studies reviewed, cancer mortality was the health outcome analyzed. There were very few cancer incidence studies; the excep-

Cohort Population (location – number, description)	Time Elapsed to Final Follow-up (+ marks earliest exposure, if known) 1900 * 1920 * 1940 * 1960 * 1980 * 2000 *	Percent Original Cohort Dead
Patients with Asbestos-Related Disease		
London Hospital, UK – 41 patients with asbestosis (Keal 1960)		73%
London, Cardiff, and Swansea, UK – 665 men with asbestosis (Berry 1981)		43%
Finland – 122 asbestos sprayers and 128 asbestosis patients (Oksa et al. 1997)	---------------	
Czech Republic – people with pleural plaques (Navratil et al. 1988)		
Osaka, Japan – 296 asbestos workers and 107 patients with asbestosis (Sera and Kang 1981)	----------	14%
Mining		
New York State, US – 260 talc miners and millers (Kleinfeld et al. 1974)	---------------	42%
Lead, SD, US – 440 hard rock gold miners (Gillam et al. 1976)	----------	16%
Enoree, SC, US – 194 male vermiculite miners and millers (McDonald et al. 1988)	+ --------	26%
Italy – 487 rock salt mine workers (Tarchi et al. 1994)	------------	21%
Via Chisone, Italy – 1795 male talc miners and millers (Coggiola et.al 2003)	------------------------	
Cape Province, South Africa – crocidolite miners and residents (Wagner et al. 1960)		
South Africa – miners and asbestos-cement workers (Goldstein et al. 1975)		
Wittenoom Gorge, Western Australia – 1,203 miners and millers (Musk et al. 1998)	+ --	

1900 * 1920 * 1940 * 1960 * 1980 * 2000 *

continues

FIGURE 6.2 Follow-up on asbestos-exposed cohorts without information on selected cancers.

Cohort Population (location – number, description)	1900 * 1920 * 1940 * 1960 * 1980 * 2000 * **Time Elapsed to Final Follow-up** (+ marks earliest exposure, if known)	**Percent Original Cohort Dead**
Insulation Manufacture and Insulators (Laggers)		
Asbestos insulators by union records (Kleinfeld et al. 1967)	-	
Amosite insulation plant (Joubert et al. 1991)	+ ---------	
Belfast, Northern Ireland – 170 male insulation workers (Elmes and Simpson 1977)	-----------------	72%
Italy – 893 insulation workers (Menegozzo et al. 2002)	-----------------	
Sweden – 269 male insulation workers (Jarvholm and Sanden 1998)	------------	32%
Denmark – 953 male insulation workers (Petersen and Venstrup-Nielsen 1982)	---	
Asbestos Textile Workers		
London, UK – 379 male asbestos-textile factory workers (Berry et al. 1979)	--------------------	
Lodz, Poland – asbestos-textile factory (Selikoff 1989)		
Lodz, Poland – asbestos processing plant (Wilczynska et al. 1990)		
Gas Mask Manufacture		
UK – gas-mask manufacturing (WWII) (Jones et al. 1980)		
Canada – 199 gas mask manufacturers (McDonald and McDonald 1978)	-----------------	28%
Friction Materials		
New York State, US – 2,057 male friction products manufacturers (Parnes 1990)	-------------------	
USSR – workers on machines processing brakes (Latsenko and Kogan 1990)		
	1900 * 1920 * 1940 * 1960 * 1980 * 2000 *	

continues

FIGURE 6.2 Continued

Cohort Population (location – number, description)	1900 * 1920 * 1940 * 1960 * 1980 * 2000 * Time Elapsed to Final Follow-up (+ marks earliest exposure, if known)	Percent Original Cohort Dead
Asbestos Cement		
US – 4,231 male cement-plant and quarry workers (Amandus 1986)	---------------	
Paray-Le-Monial factory, France – 1,506 males (Alies-Patin and Valleron 1985)	----------------------	14%
Belgium – 1,973 asbestos cement workers (Lacquet et al. 1980)		
Casale Monferrato, Italy – 1,964 wives of asbestos cement workers (Magnani et al. 1993)	------------------	14%
Sweden – 1,176 males (Ohlson and Hogstedt 1985)	------------	
Austria – 2,816 males (Neuberger and Kundi 1990)	----------------	19%
Lithuania, Akmene factory – 2,498 Portland cement workers (not asbestos) (Smailyte et al. 2004b)	----------------------	18%
Poland – 4,712 workers at four cement plants (Szeszenia-Dabrowska et al. 1997)	----------------------	
Poland – 3,220 workers at two cement plants (Szeszenia-Dabrowska et al. 2000)	----------	
?- asbestos cem ent workers (Gurvich et al. 1993)	------------------	
Israel – 3,608 asbestos-cement workers (Djerassi et. al 1979)	------------	
South Africa – miners and asbestos cement workers (Goldstein et al. 1975)		
Generic "Asbestos Workers"		
New Jersey, US – 878 household contacts of asbestos factory workers (Joubert et al. 1991)	--------	13%
US – asbestos plant (Mancuso and Coulter 1963)		
US – 1,493 asbestos plant workers (Mancuso and el-Attar 1967)	------------	24%
US – 264 males in asbestos-products factory (Weiss 1977)	+ ---------	25%
US – textile, friction, and packing products (Robinson et al. 1979)		
	1900 * 1920 * 1940 * 1960 * 1980 * 2000 *	

continues

FIGURE 6.2 Continued

Cohort Population (location – number, description)	1900 * 1920 * 1940 * 1960 * 1980 * 2000 * **Time Elapsed to Final Follow-up** (+ marks earliest exposure, if known)	**Percent Original Cohort Dead**
Other Occupations with Substantial Asbestos Exposure		
Poland – 1,190 female asbestos producing plant workers (Szeszenia-Dabrowska et al. 1986a)	------------------	11%
Poland – 2,403 male asbestos-products workers (Szeszenia-Dabrowska et al. 1986b)	---------------------	
Urals, USSR – asbestos industry (Kogan et al. 1972)	--------	
China – asbestos workers (Zhou et al. 1996)		
Tianjin, China – 1,172 asbestos workers (textile friction cement) (Cheng and Kong 1992)	----------	
Chongqin, China – 515 male asbestos plant (material mined in Sichuan) workers (Yano et al. 2001)	-------------	
Osaka, Japan – 296 asbestos workers and 107 patients with asbestosis (Sera and Kang 1981)	----------	14%
Osaka, Japan – asbestos factory (mainly textile) (Morinaga et al. 1990)	---------	
Osaka, Japan – 789 workers in small asbestos industries (Morinaga et al. 1991)	-----	8%
Ship, Rail, Plane, Car - Manufacture and Maintenance		
Northeast England – 3,489 shipyard workers (Newhouse et al. 1985a)	--------------------	16%
Plymouth, UK – 1,377 dockyard workers (Lumley 1976)	-----	
Devonport, UK – 6,292 male dockyard workers (Rossiter and Coles 1980)	-----------------	17%
Northern Italy – 8,626 aircraft manufacturers (Costa et al. 1989)	------------	8%
Italy – 1,534 male railroad-car maintenance workers (Menegozzo et al. 1993)	+	13%
	1900 * 1920 * 1940 * 1960 * 1980 * 2000 *	

continues

FIGURE 6.2 Continued

Cohort Population (location – number, description)	Time Elapsed to Final Follow-up (+ marks earliest exposure, if known) 1900 * 1920 * 1940 * 1960 * 1980 * 2000 *	Percent Original Cohort Dead
Italy – railroad repair shop (Magnani et al. 1986)		
Colleferro, Italy – 276 railroad equipment manufacturers (Blasetti et al. 1990)	----------	
Finland – 7,775 shipyard workers and 4,918 machine-shop workers (Tola et al. 1988)	+ -------------	
Finland – 8,391 male locomotive drivers (Nokso-Koivisto and Pukkala 1994)	---------------------	
Iceland – 6,603 male marine engineers (Rafnsson and Sulem 2003)	------------------------	
Building Materials, Construction, Carpenters, Plumbers, and Pipefitters		
Ontario, Canada – 324 male construction materials workers (Finkelstein 1989b)	-------------	13%
Sweden – 135,000 construction workers (Fletcher et al. 1993)		
Sweden – 260,052 male construction workers (Jansson et al. 2005)	---------------	
19 US states – 61,682 white males in construction industry (occupation from death certificates) (Robinson et al. 1995)	-	100%
US – 27,527 in AFL-CIO Brotherhood of Carpenters and Joiners of America (Robinson et al. 1996)	--	100%
US – 11,791 in construction labor union (Stern et al. 1995)	--	100%
US – 13,363 in bridge-construction union (Stern et al. 1997)	----	100%
US – 11,298 males in roofing and waterproofing union (Stern et al. 2000)	------------------------	100%
US – 13,020 male deaths in plastering and masonry union (Stern et al. 2001)	---- ------	100%
North Carolina, US – 29,554 male construction workers ("usual occupation" on death certificates) (Wang et al. 1999)	---	100%
US – 84,000 members of International Union of Bricklayers and Allied Craft Workers (Salg and Alterman 2005)	---	100%
	1900 * 1920 * 1940 * 1960 * 1980 * 2000 *	

continues

FIGURE 6.2 Continued

Cohort Population (location – number, description)	1900 * 1920 * 1940 * 1960 * 1980 * 2000 * **Time Elapsed to Final Follow-up** (+ marks earliest exposure, if known)	**Percent Original Cohort Dead**
California, US – 7,121 plumbers and pipefitters (Cantor et al. 1986)	----------	100%
Finland – asbestos sprayers and asbestosis patients (Oksa et al. 1997)	---------------	
Asbestos as Possible Confounding Exposure		
Sweden– 96,000 construction workers (Albin et al. 1998)		
Sweden – 1,932 male ferrochromium workers (Axelsson et al. 1980)	+ -----------	20%
USA – 9,028 cable manufacturers (Ward et al. 1994)	49%	
Germany – 1,221 arc welders (Becker 1999)	-----------------------	22%
Nine European countries – 11,092 male welders (shipyard, stainless steel, mild steel) (Simonato et al. 1991)	10%	
Welders (some shipyard) (Moulin et al. 1993)		
New York, NY, US – 385 sheet metal workers (Zoloth and Michaels 1985)	-	100%
New York, NY, US – 331 sheet metal workers (Michaels and Zoloth 1988)	--	100%
9,605 sheet metal workers (Welch et al. 1994)		
Tonawanda, NY, US – 8,146 males at research, engineering, & metal fabrication facility (Teta and Ott 1988)	------------------	
New Zealand – 3,522 male foundry and heavy engineering workers (Firth et al. 1999)	---------------------	28%
Norway – 3,563 boiler welders (Danielsen et al. 1996)	------------------	18%
Norway – 4,778 shipyard workers (Melkild et al. 1989)	+ ----------------	
Norway – 4,571 shipyard workers (service yard established 1900) (Danielsen et al. 1993)	+	24%
Anshan, China – 8,887 iron and steel workers (Xu et al. 1996)	+	
Norway – 6,494 male ferrosilicon and ferromanganese plant workers (Kjuus et al. 1986a)	----------------	
Norway– 790 male calcium carbide plant workers (Kjuus et al. 1986b)	-----------------	
	1900 * 1920 * 1940 * 1960 * 1980 * 2000 *	

continues

FIGURE 6.2 Continued

Cohort Population (location – number, description)	Time Elapsed to Final Follow-up (+ marks earliest exposure, if known) 1900 * 1920 * 1940 * 1960 * 1980 * 2000 *	Percent Original Cohort Dead
Finland – 42,469 seafarers (Pukkala and Saarni 1996)	------------	
England – 7,981 cancers in electric workers (Fear et al. 1996)	+	
Denmark – 32,006 from 99 utility companies (Johansen and Olsen 1998)	------------	
Multicenter, International – 29,820 males in asphalt industry (Boffetta et al. 2003)	+ ------------------------	
British Columbia, Canada – male workers at 14 pulp and paper mills (Band et al. 2001)	+	
Norway – pulp and paper industry (Langseth and Andersen 2000)		
13 countries – 62,937 male pulp and paper industry workers (Carel et al. 2002)	------------------------	
Norway – 153 electro-chemical plant workers (Hilt 1987)	-	
Norway – 1,756 male nitrate-fertilizer plant workers (Zandjani et al 1994)	+ --------------------	
	1900 * 1920 * 1940 * 1960 * 1980 * 2000 *	

FIGURE 6.2 Continued

tions were studies of Swedish insulation workers (Sanden and Jarvholm 1987) and of cement workers in Sweden (Jakobsson et al. 1994) and Denmark (Raffn et al. 1989, 1996). Consequently, disease occurrence may have been under-ascertained in some cohort studies, especially for pharyngeal, laryngeal, and colorectal cancers, which generally have higher survival rates than esophageal and stomach cancers. Although under-ascertainment would tend to diminish the power of these studies, it is unlikely to have created an important systematic bias because it is reasonable to assume that the extent of disease ascertainment was unrelated to asbestos exposure.

Cancer mortality information in the cohort studies was derived predominantly from death certificates. Death-certificate data were augmented with clinical information (such as an autopsy reports or medical-chart reviews) in studies of North American insulation workers (Selikoff and Sediman 1991) and German workers in various industries (Woitowitz and Seidman 1986) to derive "best-evidence" risk estimates. We reported those "best-evidence" relative risks (RRs) in our summary of findings, acknowledging that they may over-estimate risks somewhat because comparison rates, typically from national populations, were limited to death-certificate data.

To evaluate the individual risks of cancer of the pharynx, larynx, esophagus, stomach, colon, or rectum, one would want to consider together reported statistics for International Classification of Diseases (ICD) codes 146-148, 161, 150, 151, 153, and 154, respectively, but in practice many publications grouped their findings into broader ranges. As explained in Chapter 2, the committee determined that the only coarser groupings of sites that could be considered meaningful were pharynx with oral cavity, larynx with epilarynx (portions of the oropharynx specified as ICD codes 146.4, 146.5, and 148.2), and rectum with colon.

In addition to studies reporting on the selected cancers in acceptable categories, the assembled literature on asbestos-exposed cohorts included some papers presenting data only for "gastrointestinal" or "abdominal" cancers. Such groupings make the findings for esophagus, stomach, colon, and rectum indistinguishable, and also potentially included cancers of the pancreas, liver, gall bladder, and small intestine, which are not relevant to this review. Although the desired site-specific findings are not recoverable, for completeness, Table 6.3 presents results for aggregated gastrointestinal cancers from those cohort studies that provided their findings only in such form. The information gathered in this table could not be used by the committee in reaching its conclusions.

Data on the specific cancers of interest to the committee (cancers of the pharynx, larynx, esophagus, stomach, colon, or rectum) came from 40 major cohort populations. None of the cohort studies included data on histologic type of cancer; although many of the 36 case-control studies (discussed in the following section) involved histologic confirmation of cancer diagnosis, their results were not generally presented by histologic type. Furthermore, few of the studies provided data specific for cancer subsites. As a result, the committee did not attempt to draw conclusions at a more refined level than the groupings specified in its charge.

Exposure Assessment

Considerable attention has been given to possible differences among fiber types in their potential to cause cancer, especially in the context of examining mesothelioma risk. Recent reviews suggests that, rather than having no carcinogenic activity, chrysotile has a generally lesser degree of potency than amphibole fibers and that the various types of amphibole fiber have differing potency in the extent of their biological activity (Britton 2002, IPCS 1998, Roggli 2006, Roggli et al. 1997, Suzuki et al. 2005).

In this review, we noted predominant fiber types where information was provided. Table 6.4 provides an alphabetical listing of the informative citations and the corresponding cohort populations, which will facilitate cross-referencing from the citations listed in the summary figures of site-

TABLE 6.3 Cohort—Study Results on Various Groupings of Gastrointestinal Cancers (Grouped)

Source Citation	Location	Industry Type or Occupation	Fiber Type (primary)	Population	Overall Cohort Results No. cases RR (95% CI)	Highest Exposed Results No. cases RR (95% CI)	Comments
McDonald et al. (1986)	Libby, Montana, US Overlap with NIOSH cohort in Amandus and Wheeler (1987)?	Mining	Vermiculite	406 men	7 SMR = 0.88 (no CI or p-value)	5 SMR = 1.11 (no CI or p-value)	ICD8 150-159; highest exposed: ≥20 yrs since first exposure
Sluis-Cremer et al. (1992)	South Africa	Mining	Amosite, crocidolite	7,317 men	36 SMR = 0.88 (0.62-1.22)	—	ICD9 150-159 digestive + peritoneum
Thomas et al. (1982)	Wales	Cement	Chrysotile, some crocidolite	1,592 men	18 SMR = 0.92 (no CI or p-value)	6 SMR = 1.20 (no CI or p-value)	ICD8 151-154; highest exposed: employed 1935-36
Finkelstein (1984)	Ontario, Canada	Cement	Chrysotile?	535 men	8 SMR = 2.85 (no CI or p-value)	2 (or 1 best evidence) SMR = 5.00 (no CI or p-value)	ICD? 150-154; highest exposed: 30-34 yrs since first exposure
Giaroli et al. (1994)	Italy	Cement	Chrysotile, crocidolite	3,341	28 SMR = 0.91 (0.65-1.25)	—	Digestive tract + peritoneum (1)

Hughes and Weill (1991)	New Orleans, Louisiana, US	Cement	??	839 men	6 SMR = 0.65 (no CI or p-value)	—	ICD8 150-159
McDonald et al. (1983)	South Carolina, US Overlap with cohort population in Dement et al. (1994)	Textile	Chrysotile	2,543 men	26 SMR = 1.52 (no CI or p-value)	0 SMR = 0 (irregular d-r trend, increase until last stratum, then 0 cases)	ICD? 150-159; highest exposed: ≥80 mppcfy
McDonald et al. (1982a)	Pennsylvania US	Textile, friction products	Chrysotile	1,200 men + women	54 SMR = 1.13 (no CI or p-value)	7 SMR = 2.37 (no CI or p-value) RR = 2.85 from nested c-c analysis (no CI or p-value)	ICD? 150-159; highest exposed: ≥80 mppcfy
McDonald et al. (1984)	Connecticut, US	Friction materials	Chrysotile	3,641 men	59 SMR = 1.14 (no CI or p-value)	3 SMR = 1.27 (no CI or p-value)	ICD? 150-159; highest exposed: ≥80 mppcfy
Newhouse et al. (1985b) vs Berry et al. (1985)	England	Friction materials	Chrysotile	8,404 men 4,167 women	men: 156 SMR = 0.93 (0.81-1.06) women: 46 SMR = 0.98 (0.74-1.22)	men: 56 SMR = 0.89 (0.70-1.09) women: 13 SMR = 1.23 (0.73-1.96)	highest exposed: ≥10 yrs employed, ≥20 yrs since first exposure

continues

TABLE 6.3 Continued

Source Citation	Location	Industry Type or Occupation	Fiber Type (primary)	Population	Overall Cohort Results No. cases RR (95% CI)	Highest Exposed Results No. cases RR (95% CI)	Comments
Finkelstein (1989b)	Ontario, Canada	Friction materials	Chrysotile	1,194 men	6 SMR = 0.81 (no CI or p-value)	5 SMR = 0.92 (no CI or p-value)	ICD9 150-159; data presented for ≥20 yr since first exposure; highest exposure: ≥20 yr employed
Enterline and Kendrick (1967)	US	Various Building, friction, textile products	???	21,755 men	building products: 36 SMR = 0.89 (no CI or p-value) friction materials: 36 SMR = 1.19 (no CI or p-value) textile: 11 SMR = 1.46 (no CI or p-value)	—	ICD7 150-159; cohort age 15-64 years, multiple companies; cotton-mill worker comparison group

Kolonel et al. (1985)	Hawaii, US	Shipyard	??	7,971 men	63 SMR = 0.87 estimated from Table 6 (no CI or p-value)	10 SMR = 1.0 (0.5-1.9)	Esophagus + stomach + colon + rectum; highest exposed: ≥15 yr exposed, ≥30 yr since first exposure
Jarvholm and Sanden (1998)	Gothenburg, Sweden	Shipyard workers	Amosite, crocidolite	248 men; subset of 3,900 in Sanden and Jarvholm (1987)	1970-1979: SIR = 2.9 (0.95-6.9) 1980-1992: 8 SIR = 2.2 (0.96-1.4)	—	ICD8 150-159 results SIRs for pancreatic cancer (10.0, 6.0)

NOTE: c-c = case-control; CI = Confidence interval; d-r = dose-response; ICD = International Classification of Diseases; mppcfy = millions particles per cubic foot per year; RR = relative risk; SIR = standardized incidence ratio; SMR = standardized mortality ratio.

TABLE 6.4 Asbestos Types Associated with Exposures of Cohorts Informative for Selected Cancers (alphabetical order by author to correspond with plots in Chapters 7-11)

		Type(s) of Asbestos Comprising Exposure					
			Amphibole				
Source Citation	Cohort Population (location—number, description)	Serpentine Chrysotile	Crocidolite	Amosite	Anthophyllite	Tremolite-Actinolite	Mixed (M) or Not Stated (?)
Acheson et al. (1982)	33. Lancashire, UK—gas mask manufacture	X	X				
Acheson et al. (1984)	12. Uxbridge, UK—Cape [insulation] Boards Plant			X			
Aliyu et al. (2005)	4. US clinical trial monitoring asbestos-exposed men						?
Amandus and Wheeler (1987)	10. Libby, MT, US—NIOSH sample—miners					X	
Armstrong et al. (1988)	5a. Wittenoom Gorge, Western Australia—miners [deaths before 1980]		X				
Battista et al. (1999)	38. Tuscany, Italy—railway-carriage construction and repair	X	X				
Berry (1994)	26. Ferodo, UK—friction materials factory	X mainly	X				
Berry et al. (2000)	13. East London, UK—1400 male laggers	X	X	X			

Berry et al. (2000)	32. East London, UK—3,000 male and 700 female asbestos factory workers	X mainly	X	X	
Botta et al. (1991)	20. Casale Monferrato, Italy—asbestos cement production	X	X		
Dement et al. (1994)	17. Charleston, SC, US—asbestos textile workers	X			
Enterline et al. (1987)	35. USA—asbestos industry retirees	X	X	X	
Finkelstein (1989a)	25. Ontario, Canada—two automotive parts factories				?
Finkelstein and Verma (2004)	36. Ontario, Canada—members of plumbers' and pipefitters' union				?
Gardner et al. (1986)	23. Tamworth, England, UK—TAC Construction Materials Ltd.	X			
Germani et al. (1999)	1. Italy—631 women compensated for asbestosis	X	X		
Giaroli et al. (1994)	19. Emilia Romagna, Italy—10 cement factories	X	X		
Hodgson and Jones (1986)	34. England and Wales, UK—national survey of asbestos workers				M
Hughes et al. (1987)	24. New Orleans, LA, US—workers at two asbestos cement plants	X mainly	X	X	
Jakobsson et al. (1994)	22. Southern Sweden—asbestos cement plant	X mainly	X	X	

continues

TABLE 6.4 Continued

Source Citation	Cohort Population (location—number, description)	Type(s) of Asbestos Comprising Exposure					
			Amphibole				
		Serpentine Chrysotile	Crocidolite	Amosite	Anthophyllite	Tremolite-Actinolite	Mixed (M) or Not Stated (?)
Karjalainen et al. (1999)	2. Finland— a. 1,376 asbestosis patients b. 4,887 patients with pleural disease						?
Kogan et al. (1993)	27. USSR	X					
Levin et al. (1998)	14. Tyler, TX, US—753 white male asbestos pipe-insulation plant workers			X			
Liddell et al. (1997) and McDonald et al. (1993)	6. Quebec, Canada—Asbestos and Thetford Mines—miners	X					
Meurman et al. (1994)	7. Finland—Paakkila and Maljasalmi Mines—miners				X		
Pang et al. (1997)	30. Qingdao, China—asbestos plant	X					
Parnes (1990)	28. New York, USA—friction products manufacture	X					
Peto et al. (1985)	16. Rochdale, Northern England	X	X				

Piolatto et al. (1990)	8. Balangero, Italy—miners	X			
Pira et al. (2005)	15. Italy—889 male and 1,077 female textile workers				?
Puntoni et al. (2001)	39. Genoa, Italy—ship repair, refitting, and construction				?
Raffn et al. (1989)	18. Denmark—Danish Eternit Ltd. cement factory	X mainly	X	X	
Reid et al. (2004)	5b. Wittenoom Gorge, Western Australia—miners [incidence 1979-2000]		X		
Sanden and Jarvholm (1987)	40. Gothenburg, Sweden—shipyard workers	X mainly	X	X	
Seidman et al. (1986)	11. b. Paterson, NJ, US—820 men producing insulation for shipbuilding			X	
Selikoff et al. (1979)	11. a. 632 male insulation workers before 1943 in NY/NJ				?
Selikoff and Seidman (1991)	11. Canada/USA c. 17,800 male members of asbestos insulation unions in 1967				?
Sluis-Cremer et al. (1992)	9. Northern Transvaal, South Africa—North West Cape Blue and Penge Mines—miners		X	X	
Smailyte et al. (2004a)	21. Lithuainia—Daugeliai and Akmene Factories	X			

continues

TABLE 6.4 Continued

Source Citation	Cohort Population (location—number, description)	Type(s) of Asbestos Comprising Exposure					
			Amphibole				
		Serpentine Chrysotile	Crocidolite	Amosite	Anthophyllite	Tremolite-Actinolite	Mixed (M) or Not Stated (?)
Szeszenia-Dabrowska et al. (2002)	3. Poland— a. 907 men with asbestosis b. 490 women with asbestosis						?
Tola et al. (1988)	37. Finland—7,775 male shipyard workers						?
Woitowitz et al. (1986)	31. Federal Republic of Germany—asbestos-related workers from national register						?
Zhu and Wang (1993)	29. China—eight asbestos factories	X					

NOTE: Column 1 of Tables 6.1-6.2 reordered by source citation.

specific Chapters 7-11. Table 6.4 also specifies the types of asbestos to which the cohorts were exposed. The contents of Table 6.4, however, demonstrate for workers in these cohorts that exposures have often been mixed, with one type of asbestos commonly being contaminated by others and with some industrial processes intentionally involving mixtures. If inferences could only be drawn from studies of exposure to a single type of asbestos, the database would be inadequate to draw any conclusions. There was only one informative cohort population for exposure to anthophyllite and one for exposure to tremolite or actinolite; two separate populations were said to have been exposed to amosite exclusively; two populations divided only by time from Wittenoom Gorge were the only ones considered as exposed only to crocidolite; while 10 of the 45 citations reported only exposure to serpentine chrysotile. For the remainder, the researchers stated the exposure was mixed or did not attempt to characterize it beyond "asbestos." Predictably, chrysotile was the most frequently mentioned type. There were too few studies of single forms of asbestos to support separate evaluations according to fiber type and inclusion of studies with exposure to mixed or unknown fiber types would have generated fiber-type-specific associations subject to considerable uncertainty; consequently the committee did not characterize associations by fiber type.

The type and quantity of data available for assessing asbestos exposures varied considerably among studies. The committee partitioned these methods of exposure assessment into categories of relative quality. Although the underlying data may have been gathered with a variety of methods having different sensitivities, the highest category of relative quality was quantitative estimates of the concentration of asbestos fibers based on workplace measurements. The optimal, but rarely available, exposure metric was deemed to be cumulative exposure, in which concentrations measured with reliable industrial-hygiene techniques would be combined with each individual's job history to obtain years of exposure to concentrations expressed as mppcf (million particles per cubic foot) or f/cm^3 (fibers per cubic centimeter) of air. Such estimates of cumulative exposure were derived only in studies of South Carolina textile workers (Dement et al. 1994; McDonald et al. 1982, 1983), Quebec chrysotile miners (McDonald and McDonald 1997), Italian chrysotile miners (Rubino et al. 1979), Wittenoom Gorge, Australia crocidolite miners (Reid et al. 2004), and Louisiana cement-factory workers (Hughes et al. 1987).

A second tier of exposure assessment quality consisted of more qualitative approaches to deriving scales for dose-response analyses. In numerous studies, less specific data, such as duration of employment in the industry or occupation or ordinal rankings of jobs (for example, "heavy" and "light"), served as surrogates in dose estimation.

In the remaining studies, absence of any sort of detailed exposure data from which gradients could be defined limited risk estimation to contrasts between exposed and non-exposed ("any vs none" in the meta-analyses), typically formulated as risk comparisons between an entire cohort and the general population. In practice, even studies in which quantitative exposure data had been gathered seldom reported dose-response gradients for the selected cancers of interest in this review. Lung cancer, which is far more common, was the principal focus in those studies; perhaps concerns about limitations of statistical power prevented partitioning the small observed number of these other cancers into exposure categories. Consequently, many of the cohorts in which exposure had been extensively assessed contributed no more to this evaluation for the selected cancers than an "any vs none" comparison with the general population. The dearth of quantitative dose-response data is clearly a limitation of the literature on the selected cancers.

As reflected in the results tables in Appendix D, for each cohort study, we transcribed estimates of RR for the entire cohort compared with the general population (a contrast of any exposure vs no exposure) and, when exposure gradients were defined, for the subgroup in the most extreme exposure category (a contrast of high exposure vs no exposure).

CASE-CONTROL STUDIES

Reports Included in the Evaluation of Cancer Risks

The committee's search for relevant case-control studies first screened the literature for investigations of the selected cancers that included occupation among the risk factors considered and then retained those that actually assessed and reported asbestos exposure. Table 6.5 summarizes the 36 case-control studies that were found to be informative for any of the cancer sites of interest, ordered by the quality of the method of exposure assessment used (as described below). Details about the design characteristics of the studies can be found in Table C.1 in Appendix C.

Although multiple publications may result from a single case-control investigation, in general they do not have as complex histories as do cohort studies carried out over several decades. This chapter's presentation of the case-control studies evaluated in a single one-page table, in contrast to the several multipage tables and figures shown concerning the cohort studies, is not a reflection of the relative importance of these two study designs in the committee's evaluation. Both designs have their merits, and the results from both are complementary.

The case-control method has several specific strengths in comparison to the cohort study design, some of which may be particularly advantageous for studies of asbestos. First, case ascertainment can be accompanied by pathological review of cancers, thus validating the cancer type and allowing

TABLE 6.5 Summary of Case-Control Studies Addressing Selected Cancers

Quality of Exposure Characterization	Type of Cancer Investigated				
	Pharyngeal	Laryngeal	Esophageal	Stomach	Colorectal
High					
11 unique citations	Berrino et al. (2003)	Berrino et al. (2003)			
		Dietz et al. (2004)			Dumas et al. (2000)
	Gustavsson et al. (1998)	Gustavsson et al. (1998)	Gustavsson et al. (1998)		Goldberg et al. (2001)
	Marchand et al. (2000)	Marchand et al. (2000)	Parent et al. (2000)	Parent et al. (1998)	
	Merletti et al. (1991)	Muscat and Wynder (1992)			
		Wortley et al. (1992)			
Medium					
15 unique citations		Brown et al. (1988)		Cocco et al. (1994)	Demers et al. (1994)
		Burch et al. (1981)		Krstev et al. (2005)	Fredriksson et al. (1989)
		De Stefani et al. (1998)			Garabrant et al. (1992)
		Elci et al. (2002)			Hardell (1981)
		Hinds et al. (1979)			Neugut et al. (1991)
	Luce et al. (2000)	Luce et al. (2000)			Spiegelman and Wegman (1985)
		Zagraniski et al. (1986)			

continues

TABLE 6.5 Continued

Quality of Exposure Characterization	Type of Cancer Investigated: Pharyngeal	Laryngeal	Esophageal	Stomach	Colorectal
Low					
10 unique citations		Ahrens et al. (1991)		Ekstrom et al. (1999)	Gerhardsson de Verdier et al. (1992)
		Olsen and Sabroe (1984)	Hillerdal (1980)	Hillerdal (1980)	Hillerdal (1980)
		Shettigara and Morgan (1975)			Vineis et al. (1993)
		Stell and McGill (1973)			
	Zheng et al. (1992b)	Zheng et al. (1992a)			
36 unique citations	6	18	3	5	11

differentiation among histologic types. For example (although not specifically considered in the studies gathered for this review), esophageal cancer can be squamous or it can be adenocarcinomatous; the types are biologically and epidemiologically distinct. Second, cases can be (and generally are) studied shortly after diagnosis, and so survival rates do not so strongly influence case inclusion, as they do in occupational cohorts that rely on mortality records to define outcomes. Incidence-based case-control studies would be expected to be useful for investigating all the cancers in this review aside from esophageal cancer. Third, case-control studies are well suited to less common diseases, which would not occur in enough subjects in a typically sized cohort to permit any detailed analysis. This characteristic applies to laryngeal, pharyngeal, esophageal, and stomach cancers. Finally, case-control studies are well suited to exposures that cause disease only after a long latent period, as is presumed to occur between asbestos exposure and cancer.

Case-control studies also have disadvantages. First, there is a potential of unanticipated selection factors in choosing controls, leading to selection bias. Second, because the design is retrospective, it can be unclear whether exposure preceded or concurred with the outcome of cancer, although this is unlikely to be an issue for health effects arising from asbestos exposure, which typically have long latency periods. Third, recall bias poses some concern, but the greatest disadvantage and challenge of case-control studies is the overall difficulty of validly and reliably assessing exposure.

Health Outcome Data

Case-control studies examine the association between asbestos and cancer by identifying people with cancer (cases) and comparing their asbestos exposure with that of people without cancer (controls). Because exposures occurred in the past, the case-control design is termed retrospective. Cases can be ascertained over a specified period from a hospital or medical practice where cancer is treated. When cases are selected that way, the case-control study is called a hospital-based case-control study and typically involves as controls people who were treated at the same institutions for noncancer conditions. Cases can also be ascertained from a source that allows identification of all cancer occurring within a defined geographic area over some period, often through a hospital network or cancer registry. This type of case-control study is called a population-based case-control study and typically involves as controls people sampled in the underlying community from which cases arose. For example, controls may be selected from driver's-license or voter-registration lists, by random dialing of telephone numbers, or by random contacting of neighbors.

In either the hospital-based or the population-based design, the strategy is to find controls that differ from cases only with regard to asbestos exposure. Cases and controls should not systematically differ in other important respects. For that reason, the population-based case-control method is sometimes considered methodologically superior to the hospital-based method. In the latter, controls with diseases other than cancer may have nonrandom patterns of asbestos exposure. Every attempt is made to avoid selection of controls who would have been systematically exposed to asbestos, such as hospital-based people with pleural plaques or mesotheliomas. Similarly, every attempt is made to avoid controls who systematically would not have been exposed to asbestos. For example, one would avoid a comparison of men with cancer to women without cancer, because women are less likely to have worked in an asbestos-exposed occupation.

Exposure Assessment

Unlike cohort studies, which have access to workplace data, assessment of exposure in occupational case-control studies almost always relies on subject recall. Information on the type of asbestos fiber to which subjects were exposed was uniformly unavailable in the case-control studies. The quality of an exposure assessment is determined by the type and amount of data collected, how the information was collected, and how it is used to assign exposure.

The best case-control studies collected detail lifetime work histories by using a structured interview or extensive questionnaires and assigned exposure on the basis of a review of the data by an "expert" in exposure or the use of a job-exposure matrix (JEM) created specifically to look at asbestos exposure. Those methods avoid some of the limitations of recall bias because exposure is not directly self-assessed, and they greatly improve the quality of the assessment.

Moderate-quality studies collected less detailed or more limited work-history information (for example, relied on proxy respondents or collected information on only the longest held jobs) or assigned exposure by using a multipurpose JEM that did not consider level of exposure. The best- and moderate-quality studies were combined in the exposure-assessment method (EAM) category "EAM = 1" for the meta-analyses.

The lowest-quality studies ("EAM = 2" for the meta-analyses) considered in this review used self-ascribed exposure based on direct questions or had very limited work-history information, as was the case for the lowest tier of studies in Table 6.5.

The method used to measure exposure to asbestos was an important criterion in reviewing the case-control studies. Case-control studies that used job information abstracted from death certificates were excluded from this evaluation, and none of those retained happened to have gathered exposure information from workplace records. They all used some sort of structured or semi-structured interview administered in person, over the telephone, or by mail (with or without the option of follow-up by telephone); these are listed in decreasing order of desirability. The committee decided to set aside case-control studies in which exposure to asbestos could only be inferred from an occupational category (such as insulator or ship repair) rather than from the original researchers' explicit attribution of asbestos exposure.

The ability to assess dose-response relationships depends heavily on the quality of the underlying data. For example, dose-response relationships cannot be analyzed if the data collected were too crude to assign a level of exposure or some surrogate of dose. Therefore, the quality of exposure assessment correlates with the thoroughness and overall quality of analyses ultimately possible.

INTEGRATION OF EPIDEMIOLOGIC EVIDENCE WITH NON-EPIDEMIOLOGIC EVIDENCE

Results from epidemiologic studies of both cohort and case-control designs constitute an important component, but not the only type of evidence considered in the approach applied in Chapters 7-11 to assess the likelihood and strength of causal associations between asbestos and cancer at the selected sites. The committee's strategy for integrating all the evidence closely follows that used by the surgeon general's report on health risks related to tobacco-smoking (HHS 2004). To illustrate, we would characterize as strongly supportive epidemiologic evidence those datasets that contain consistently increased risks with increasing dose-response gradients from both case-control studies performed in different places and cohort studies conducted in various industries. The magnitude of observed risks and their statistical precision also entered into the committee's evaluations. Many of the case-control studies addressed potential confounding by non-occupational risk factors (such as smoking, alcohol use, and diet), but this was not possible in most cohort studies; these factors are seldom correlated with exposure strongly enough to greatly bias estimated risks through confounding (Axelson 1989, Kriebel et al. 2004). Consequently, the impossibility of controlling for potential confounding by risk factors not related to occupation was not considered a major concern for evaluation of the cohort studies. The epidemiologic evidence thus distilled is then considered in the context of the available non-epidemiologic information in reaching a determination about a causal role for asbestos exposure on a site-specific basis.

REFERENCES
(including references cited in Appendices B–F)

Acheson ED, Gardner MJ, Pippard EC, Grime LP. 1982. Mortality of two groups of women who manufactured gas masks from chrysotile and crocidolite asbestos: A 40-year follow-up. *British Journal of Industrial Medicine* 39(4): 344-348.

Acheson ED, Gardner MJ, Winter PD, Bennett C. 1984. Cancer in a factory using amosite asbestos. *International Journal of Epidemiology* 13(1): 3-10.

Ahrens W, Jockel K, Patzak W, Elsner G. 1991. Alcohol, smoking, and occupational factors in cancer of the larynx: A case-control study. *American Journal of Industrial Medicine* 20(4): 477-493.

Albin M, Attewell R, Jakobsson K, Johansson L, Welinder H. 1988. [Total and cause-specific mortality in cohorts of asbestos-cement workers and referents between 1907 and 1985]. *Arh Hig Rada Toksikol* 39 (4): 461-467.

Albin M, Jakobsson K, Attewell R, Johansson L, Welinder H. 1990. Mortality and cancer morbidity in cohorts of asbestos cement workers and referents. *British Journal of Industrial Medicine* 47(9): 602-610.

Albin M, Engholm G, Hallin N, Hagmar L. 1998. Impact of exposure to insulation wool on lung function and cough in Swedish construction workers. *Occupational and Environmental Medicine* 55(10): 661-667.

Alies-Patin AM, Valleron AJ. 1985. Mortality of workers in a French asbestos cement factory 1940-82. *British Journal of Industrial Medicine* 42(4): 219-225.

Aliyu OA, Cullen MR, Barnett MJ, Balmes JR, Cartmel B, Redlich CA, Brodkin CA, Barnhart S, Rosenstock L, Israel L, Goodman GE, Thornquist MD, Omenn GS. 2005. Evidence for excess colorectal cancer incidence among asbestos-exposed men in the Beta-Carotene and Retinol Efficacy Trial. *American Journal of Epidemiology* 162(9): 868-878.

Amandus HE. 1986. Mortality from stomach cancer in United States cement plant and quarry workers, 1950-80. *British Journal of Industrial Medicine* 43(8): 526-528.

Amandus HE, Wheeler R. 1987. The morbidity and mortality of vermiculite miners and millers exposed to tremolite-actinolite: Part II. Mortality. *American Journal Industrial Medicine* 11(1): 15-26.

Amandus HE, Wheeler R, Jankovic J, Tucker J. 1987. The morbidity and mortality of vermiculite miners and millers exposed to tremolite-actinolite: Part I. Exposure estimates. *American Journal of Industrial Medicine* 11(1): 1-14.

Amandus HE, Wheeler R, Armstong BG, McDonald AD, Sebastien P. 1988. Mortality of vermiculite miners exposed to tremolite. *Annals of Occupational Hygiene* 32: 459-467.

Armstrong BK, de Klerk NH, Musk AW, Hobbs MS. 1988. Mortality in miners and millers of crocidolite in Western Australia. *British Journal of Industrial Medicine* 45(1): 5-13.

Axelson O. 1989. Confounding from smoking in occupational epidemiology. *British Journal of Industrial Medicine* 46(8): 505-507.

Axelsson G, Rylander R, Schmidt A. 1980. Mortality and incidence of tumours among ferrochromium workers. *British Journal of Industrial Medicine* 37(2): 121-127.

Band PR, Le ND, Fang R, Astrakianakis G, Bert J, Keefe A, Krewski D. 2001. Cohort cancer incidence among pulp and paper mill workers in British Columbia. *Scandinavian Journal of Work, Environment and Health* 27(2): 113-119.

Battista G, Belli S, Comba P, Fiumalbi C, Grignoli M, Loi F, Orsi D, Paredes I. 1999. Mortality due to asbestos-related causes among railway carriage construction and repair workers. *Occupation Medicine (London)* 49(8): 536-539.

Becker N. 1999. Cancer mortality among arc welders exposed to fumes containing chromium and nickel: Results of a third follow-up: 1989-1995. *Journal of Occupational and Environmental Medicine* 41(4): 294-303.

Berrino F, Richiardi L, Boffetta P, Esteve J, Belletti I, Raymond L, Troschel L, Pisani P, Zubiri L, Ascunce N, Guberan E, Tuyns A, Terracini B, Merletti F. 2003. Occupation and larynx and hypopharynx cancer: A job-exposure matrix approach in an international case-control study in France, Italy, Spain and Switzerland. *Cancer Causes and Control* 14(3): 213-223.

Berry G. 1981. Mortality of workers certified by pneumoconiosis medical panels as having asbestosis. *British Journal of Industrial Medicine* 38(2): 130-137.

Berry G. 1994. Mortality and cancer incidence of workers exposed to chrysotile asbestos in the friction-products industry. *Annals of Occupational Hygiene* 38(4): 539-546.

Berry G, Newhouse ML. 1983. Mortality of workers manufacturing friction materials using asbestos. *British Journal of Industrial Medicine* 40(1): 1-7.

Berry G, Gilson JC, Holmes S, Lewinsohn HC, Roach SA. 1979. Asbestosis: A study of dose-response relationships in an asbestos textile factory. *British Journal of Industrial Medicine* 36(2): 98-112.

Berry G, Newhouse ML, Antonis P. 1985. Combined effect of asbestos and smoking on mortality from lung cancer and mesothelioma in factory workers. *British Journal of Industrial Medicine* 42(1): 12-18.

Berry G, Newhouse ML, Wagner JC. 2000. Mortality from all cancers of asbestos factory workers in east London 1933-80. *Occupational and Environmental Medicine* 57(11): 782-785.

Berry G, de Klerk NH, Reid A, Ambrosini GL, Fritschi L, Olsen NJ, Merler E, Musk AW. 2004. Malignant pleural and peritoneal mesotheliomas in former miners and millers of crocidolite at Wittenoom, Western Australia. *Occupational and Environmental Medicine* 61(4): e14.

Blasetti F, Bruno C, Comba P, Fantini F, Grignoli M. 1990. [Mortality study of workers employed in the construction of railway cars in Collefero]. *Medicina del Lavoro* 81(5): 407-413.

Boffetta P, Burstyn I, Partanen T, Kromhout H, Svane O, Langard S, Jarvholm B, Frentzel-Beyme R, Kauppinen T, Stucker I, Shaham J , Heederik D, Ahrens W, Bergdahl IA, Cenee S, Ferro G, Heikkila P, Hooiveld M, Johansen C, Randem BG, Schill W. 2003. Cancer mortality among European asphalt workers: An international epidemiological study. II. Exposure to bitumen fume and other agents. *American Journal of Industrial Medicine* 43(1): 28-39.

Botta M, Magnani C, Terracini B, Bertolone GP, Castagneto B, Cocito V, DeGiovanni D, Paglieri P. 1991. Mortality from respiratory and digestive cancers among asbestos cement workers in Italy. *Cancer Detection and Prevention* 15(6): 445-447.

Braun DC, Truan TD. 1958. An epidemiological study of lung cancer in asbestos miners. *AMA Archives of Industrial Health* 17 (6): 634-653.

Britton M. 2002. The epidemiology of mesothelioma. *Seminars in Oncology* 29(1): 18-25.

Brown LM, Mason TJ, Pickle LW, Stewart PA, Buffler PA, Burau K, Ziegler RG, Fraumeni JF Jr. 1988. Occupational risk factors for laryngeal cancer on the Texas Gulf Coast. *Cancer Research* 48(7): 1960-1964.

Brown DP, Dement JM, Okun A. 1994. Mortality patterns among female and male chrysotile asbestos textile workers. *Journal of Occupational Medicine* 36(8): 882-888.

Burch JD, Howe GR, Miller AB, Semenciw R. 1981. Tobacco, alcohol, asbestos, and nickel in the etiology of cancer of the larynx: A case-control study. *Journal of the National Cancer Institute* 67(6): 1219-1224.

Cantor KP, Sontag JM, Heid MF. 1986. Patterns of mortality among plumbers and pipefitters. *American Journal of Industrial Medicine* 10(1): 73-89.

Carel R, Boffetta P, Kauppinen T, Teschke K, Andersen A, Jappinen P, Pearce N, Rix BA, Bergeret A, Coggon D, Persson B, Szadkowska-Stanczyk I, Kielkowski D, Henneberger P, Kishi R, Facchini LA, Sala M, Colin D, Kogevinas M. 2002. Exposure to asbestos and lung and pleural cancer mortality among pulp and paper industry workers. *Journal of Occupational and Environmental Medicine* 44(6): 579-584.

Cheng WN, Kong J. 1992. A retrospective cohort study of chrysotile asbestos products workers in Tianjin 1972-1987. *Environmental Research* 59(1): 271-278.

Clemmensen J, Hjalgrim-Jensen S. 1981. Cancer incidence among 5686 asbestos-cement workers followed from 1943 through 1976. *Ecotoxicology Environment Safety* 5(1): 15-23.

Cocco P, Palli D, Buiatti E, Cipriani F, DeCarli A, Manca P, Ward MH, Blot WJ, Fraumeni JF Jr. 1994. Occupational exposures as risk factors for gastric cancer in Italy. *Cancer Causes and Control* 5(3): 241-248.

Coggiola M, Bosio D, Pira E, Piolatto PG, La Vecchia C, Negri E, Michelazzi M, Bacaloni A. 2003. An update of a mortality study of talc miners and millers in Italy. *American Journal of Industrial Medicine* 44(1): 63-69.

Costa G, Merletti F, Segnan N. 1989. A mortality cohort study in a north Italian aircraft factory. *British Journal of Industrial Medicine* 46(10): 738-743.

Danielsen TE, Langard S, Andersen A, Knudsen O. 1993. Incidence of cancer among welders of mild steel and other shipyard workers. *British Journal of Industrial Medicine* 50(12): 1097-1103.

Danielsen TE, Langard S, Andersen A. 1996. Incidence of cancer among Norwegian boiler welders. *Occupational and Environmental Medicine* 53(4): 231-234.

de Klerk NH, Armstrong BK, Musk AW, Hobbs MS. 1989. Cancer mortality in relation to measures of occupational exposure to crocidolite at Wittenoom Gorge in Western Australia. *British Journal of Industrial Medicine* 46(8): 529-536.

De Stefani E, Boffetta P, Oreggia F, Ronco A, Kogevinas M, Mendilaharsu M. 1998. Occupation and the risk of laryngeal cancer in Uruguay. *American Journal of Industrial Medicine* 33(6): 537-542.

Dement JM, Harris RL Jr, Symons MJ, Shy C. 1982. Estimates of dose-response for respiratory cancer among chrysotile asbestos textile workers. *Annals of Occupational Hygiene* 26(1-4): 869-887.

Dement JM, Harris RL Jr, Symons MJ, Shy C. 1983a. Exposures and mortality among chrysotile asbestos workers. Part I: Exposure estimates. *American Journal of Industrial Medicine* 4(3): 399-419.

Dement JM, Harris RL Jr, Symons MJ, Shy C. 1983b. Exposures and mortality among chrysotile asbestos workers. Part II: Mortality. *American Journal of Industrial Medicine* 4(3): 421-433.

Dement JM, Brown DP, Okun A. 1994. Follow-up study of chrysotile asbestos textile workers: Cohort mortality and case-control analyses. *American Journal of Industrial Medicine* 26(4): 431-447.

Demers RY, Burns PB, Swanson GM. 1994. Construction occupations, asbestos exposure, and cancer of the colon and rectum. *Journal of Occupational Medicine* 36(9): 1027-1031.

Dietz A, Ramroth H, Urban T, Ahrens W, Becher H. 2004. Exposure to cement dust, related occupational groups and laryngeal cancer risk: Results of a population based case-control study. *International Journal of Cancer* 108(6): 907-911.

Djerassi L, Kaufmann G, Bar-Nets M. 1979. Malignant disease and environmental control in an asbestos cement plant. *Annals of the New York Academy of Sciences* 330: 243-253.

Doll R. 1955. Mortality from lung cancer in asbestos workers. *British Journal of Industrial Medicine* 12(2): 81-86.

Dumas S, Parent ME, Siemiatycki J, Brisson J. 2000. Rectal cancer and occupational risk factors: A hypothesis-generating, exposure-based case-control study. *International Journal of Cancer* 87(6): 874-879.

Ekstrom AM, Eriksson M, Hansson LE, Lindgren A, Signorello LB, Nyren O, Hardell L. 1999. Occupational exposures and risk of gastric cancer in a population-based case-control study. *Cancer Research* 59(23): 5932-5937.

Elci OC, Akpinar-Elci M, Blair A, Dosemeci M. 2002. Occupational dust exposure and the risk of laryngeal cancer in Turkey. *Scandinavian Journal of Work, Environment and Health* 28(4): 278-284.

Elmes PC, Simpson MJ. 1977. Insulation workers in Belfast: A further study of mortality due to asbestos exposure (1940-75). *British Journal of Industrial Medicine* 34(3): 174-180.

Enterline PE, Henderson V. 1973. Type of asbestos and respiratory cancer in the asbestos industry. *Archives of Environmental Health* 27(5): 312-317.

Enterline PE, Kendrick MA. 1967. Asbestos-dust exposures at various levels and mortality. *Archives of Environmental Health* 15(2): 181-186.

Enterline P, de Coufle P, Henderson V. 1972. Mortality in relation to occupational exposure in the asbestos industry. *Journal of Occupational Medicine* 14(12): 897-903.

Enterline P, de Coufle P, Henderson V. 1973. Respiratory cancer in relation to occupational exposures among retired asbestos workers. *British Journal of Industrial Medicine* 30(2): 162-166.

Enterline PE, Hartley J, Henderson V. 1987. Asbestos and cancer: A cohort followed up to death. *British Journal of Industrial Medicine* 44(6): 396-401.

Fear NT, Roman E, Carpenter LM, Newton R, Bull D. 1996. Cancer in electrical workers: An analysis of cancer registrations in England, 1981-1987. *British Journal of Cancer* 73(7): 935-939.

Finkelstein MM. 1984. Mortality among employees of an Ontario asbestos-cement factory. *American Review of Respiratory Disease* 129(5): 754-761.

Finkelstein MM. 1989a. Mortality rates among employees potentially exposed to chrysotile asbestos at two automotive parts factories. *Canadian Medical Association Journal* 141(2): 125-130.

Finkelstein MM. 1989b. Mortality among employees of an Ontario factory that manufactured construction materials using chrysotile asbestos and coal tar pitch. *American Journal of Industrial Medicine* 16(3): 281-287.

Finkelstein MM, Verma DK. 2004. A cohort study of mortality among Ontario pipe trades workers. *Occupational and Environmental Medicine* 61(9): 736-742.

Firth HM, Elwood JM, Cox B, Herbison GP. 1999. Historical cohort study of a New Zealand foundry and heavy engineering plant. *Occupational and Environmental Medicine* 56(2): 134-138.

Fletcher AC, Engholm G, Englund A. 1993. The risk of lung cancer from asbestos among Swedish construction workers: Self-reported exposure and a job exposure matrix compared. *International Journal of Epidemiology* 22 (Supplement 2): S29-35.

Fredriksson M, Bengtsson NO, Hardell L, Axelson O. 1989. Colon cancer, physical activity, and occupational exposures: A case-control study. *Cancer* 63(9): 1838-1842.

Garabrant DH, Peters RK, Homa DM. 1992. Asbestos and colon cancer: Lack of association in a large case-control study. *American Journal of Epidemiology* 135(8): 843-853.

Gardner MJ, Winter PD, Pannett B, Powell CA. 1986. Follow up study of workers manufacturing chrysotile asbestos cement products. *British Journal of Industrial Medicine* 43(11): 726-732.

Gardner MJ, Powell CA, Gardner AW, Winter PD, Fletcher AC. 1988. Continuing high lung cancer mortality among ex-amosite asbestos factory workers and a pilot study of individual anti-smoking advice. *Journal of the Society of Occupational Medicine* 38(3): 69-72.

Gerhardsson de Verdier M, Plato N, Steineck G, Peters JM. 1992. Occupational exposures and cancer of the colon and rectum. *American Journal of Industrial Medicine* 22(3): 291-303.

Germani D, Belli S, Bruno C, Grignoli M, Nesti M, Pirastu R, Comba P. 1999. Cohort mortality study of women compensated for asbestosis in Italy. *American Journal of Industrial Medicine* 36(1): 129-134.

Giaroli C, Belli S, Bruno C, Candela S, Grignoli M, Minisci S, Poletti R, Ricco G, Vecchi G, Venturi G, Ziccardi A, Combra P. 1994. Mortality study of asbestos cement workers. *International Archives of Occupational and Environmental Health* 66(1): 7-11.

Gibbs AR, Gardner MJ, Pooley FD, Griffiths DM, Blight B, Wagner JC. 1994. Fiber levels and disease in workers from a factory predominantly using amosite. *Environmental Health Perspectives* 102 (Supplement 5): 261-263.

Gillam JD, Dement JM, Lemen RA, Wagoner JK, Archer VE, Blejer HP. 1976. Mortality patterns among hard rock gold miners exposed to an asbestiform mineral. *Annals of the New York Academy of Sciences* 271: 336-344.

Goldberg MS, Parent ME, Siemiatycki J, Desy M, Nadon L, Richardson L, Lakhani R, Latreille B, Valois MF. 2001. A case-control study of the relationship between the risk of colon cancer in men and exposures to occupational agents. *American Journal of Industrial Medicine* 39(6): 531-546.

Goldstein B, Webster I, Harrison WO, Talent J. 1975. Epidemiological studies on asbestos-exposed workers in South Africa. *Hefte Unfallheilkd* (126): 538-542.

Gurvich EB, Gladkova EV, Gutnikova OV, Kostiukovskaia AV, Kuzina LE, Saprykova VV. 1993. [Epidemiology of chronic, precancerous and oncologic diseases in workers of asbestos and cement industry]. *Meditsina Truda i Promyshlennaia Ekologiia* 5-6: 4-6.

Gustavsson P, Jakobsson R, Johansson H, Lewin F, Norell S, Rutkvist LE. 1998. Occupational exposures and squamous cell carcinoma of the oral cavity, pharynx, larynx, and oesophagus: A case-control study in Sweden. *Occupational and Environmental Medicine* 55(6): 393-400.

Hardell L. 1981. Relation of soft-tissue sarcoma, malignant lymphoma and colon cancer to phenoxy acids, chlorophenols and other agents. *Scandinavian Journal of Work, Environment and Health* 7(2): 119-130.

Henderson VL, Enterline PE. 1979. Asbestos exposure: Factors associated with excess cancer and respiratory disease mortality. *Annals of the New York Academy of Sciences* 330: 117-126.

HHS (US Department of Health and Human Services). 2004. *The Health Effects of Active Smoking: A Report of the Surgeon General.* Washington, DC: US Government Printing Office.

Hill ID, Doll R, Knox JF. 1966. Mortality among asbestos workers. *Proceedings of the Royal Society of Medicine* 59(1): 59-60.

Hillerdal G. 1980. Gastrointestinal carcinoma and occurrence of pleural plaques on pulmonary X-ray. *Journal of Occupational Medicine* 22(12): 806-809.

Hilt B. 1987. Non-malignant asbestos diseases in workers in an electrochemical plant. *British Journal of Industrial Medicine* 44(9): 621-626.

Hilt B, Andersen A, Rosenberg J, Langard S. 1991. Cancer incidence among asbestos-exposed chemical industry workers: An extended observation period. *American Journal of Industrial Medicine* 20(2): 261-264.

Hinds MW, Thomas DB, O'Reilly HP. 1979. Asbestos, dental X-rays, tobacco, and alcohol in the epidemiology of laryngeal cancer. *Cancer* 44(3): 1114-1120.

Hobbs MS, Woodward SD, Murphy B, Musk AW, Elder JE. 1980. The incidence of pneumoconiosis, mesothelioma and other respiratory cancer in men engaged in mining and milling crocidolite in Western Australia. *IARC Scientific Publications* 30: 615-625.

Hodgson J, Jones R. 1986. Mortality of asbestos workers in England and Wales 1971-1981. *British Journal of Industrial Medicine* 43(3): 158-164.

Hughes JM, Weill H. 1991. Asbestosis as a precursor of asbestos related lung cancer: Results of a prospective mortality study. *British Journal Industrial Medicine* 48(4): 229-233.

Hughes JM, Weill H, Hammad YY. 1987. Mortality of workers employed in two asbestos cement manufacturing plants. *British Journal of Industrial Medicine* 44(3): 161-174.

IPCS (International Programme on Chemical Safety). 1998. *Chrysotile Asbestos: Environmental Health Criteria 203.* Geneva: World Health Organization.

Jakobsson K, Albin M, Hagmar L. 1994. Asbestos, cement, and cancer in the right part of the colon. *Occupational and Environmental Medicine* 51(2): 95-101.

Jansson C, Johansson AL, Bergdahl IA, Dickman PW, Plato N, Admai J, Boffetta P, Lagergren J. 2005. Occupational exposures and risk of esophageal and gastric cardia cancers among male Swedish construction workers. *Cancer Causes and Control* 16(6): 755-764.

Jarvholm B, Sanden A. 1988. Asbestos-associated diseases in Swedish shipyard workers. *Arh Hig Rada Toksikol* 39(4): 437-440.

Jarvholm B, Sanden A. 1998. Lung cancer and mesothelioma in the pleura and peritoneum among Swedish insulation workers. *Occupational and Environmental Medicine* 55(11): 766-770.

Johansen C, Olsen JH. 1998. Risk of cancer among Danish utility workers: A nationwide cohort study. *American Journal of Epidemiology* 147(6): 548-555.

Jones JS, Smith PG, Pooley FD, Berry G, Sawle GW, Madeley RJ, Wignall BK, Aggarwal A. 1980. The consequences of exposure to asbestos dust in a wartime gas-mask factory. *IARC Scientific Publications* 30: 637-653.

Joubert L, Seidman H, Selikoff IJ. 1991. Mortality experience of family contacts of asbestos factory workers. *Annals of the New York Academy of Sciences* 643: 416-418.

Karjalainen A, Pukkala E, Kauppinen T, Partanen T. 1999. Incidence of cancer among Finnish patients with asbestos-related pulmonary or pleural fibrosis. *Cancer Causes and Control* 10(1): 51-57.

Keal EE. 1960. Asbestosis and abdominal neoplasms. *Lancet* 2: 1214-1216.

Kjuus H, Andersen A, Langard S, Knudsen KE. 1986a. Cancer incidence among workers in the Norwegian ferroalloy industry. *British Journal of Industrial Medicine* 43(4): 227-236.

Kjuus H, Andersen A, Langard S. 1986b. Incidence of cancer among workers producing calcium carbide. *British Journal of Industrial Medicine* 43(4): 237-242.

Kleinfeld M, Messite J, Kooyman O. 1967. Mortality experience in a group of asbestos workers. *Archives Environmental Health* 15(2): 177-180.

Kleinfeld M, Messite J, Zaki MH. 1974. Mortality experiences among talc workers: A follow-up study. *Journal of Occupational and Environmental Medicine* 16(5): 345-349.

Knox JF, Doll RS, Hill ID. 1965. Cohort analysis of changes in incidence of bronchial carcinoma in a textile asbestos factory. *Annals of the New York Academy of Sciences* 132(1): 526-535.

Knox JF, Holmes S, Doll R, Hill ID. 1968. Mortality from lung cancer and other causes among workers in an asbestos textile factory. *British Journal of Industrial Medicine* 25(4): 293-303.

Kogan FM, Gusel'nikova NA, Gulevskaia MR. 1972. [Cancer mortality among workers in the asbestos industry of the Urals]. *Gigiena I Sanitariia (Moskva)* 37(7): 29-32.

Kogan PM, Yatsenko AS, Tregubov ES, Gurvich EB, Kuzina LE. 1993. Evaluation of carcinogenic risk in friction product workers. *Medicina del Lavoro* 84(4): 290-296.

Kolonel LN, Yoshizawa CN, Hirohata T, Myers BC. 1985. Cancer occurrence in shipyard workers exposed to asbestos in Hawaii. *Cancer Research* 45(8): 3924-3928.

Kriebel D, Zeka A, Eisen EA, Wegman DH. 2004. Quantitative evaluation of the effects of uncontrolled confounding by alcohol and tobacco in occupational cancer studies. *International Journal of Epidemiology* 33(5): 1040-1045.

Krstev S, Dosemeci M, Lissowska J, Chow WH, Zatonski W, Ward MH. 2005. Occupation and risk of stomach cancer in Poland. *Occupational and Environmental Medicine* 62(5): 318-324.

Lacquet LM, van der Linden L, Lepoutre J. 1980. Roentgenographic lung changes, asbestosis and mortality in a Belgian asbestos-cement factory. *IARC Scientific Publications* 30: 783-793.

Langseth H, Andersen A. 2000. Cancer incidence among male pulp and paper workers in Norway. *Scandinavian Journal of Work, Environment and Health* 26(2): 99-105.

Latsenko AS, Kogan FM. 1990. [Occupational morbidity and mortality in malignant neoplasms among persons professionally exposed to asbestos dust]. *Gigiena Truda I Professionalnye Zabolevaniia (Moskva)* (2): 10-12.

Levin J, McLarty J, Hurst GA, Smith A, Frank AL. 1998. Tyler asbestos workers: Mortality experience in a cohort exposed to amosite. *Occupational and Environmental Medicine* 55(3): 155-160.

Liddell FD, Thomas DC, Gibbs GW, McDonald JC. 1984. Fibre exposure and mortality from pneumoconiosis, respiratory and abdominal malignancies in chrysotile production in Quebec, 1926-75. *Annals of the Academy of Medicine, Singapore* 13 (2 Supplement): 340-344.

Liddell FD, McDonald AD, McDonald JC. 1997. The 1891-1920 birth cohort of Quebec chrysotile miners and millers: Development from 1904 and mortality to 1992. *Annals of Occupational Hygiene* 41(1): 13-36.

Luce D, Bugel I, Goldberg P, Goldberg M, Salomon C, Billon-Galland MA, Nicolau J, Quenel P, Fevotte J, Brochard P. 2000. Environmental exposure to tremolite and respiratory cancer in New Caledonia: A case-control study. *American Journal of Epidemiology* 151(3): 259-265.

Lumley KP. 1976. A proportional study of cancer registrations of dockyard workers. *British Journal of Industrial Medicine* 33(2): 108-114.

Magnani C, Nardini I, Governa M, Serio A. 1986. [A cohort study of the personnel assigned to a state railroad repair shop]. *Medicina del Lavoro* 77(2): 154-161.

Magnani C, Terracini B, Ivaldi C, Botta M, Budel P, Mancini A, Zanetti R. 1993. A cohort study on mortality among wives of workers in the asbestos cement industry in Casale Monferrato, Italy. *British Journal of Industrial Medicine* 50(9): 779-784.

Mancuso TF, Coulter EJ. 1963. Methodology in industrial health studies: The cohort approach with special reference to an asbestos company. *Archives of Environmental Health* 6: 36-52.

Mancuso TF, el-Attar AA. 1967. Mortality pattern in a cohort of asbestos workers: A study on employment experience. *Journal of Occupational Medicine* 9(4): 147-162.

Marchand JL, Luce D, Leclerc A, Goldberg P, Orlowski E, Bugel I, Brugere J. 2000. Laryngeal and hypopharyngeal cancer and occupational exposure to asbestos and man-made vitreous fibers: Results of a case-control study. *American Journal of Industrial Medicine* 37(6): 581-589.

McDonald AD, McDonald JC. 1978. Mesothelioma after crocidolite exposure during gas mask manufacture. *Environmental Research* 17(3): 340-346.

McDonald AD, Fry JS, Woolley AJ, McDonald JC. 1982. Dust exposure and mortality in an American factory using chrysotile, amosite, and crocidolite in mainly textile manufacture. *British Journal of Industrial Medicine* 39(4): 368-374.

McDonald AD, Fry JS, Woolley AJ, McDonald J. 1983. Dust exposure and mortality in an American chrysotile textile plant. *British Journal of Industrial Medicine* 40(4): 361-367.

McDonald AD, Fry JS, Woolley AJ, McDonald JC. 1984. Dust exposure and mortality in an American chrysotile asbestos friction products plant. *British Journal of Industrial Medicine* 41(2): 151-157.

McDonald JC, Liddell FD. 1979. Mortality in Canadian miners and millers exposed to chrysotile. *Annals of the New York Academy of Sciences* 330: 1-9.

McDonald JC, McDonald AD. 1997. Chrysotile, tremolite and carcinogenicity. *Annals of Occupational Hygiene* 41(6): 699-705.

McDonald JC, McDonald AD, Gibbs GW, Siemiatycki J, Rossiter CE. 1971. Mortality in the chrysotile asbestos mines and mills of Quebec. *Archives of Environmental Health* 22(6): 677-686.

McDonald JC, Liddell FD, Gibbs GW, Eyssen GE, McDonald AD. 1980. Dust exposure and mortality in chrysotile mining, 1910-75. *British Journal of Industrial Medicine* 37(1): 11-24.

McDonald JC, McDonald AD, Armstrong B, Sebastien P. 1986. Cohort study of mortality of vermiculite miners exposed to tremolite. *British Journal of Industrial Medicine* 43(7): 436-444.

McDonald JC, McDonald AD, Sebastien P, Moy K. 1988. Health of vermiculite miners exposed to trace amounts of fibrous tremolite. *British Journal of Industrial Medicine* 45(9): 630-634.

McDonald JC, Liddell FD, Dufresne A, McDonald AD. 1993. The 1891-1920 birth cohort of Quebec chrysotile miners and millers: Mortality 1976-88. *British Journal of Industrial Medicine* 50(12): 1073-1081.

Melkild A, Langard S, Andersen A, Tonnessen JN. 1989. Incidence of cancer among welders and other workers in a Norwegian shipyard. *Scandinavian Journal of Work, Environment and Health* 15(6): 387-394.

Menegozzo M, Belli S, Bruno C, Canfora V, Costigliola A, Di Cintio P, Di Liello L, Grignoli M, Palumbo F, Sapio P, et al. 1993. [Mortality due to causes correlatable to asbestos in a cohort of workers in railway car construction]. *Medicina del Lavoro* 84(3): 193-200.

Menegozzo M, Belli S, Borriero S, Bruno C, Carboni M, Grignoli M, Menegozzo S, Olivieri N, Comba P. 2002. [Mortality study of a cohort of insulation workers]. *Epidemiology Prevention* 26(2): 71-75.

Merletti F, Boffetta P, Ferro G, Pisani P, Terracini B. 1991. Occupation and cancer of the oral cavity or oropharynx in Turin, Italy. *Scandinavian Journal of Work, Environment and Health* 17(4): 248-254.

Meurman LO, Kiviluoto R, Hakama M. 1974. Mortality and morbidity among the working population of anthophyllite asbestos miners in Finland. *British Journal of Industrial Medicine* 31(2): 105-112.

Meurman LO, Kiviluoto R, Hakama M. 1979. Combined effect of asbestos exposure and tobacco smoking on Finnish anthophyllite miners and millers. *Annals of the New York Academy of Sciences* 330: 491-495.

Meurman LO, Pukkala E, Hakama M. 1994. Incidence of cancer among anthophyllite asbestos miners in Finland. *Occupational and Environmental Medicine* 51(6): 421-425.

Michaels D, Zoloth S. 1988. Asbestos disease in sheet metal workers: Proportional mortality update. *American Journal of Industrial Medicine* 13(6): 731-734.

Morinaga K, Hara I, Yasui I, Yokoyama K, Sera Y. 1990. [Twenty years' follow-up study of asbestos workers]. *Sangyo Igaku* 32(4): 265-268.

Morinaga K, Hanai A, Fujimoto I, Ohtsuka J, Matsumura T, Sakato J, Hara I, Yokoyama K, Sera Y. 1991. [A retrospective cohort study of workers in small asbestos industries in south Osaka]. *Nippon Koshu Eisei Zasshi* 38(4): 267-271.

Moulin JJ, Wild P, Haguenoer JM, Faucon D, De Gaudemaris R, Mur JM, Mereau M, Gary Y, Toamain JP, Birembaut Y, Blanc M, Debiolles M, Jegaden D, Laterrier B, Leonard M, Marini F, Massardier C, Moulin M, Reure M, Rigal L, Robert G, Viossat M. 1993. A mortality study among mild steel and stainless steel welders. *British Journal of Industrial Medicine* 50(3): 234-243.

Muscat J, Wynder E. 1992. Tobacco, alcohol, asbestos, and occupational risk factors for laryngeal cancer. *Cancer* 69(9): 2244-2251.

Musk AW, de Klerk NH, Ambrosini GL, Eccles JL, Hansen J, Olsen NJ, Watts VL, Lund HG, Pang SC, Beilby J, Hobbs MS. 1998. Vitamin A and cancer prevention I: Observations in workers previously exposed to asbestos at Wittenoom, Western Australia. *International Journal of Cancer* 75(3): 355-361.

Navratil M, Moravkova K, Gafronova M, Hruska F. 1988. The fate of people with pleural hyalinosis (plaques): Relationship to direct and indirect asbestos exposure. *Czechoslovak Medicine (Prague)* 11(3): 146-156.

Neuberger M, Kundi M. 1990. Individual asbestos exposure: Smoking and mortality. A cohort study in the asbestos cement industry. *British Journal of Industrial Medicine* 47(9): 615-620.

Neugut AI, Murray TI, Garbowski GC, Treat MR, Forde KA, Waye JD, Fenoglio-Preiser C. 1991. Association of asbestos exposure with colorectal adenomatous polyps and cancer. *Journal of the National Cancer Institute* 83(24): 1827-1828.

Newhouse ML. 1969. A study of the mortality of workers in an asbestos factory. *British Journal of Industrial Medicine* 26(4): 294-301.

Newhouse ML, Berry G. 1973. Abestos and laryngeal carcinoma. *Lancet* 2(7829): 615.

Newhouse ML, Berry G. 1979. Patterns of mortality in asbestos factory workers in London. *Annals of the New York Academy of Sciences* 330: 53-60.

Newhouse ML, Sullivan KR. 1989. A mortality study of workers manufacturing friction materials: 1941-86. *British Journal of Industrial Medicine* 46(3): 176-179.

Newhouse ML, Thompson H. 1965. Epidemiolgy of mesothelial tumors in the London area. *Annals of the New York Academy of Sciences* 132(1): 579-588.

Newhouse ML, Berry G, Wagner JC, Turok ME. 1972. A study of the mortality of female asbestos workers. *British Journal of Industrial Medicine* 29(2): 134-141.

Newhouse ML, Berry G, Skidmore JW. 1982. A mortality study of workers manufacturing friction materials with chrysotile asbestos. *Annals of Occupational Hygiene* 26(1-4): 899-909.

Newhouse ML, Oakes D, Woolley AJ. 1985a. Mortality of welders and other craftsmen at a shipyard in NE England. *British Journal of Industrial Medicine* 42(6): 406-410.

Newhouse ML, Berry G, Wagner JC. 1985b. Mortality of factory workers in east London 1933-1980. *British Journal of Industrial Medicine* 42(1): 4-11.

Nicholson WJ, Selikoff IJ, Seidman H, Lilis R, Formby P. 1979. Long-term mortality experience of chrysotile miners and millers in Thetford Mines, Quebec. *Annals of the New York Academy of Sciences* 330: 11-21.

Nokso-Koivisto P, Pukkala E. 1994. Past exposure to asbestos and combustion products and incidence of cancer among Finnish locomotive drivers. *Occupational and Environmental Medicine* 51(5): 330-334.

Ohlson CG, Hogstedt C. 1985. Lung cancer among asbestos cement workers. A Swedish cohort study and a review. *British Journal of Industrial Medicine* 42(6): 397-402.

Oksa P, Pukkala E, Karjalainen A, Ojajarvi A, Huuskonen MS. 1997. Cancer incidence and mortality among Finnish asbestos sprayers and in asbestosis and silicosis patients. *American Journal of Industrial Medicine* 31(6): 693-698.

Olsen J, Sabroe S. 1984. Occupational causes of laryngeal cancer. *Journal of Epidemiology and Community Health* 38(2): 117-121.

Pang ZC, Zhang Z, Wang Y, Zhang H. 1997. Mortality from a Chinese asbestos plant: Overall cancer mortality. *American Journal of Industrial Medicine* 32(5): 442-444.

Parent ME, Siemiatycki J, Fritschi L. 1998. Occupational exposures and gastric cancer. *Epidemiology* 9(1): 48-55.

Parent ME, Siemiatycki J, Fritschi L. 2000. Workplace exposures and oesophageal cancer. *Occupational and Environmental Medicine* 57(5): 325-334.

Parnes SM. 1990. Asbestos and cancer of the larynx: Is there a relationship? *Laryngoscope* 100(3): 254-261.

Petersen R, Venstrup-Nielsen SE. 1982. [Mortality among Danish insulation workers during 1970-1975]. *Ugeskrift for Laeger* 144(13): 967-970.

Peto J, Doll R, Howard SV, Kinlen LJ, Lewinsohn HC. 1977. A mortality study among workers in an English asbestos factory. *British Journal of Industrial Medicine* 34(3): 169-173.

Peto J, Doll R, Hermon C, Binns W, Clayton R, Goffe T. 1985. Relationship of mortality to measures of environmental asbestos pollution in an asbestos textile factory. *Annals of Occupational Hygiene* 29(3): 305-355.

Piolatto G, Negri E, La Vecchia C, Pira E, Decarli A, Peto J. 1990. An update of cancer mortality among chrysotile asbestos miners in Balangero, northern Italy. *British Journal of Industrial Medicine* 47(12): 810-814.

Pira E, Pelucchi C, Buffoni L, Palmas A, Turbiglio M, Negri E, Piolatto PG, La Vecchia C. 2005. Cancer mortality in a cohort of asbestos textile workers. *British Journal of Cancer* 92(3): 580-586.

Pukkala E, Saarni H. 1996. Cancer incidence among Finnish seafarers, 1967-92. *Cancer Causes and Control* 7(2): 231-239.

Puntoni R, Russo L, Zannini D, Vercelli M, Gambaro RP, Valerio F, Santi L. 1977. Mortality among dock-yard workers in Genoa, Italy. *Tumori* 63(1): 91-96.

Puntoni R, Vercelli M, Merlo F, Valerio F, Santi L. 1979. Mortality among shipyard workers in Genoa, Italy. *Annals of the New York Academy of Sciences* 330: 353-377.

Puntoni R, Merlo F, Borsa L, Reggiardo G, Garrone E, Ceppi M. 2001. A historical cohort mortality study among shipyard workers in Genoa, Italy. *American Journal of Industrial Medicine* 40(4): 363-370.

Raffn E, Lynge E, Juel K, Korsgaard B. 1989. Incidence of cancer and mortality among employees in the asbestos cement industry in Denmark. *British Journal of Industrial Medicine* 46(2): 90-96.

Raffn E, Villadsen E, Lynge E. 1996. Colorectal cancer in asbestos cement workers in Denmark. *American Journal of Industrial Medicine* 30(3): 267-272.

Raffn E, Villadsen E, Engholm G, Lynge E. 1998. [Lung cancer among asbestos-cement workers in Denmark]. *Ugeskr Laeger* 160(7): 1029-1033.

Rafnsson V, Sulem P. 2003. Cancer incidence among marine engineers, a population-based study (Iceland). *Cancer Causes and Control* 14(1): 29-35.

Reid A, Ambrosini G, de Klerk N, Fritschi L, Musk B. 2004. Aerodigestive and gastrointestinal tract cancers and exposure to crocidolite (blue asbestos): Incidence and mortality among former crocidolite workers. *International Journal of Cancer* 111(5): 757-761.

Ribak J, Seidman H, Selikoff IJ. 1989. Amosite mesothelioma in a cohort of asbestos workers. *Scandinavian Journal of Work and Environmental Health* 15(2): 106-110.

Robinson C, Stern F, Halperin W, Venable H, Petersen M, Frazier T, Burnett C, Lalich N, Salg J, Sestito J. 1995. Assessment of mortality in the construction industry in the United States, 1984-1986. *American Journal of Industrial Medicine* 28(1): 49-70.

Robinson CF, Lemen RA, Wagoner JK. 1979. Morality patterns, 1940-1975 among workers employed in an asbestos textile friction and packing products manufacturing facilites. In: Lemen RA, Dement JM, eds. *Dust and Disease*. Park Forest, IL: Pathotox Publishers. Pp. 131-143.

Robinson CF, Petersen M, Sieber WK, Palu S, Halperin WE. 1996. Mortality of Carpenters' Union members employed in the US construction or wood products industries, 1987-1990. *American Journal of Industrial Medicine* 30(6): 674-694.

Roggli VL. 2006. The role of analytical SEM in the determination of causation in malignant mesothelioma. *Ultrastructal Pathology* 30(1): 31-35.

Roggli VL, Oury TD, Moffatt EJ. 1997. Malignant mesothelioma in women. *Anatomic Pathology* 2: 147-163.

Rosler JA, Woitowitz HJ. 1995. Recent data on cancer due to asbestos in Germany. *Med Lav* 86(5): 440-448.

Rosler JA, Woitowitz HJ, Lange HJ, Woitowitz RH, Ulm K, Rodelsperger K. 1994. Mortality rates in a female cohort following asbestos exposure in Germany. *Journal of Occupational Medicine* 36(8): 889-893.

Rossiter CE, Coles RM. 1980. HM Dockyard, Devonport: 1947 mortality study. *IARC Scientific Publications* 30: 713-721.

Rubino GF, Piolatto G, Newhouse ML, Scansetti G, Aresini GA, Murray R. 1979. Mortality of chrysotile asbestos workers at the Balangero Mine, northern Italy. *British Journal of Industrial Medicine* 36(3): 187-194.

Salg J, Alterman T. 2005. A proportionate mortality study of bricklayers and allied craftworkers. *American Journal of Industrial Medicine* 47(1): 10-19.

Sanden A, Jarvholm B. 1987. Cancer morbidity in Swedish shipyard workers 1978-1983. *International Archives of Occupational and Environmental Health* 59(5): 455-462.

Sanden A, Jarvholm B, Naslund PE. 1984. Mortality and morbidity of Swedish insulation workers. *Scandinavian Journal of Work and Environmental Health* 10(3): 207.

Sanden A, Naslund PE, Jarvholm B. 1985. Mortality in lung and gastrointestinal cancer among shipyard workers. *International Archives of Occupational and Environmental Health* 55(4): 277-283.

Sanden A, Jarvholm B, Larsson S, Thiringer G. 1992. The risk of lung cancer and mesothelioma after cessation of asbestos exposure: A prospective cohort study of shipyard workers. *European Respiratory Journal* 5(3): 281-285.

Seidman H, Selikoff IJ. 1990. Decline in death rates among asbestos insulation workers 1967-1986 associated with diminution of work exposure to asbestos. *Annals of the New York Academy of Sciences* 609: 300-317.

Seidman H, Selikoff IJ, Hammond EC. 1982. Mortality of brain tumors among asbestos insulation workers in the United States and Canada. *Annals of the New York Academy of Sciences* 381: 160-171.

Seidman H, Selikoff IJ, Gelb SK. 1986. Mortality experience of amosite asbestos factory workers: Dose-response relationships 5 to 40 years after onset of short-term work exposure. *American Journal of Industrial Medicine* 10(5-6): 479-514.

Selikoff IJ. 1974. Epidemiology of gastrointestinal cancer. *Environmental Health Perspectives* 9: 299-305.

Selikoff IJ. 1989. Mortality study of workers exposed to asbestos in a Lodz factory. *Polish Journal of Occupational Medicine* 2(3): 323-328.

Selikoff IJ, Seidman H. 1991. Asbestos-associated deaths among insulation workers in the United States and Canada, 1967-1987. *Annals of the New York Academy of Sciences* 643: 1-14.

Selikoff IJ., Churg J, Hammond EC. 1964. Asbestos exposure and neoplasia. *Journal of the American Medical Association* 188(1): 22-26.

Selikoff IJ, Hammond EC, Seidman H. 1979. Mortality experience of insulation workers in the United States and Canada, 1943-1976. *Annals of the New York Academy of Sciences* 330: 91-116.

Selikoff IJ, Hammond EC, Seidman H. 1980. Latency of asbestos disease among insulation workers in the United States and Canada. *Cancer* 46(12): 2736-2740.

Sera Y, Kang KY. 1981. Asbestos and cancer in the Sennan District of Osaka. *Tohoku Journal of Experimental Medicine* 133(3): 313-320.

Shettigara PT, Morgan RW. 1975. Asbestos, smoking, and laryngeal carcinoma. *Archives of Environmental Health* 30(10): 517-519.

Simonato L, Fletcher AC, Andersen A, Anderson K, Becker N, Chang-Claude J, Ferro G, Gerin M, Gray CN, Hansen KS, Kalliomaki P-L, Kurppa K, Langard S, Merlo F, Moulin J, Newhouse M, Peto J, Pukkala E, Sjogren B, Wild P, Winkelmann R, Saracci R. 1991. A historical prospective study of European stainless steel, mild steel, and shipyard welders. *British Journal of Industrial Medicine* 48(3): 145-154.

Sluis-Cremer GK, Liddell FD, Logan WP, Bezuidenhout BN. 1992. The mortality of amphibole miners in South Africa, 1946-80. *British Journal of Industrial Medicine* 49(8): 566-575.

Smailyte G, Kurtinaitis J, Andersen A. 2004a. Cancer mortality and morbidity among Lithuanian asbestos-cement producing workers. *Scandinavian Journal of Work, Environment and Health* 30(1): 64-70.

Smailyte G, Kurtinaitis J, Andersen A. 2004b. Mortality and cancer incidence among Lithuanian cement producing workers. *Occupational and Environmental Medicine* 61(6): 529-534.

Spiegelman D, Wegman DH. 1985. Occupation-related risks for colorectal cancer. *Journal of the National Cancer Institute* 75(5): 813-821.

Stell P, McGill T. 1973. Asbestos and laryngeal carcinoma. *Lancet* 2(7826): 416-417.

Stern F, Schulte P, Sweeney MH, Fingerhut M, Vossenas P, Burkhardt G, Kornak MF. 1995. Proportionate mortality among construction laborers. *American Journal of Industrial Medicine* 27(4): 485-509.

Stern FB, Sweeney MH, Ward E. 1997. Proportionate mortality among unionized construction ironworkers. *American Journal of Industrial Medicine* 31(2): 176-187.

Stern FB, Ruder AM, Chen G. 2000. Proportionate mortality among unionized roofers and waterproofers. *American Journal of Industrial Medicine* 37(5): 478-492.

Stern F, Lehman E, Ruder A. 2001. Mortality among unionized construction plasterers and cement masons. *American Journal of Industrial Medicine* 39(4): 373-88.

Straif K, Chambless L, Weiland SK, Wienke A, Bungers M, Taeger D, Keil U. 1999. Occupational risk factors for mortality from stomach and lung cancer among rubber workers: An analysis using internal controls and refined exposure assessment. *International Journal of Epidemiology* 28(6): 1037-1043.

Suzuki Y, Yuen SR, Ashley R. 2005. Short, thin asbestos fibers contribute to the development of human malignant mesothelioma: Pathological evidence. *International Journal of Hygiene and Environmental Health* 208(3): 201-210.

Szeszenia-Dabrowska N, Wilczynska U, Szymczak W. 1986a. [Risk of cancer in women occupationally exposed to asbestos dust]. *Medycyna Pracy* 37(4): 243-249.

Szeszenia-Dabrowska N, Wilczynska U, Szymczak W. 1986b. [Neoplasm risk in men occupationally exposed to asbestos dust] [Polish]. *Medycyna Pracy* 37(3): 129-138.

Szeszenia-Dabrowska N, Wilczynska U, Szymczak W. 1997. [Cancer risk in asbestos-cement industry workers in Poland]. *Medycyna Pracy* 48(5): 473-483.

Szeszenia-Dabrowska N, Wilczynska U, Szymczak W. 2000. Mortality of workers at two asbestos-cement plants in Poland. *International Journal of Occupational Medicine and Environmental Health* 13(2): 121-130.

Szeszenia-Dabrowska N, Urszula W, Szymczak W, Strzelecka A. 2002. Mortality study of workers compensated for asbestosis in Poland, 1970-1997. *International Journal Occupational Medicine and Environmental Health* 15(3): 267-278.

Tarchi M, Orsi D, Comba P, De Santis M, Pirastu R, Battista G, Valiani M. 1994. Cohort mortality study of rock salt workers in Italy. *American Journal of Industrial Medicine* 25(2): 251-256.

Teta MJ, Ott MG. 1988. A mortality study of a research, engineering, and metal fabrication facility in western New York State. *American Journal of Epidemiology* 127(3): 540-551.

Thomas HF, Benjamin IT, Elwood PC, Sweetnam PM. 1982. Further follow-up study of workers from an asbestos cement factory. *British Journal of Industrial Medicine* 39(3): 273-276.

Tola S, Kalliomaki PL, Pukkala E, Asp S, Korkala ML. 1988. Incidence of cancer among welders, platers, machinists, and pipe fitters in shipyards and machine shops. *British Journal of Industrial Medicine* 45(4): 209-218.

Tsai SP, Waddell LC, Gilstrap EL, Ransdell JD, Ross CE. 1996. Mortality among maintenance employees potentially exposed to asbestos in a refinery and petrochemical plant. *American Journal of Industrial Medicine* 29(1): 89-98.

Vineis P, Ciccone G, Magnino A. 1993. Asbestos exposure, physical activity and colon cancer: A case-control study. *Tumori* 79(5): 301-303.

Wagner JC, Sleggs CA, Marchand P. 1960. Diffuse pleural mesothelioma and asbestos exposure in the North Western Cape Province. *British Journal of Industrial Medicine* 17: 260-271.

Wang E, Dement JM, Lipscomb H. 1999. Mortality among North Carolina construction workers, 1988-1994. *Applied Occupational Environment Hygiene* 14(1): 45-58.

Ward EM, Ruder AM, Suruda A, Smith AB, Halperin W, Fessler CA, Zahm SH. 1994. Cancer mortality patterns among female and male workers employed in a cable manufacturing plant during World War II. *Journal of Occupational Medicine* 36(8): 860-866.

Weiss W. 1977. Mortality of a cohort exposed to chrysotile asbestos. *Journal of Occupational Medicine* 19(11): 737-40.

Welch LS, Michaels D, Zoloth SR. 1994. The National Sheet Metal Worker Asbestos Disease Screening Program: Radiologic findings. National Sheet Metal Examination Group. *American Journal of Industrial Medicine* 25(5): 635-648.

Wilczynska U, Szeszenia-Dabrowska N, Szymczak W. 1990. [Effect of the selection of reference population on the evaluation of the degree of the risk of death among industrial cohorts]. *Medycyna Pracy* 41(3): 175-180.

Woitowitz HJ, Lange HJ, Beierl L, Rathgeb M, Schmidt K, Ulm K, Giesen T, Woitowitz RH, Pache L, Rodelsperger K. 1986. Mortality rates in the Federal Republic of Germany following previous occupational exposure to asbestos dust. *International Archives of Occupational and Environmental Health* 57(3): 161-171.

Wortley P, Vaughan TL, Davis S, Morgan MS, Thomas DB. 1992. A case-control study of occupational risk factors for laryngeal cancer. *British Journal of Industrial Medicine* 49(12): 837-844.

Xu, Z, Pan GW, Liu LM, Brown LM, Guan DX, Xiu Q, Sheng JH, Stone BJ, Dosemeci M, Fraumeni JF Jr, Blot WJ. 1996. Cancer risks among iron and steel workers in Anshan, China, Part I: Proportional mortality ratio analysis. *American Journal of Industrial Medicine* 30(1): 1-6.

Yano E, Wang ZM, Wang XR, Wang MZ, Lan YJ. 2001. Cancer mortality among workers exposed to amphibole-free chrysotile asbestos. *American Journal of Epidemiology* 154(6): 538-543.

Zagraniski RT, Kelsey JL, Walter SD. 1986. Occupational risk factors for laryngeal carcinoma: Connecticut, 1975-1980. *American Journal of Epidemiology* 124(1): 67-76.

Zandjani F, Hogsaet B, Andersen A, Langard S. 1994. Incidence of cancer among nitrate fertilizer workers. *International Archives of Occupational and Environmental Health* 66(3): 189-193.

Zheng W, Blot WJ, Shu XO, Diamond EL, Gao YT, Ji BT, Fraumeni JF Jr. 1992a. Risk factors for oral and pharyngeal cancer in Shanghai, with emphasis on diet. *Cancer Epidemiology, Biomarkers and Prevention* 1(6): 441-448.

Zheng W, Blot WJ, Shu XO, Gao YT, Ji BT, Ziegler RG, Fraumeni JF Jr. 1992b. Diet and other risk factors for laryngeal cancer in Shanghai, China. *American Journal of Epidemiology* 136(2): 178-191.

Zhou KH, Liu P, Xuan CS, Zhao YJ. 1996. [24 years follow-up study on cancer mortality on asbestos workers]. *China Public Health* 12: 515-516 (In Chinese).

Zhu H, Wang Z. 1993. Study of occupational lung cancer in asbestos factories in China. *British Journal of Industrial Medicine* 50(11): 1039-1042.

Zoloth S, Michaels D. 1985. Asbestos disease in sheet metal workers: The results of a proportional mortality analysis. *American Journal of Industrial Medicine* 7(4): 315-321.

7

Pharyngeal Cancer and Asbestos

NATURE OF THIS CANCER TYPE

Cancers of the pharynx are frequently grouped with "head and neck cancers," which also include the oral and nasal cavities. The pharynx itself spans several sublocations: the oropharynx (ICD-9 146; ICD-O-3 C09-C10), the nasopharynx (ICD-9 147; ICD-O-3 C11), and the hypopharynx (ICD-9 148; ICD-O-3 C12-C13.9). Each of those can be further subdivided (for example, the tonsil is located within the oropharynx), and the more specific locations have somewhat differing characteristics in terms of etiologic factors. During the time when most of the studies considered in this review were conducted, cancers of the oral (or buccal) cavity (ICD-9 141-145; ICD-O-3 C00-C09) were frequently grouped with the pharynx (particularly the oropharynx), and the committee decided to include such data. Similarly, the nasal cavities (ICD-9 160.0; ICD-O-3 C30) are sometimes grouped with the nasopharynx, but this did not arise in the informative studies screened for this review. Figure 7.1 illustrates the location of cancers that arise in the upper respiratory tract and digestive tract.

The American Cancer Society (Jemal et al. 2006) has projected that about 30,990 new cases of and 7,430 deaths from cancer of the oral cavity and pharynx will occur in 2006. Those estimates include cancers of the mouth (the inside lining of the lips and cheeks, gums, tongue, and hard and soft palate), nasopharynx, oropharynx, and hypopharynx. In the study populations considered in this review, pharyngeal cancers would be expected to occur primarily in the *oropharynx*.

Cancer of the *nasopharynx* is rare in the United States, where it occurs

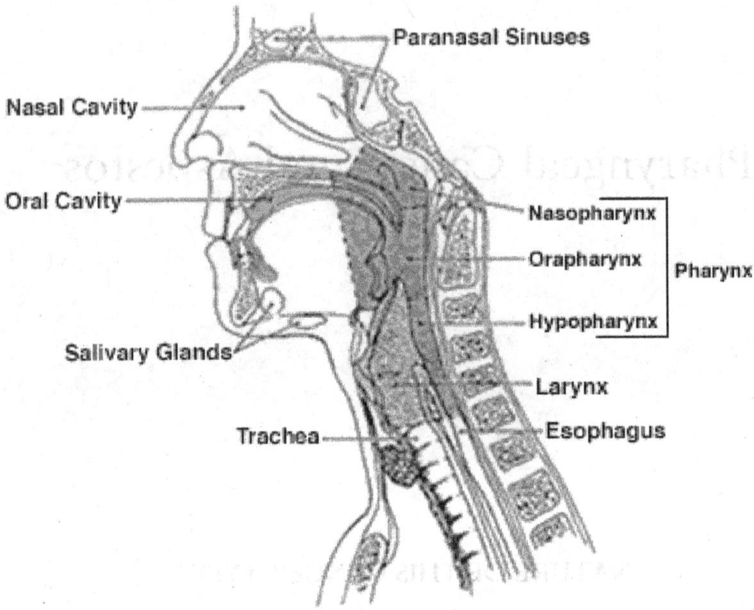

FIGURE 7.1 Anatomy of the pharynx showing its proximity to the oral and nasal cavities and to the larynx and esophagus.
SOURCE: Copyright 2005 American Cancer Society, Inc. Reprinted with permission from www.cancer.org.

at the rate of about one cancer per 100,000 per year, whereas the incidence is high in southern China (30-50 per 100,000 per year), among Eskimos in the Artic region, and among some indigenous populations in Southeast Asia. The risk is 2-3 times higher in men than in women. Risk factors include Epstein-Barr virus (Mueller 1995), consumption of salted fish (Miller et al. 1996), and occupational exposure to formaldehyde (IARC 1995). There are three histologic types: keratinizing squamous-cell carcinoma, non-keratinizing carcinoma, and undifferentiated carcinoma.

Carcinoma of the *hypopharynx* is an uncommon disease. Considered collectively with carcinomas of the cervical esophagus, they make up about 10% of all tumors of the upper respiratory tract and digestive tract and less than 1% of all cancers diagnosed in the United States each year (Pfister et al. 2004). By far the most common histology is squamous-cell carcinoma. Cervical esophageal squamous-cell cancer and hypopharyngeal cancer typically present as extremely advanced disease, and 5-year survival is about 17-30%. Standard therapy for advanced disease is a combination of chemotherapy and radiation (Lefebvre et al. 1996). The major risk factors for squamous-cell cancers of the hypopharynx and cervical esophagus are tobacco and alcohol use. Ethanol is a promoter of the mutagenic effects of tobacco-derived substances and thereby contributes to the carcinogenic synergy seen with concurrent tobacco and alcohol use. The high incidence of second primary tumors and the concomitant mucosal dysplasia that frequently surrounds primary tumors suggest the presence of a regional field effect in these diseases.

For cancers of the oral cavity and pharynx overall, the incidence rate, or rate at which new cancers are diagnosed, is nearly 3 times higher in men than in women and slightly higher in black men than in white men. Most cases occur in men who are more than 50 years old. The incidence has decreased by an average of 1.2% per year since 1981; the decrease has been larger in men than in women and larger in black than in white men. Mortality from oropharyngeal cancer has been decreasing since the late 1970s, with more rapid improvement since 1993.

Most cancers of the oral cavity and pharynx are squamous-cell carcinomas. Development of cancers in the mouth may be preceded by the onset and progression of premalignant lesions, such as leukoplakia (raised white patches on the oral mucosa that measure at least 5 mm and cannot be scraped off) or erythroplasia (leukoplakia with an erythematous or red component).

Radiation therapy and surgery are standard treatments for cancer of the oral cavity and pharynx; in advanced disease, chemotherapy may be a useful addition. Survival varies with stage at diagnosis. For all stages combined, about 85% of persons with oral cavity or pharynx cancer survive 1 year after diagnosis. The 5-year and 10-year survival rates are 59% and 44%, respectively.

Known risk factors for cancers of the oral cavity and pharynx include all forms of tobacco-smoking (cigarettes, cigars, pipes, and bidis), use of chewing tobacco or snuff, and excessive consumption of alcohol. The combination of tobacco use and alcohol consumption potentiates the risk of either factor alone. Premalignant lesions often regress after the discontinuation of smoking or using smokeless tobacco. Other factors that may contribute to risk are chronic irritation and infection with some strains of human papillomavirus.

EPIDEMIOLOGIC EVIDENCE CONSIDERED

Information on the association between asbestos exposure and cancer of the pharynx was available on 16 cohort populations with results presented in 14 articles and from six case-control studies. Cohort studies offer the opportunity to examine exposure-response trends, but the number of pharyngeal cancers in the cohort studies was generally too small to permit examination by magnitude of exposure. Case-control studies are often based on larger numbers of cases, which tends to give them greater statistical power and the potential for stratification on tobacco or alcohol use. Both types of studies contributed evidence for the evaluation of asbestos and pharynx cancer.

Cohort Studies

The cohorts that presented usable information about the risk of pharyngeal cancer were indicated in Table 6.1. Their histories and design properties are described in Table B.1, and the details of their results concerning cancer at this site are abstracted in Table D.1. The results of the cohort and case-control studies are summarized in Table 7.1, and Figures 7.2 and 7.3

TABLE 7.1 Summary of Epidemiologic Findings Regarding Cancer of the Pharynx

Study Type	Figure	Comparison	Study Populations Included	No. Study Populations	Summary RR (95% CI)	Between-Study SD
Cohort	7.2	Any vs none	All	16	1.44 (1.04-2.00)	—
	7.3	High vs none[a]		3	0.93 (0.21-4.15)	—
Case-Control	7.4	Any vs none	All	4	1.47 (1.10-1.96)	0.00
	7.5	Any vs none	EAM = 1	3	1.37 (0.94-1.99)	0.12
			EAM = 2	1		
	7.6	Any vs none	EAM = 1 Adjusted[b]	2	1.39 (0.86-2.25)	0.25
			EAM = 1 Unadjusted[b]	1		
	7.7	High vs none[a]	EAM = 1	4	1.25 (0.68-2.30)	0.46

NOTE: CI = Confidence interval; EAM = exposure-assessment method; high quality, EAM = 1; lower quality, EAM = 2; RR = relative risk; SD = standard deviation.

[a]Used studies that reported dose-response relationship (RR on an exposure gradient).
[b]Adjusted: RR was adjusted for both smoking and alcohol use.

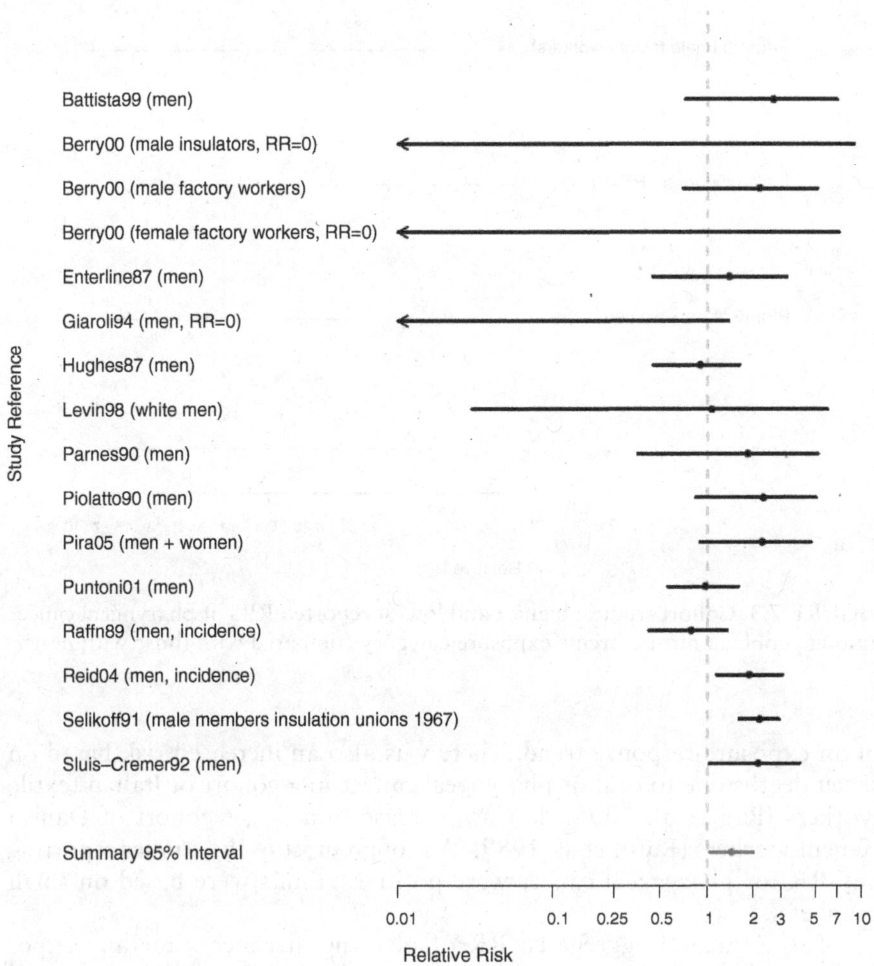

FIGURE 7.2 Cohort studies: RR of pharyngeal cancer in people with "any" exposure to asbestos compared with people who report none.

are plots of relative risks (RRs) for overall exposure and for exposure-response gradients from the cohort studies reviewed.

There were 16 cohort populations that had reported findings for this rare cause of death. The strongest evidence of an association comes from a study of insulation workers (Selikoff and Seidman 1991) with a standardized mortality ratio (SMR) of 2.2 based on 48 cases of oropharyngeal cancer. The rest of the studies were based fewer than 10 cases. RRs were increased in a mining cohort (Piolatto et al. 1990), but there was no indication

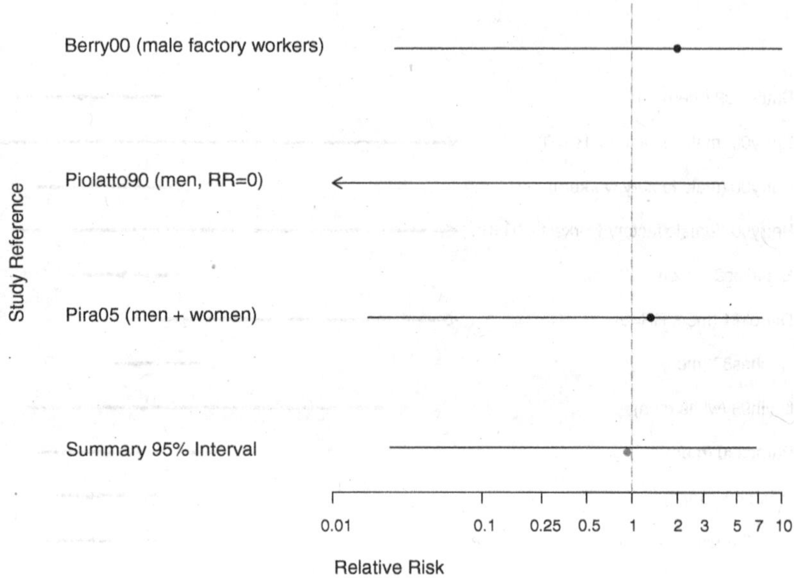

FIGURE 7.3 Cohort studies: highest and lowest reported RRs of pharyngeal cancer among people in most extreme exposure category compared with those with none.

of an exposure-response trend. There was also an increased risk based on seven deaths due to oral or pharyngeal cancer in a cohort of Italian textile workers (Pira et al. 2005), but no increase in a larger cohort of Danish cement workers (Raffn et al. 1989). Although most of the studies reporting any RR for pharyngeal cancer were positive, results were based on small numbers.

The estimated aggregated RR of pharyngeal cancers for any exposure to asbestos was 1.44 (95% CI 1.04-2.00). Few studies evaluated exposure-response trends, and there was no indication of higher risk associated with more extreme exposures (RR = 0.93, 95% CI 0.21-4.15).

Case-Control Studies

The six case-control studies retained for thorough evaluation after exclusion of studies that did not assess exposure to asbestos or did not meet other exclusion criteria are listed in Table 6.5 according to quality of their exposure assessment. The details of the design aspects of those studies are presented in Table C.1, and their detailed results are abstracted in Table E.1. The findings of those studies are summarized in Table 7.1 and in the plots presented in Figures 7.4-7.7.

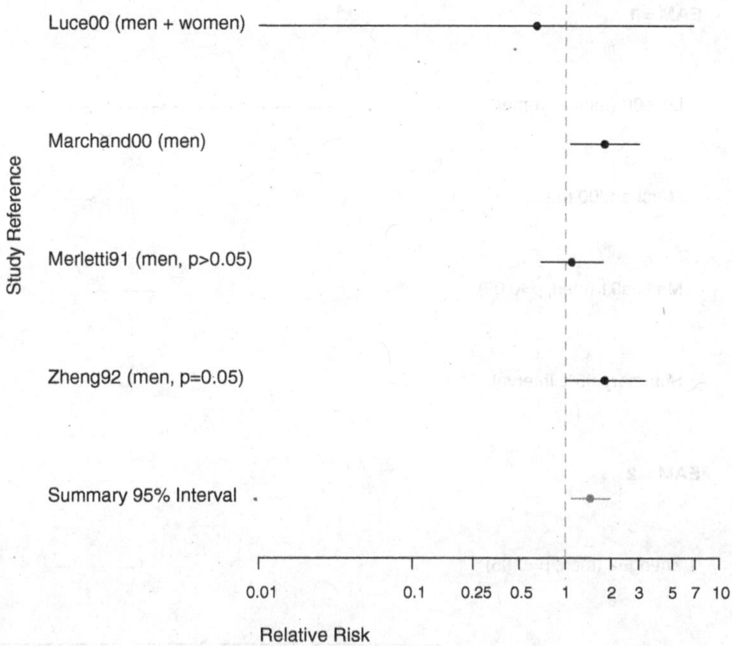

FIGURE 7.4 Case-control studies: RR of pharyngeal cancer in people with "any" exposure to asbestos compared with people with none.

The committee found only six case-control studies that assessed the association between pharyngeal cancer and asbestos exposure. Of the four studies with contrasts of any versus no asbestos exposure, one had only a yes-no exposure classification; of the other three studies, two gathered data on potential confounders and adjusted the risk estimates associated with asbestos exposure accordingly. Two of these four studies also had results from dose-response gradients. Two additional studies (Berrino et al. 2003, Gustavsson et al. 1998) had information on gradients without combined results for all asbestos-exposed cases.

Four of the studies adjusted for alcohol use and smoking. Of those, the largest was by Marchand et al. (2000), whose hospital-based study of 206 total hypopharynx cases and 305 controls was designed to assess the effects of occupational exposures to asbestos and man-made mineral fibers. They reported an RR of 1.80 (95% CI 1.08-2.99) for those ever exposed to asbestos, adjusted for smoking and alcohol consumption. In an analysis by magnitude of exposure, the RR was increased in all categories, but there was little evidence of a trend with increasing exposure. Marchand et al. (2000) also estimated the joint effects of smoking and asbestos. When the

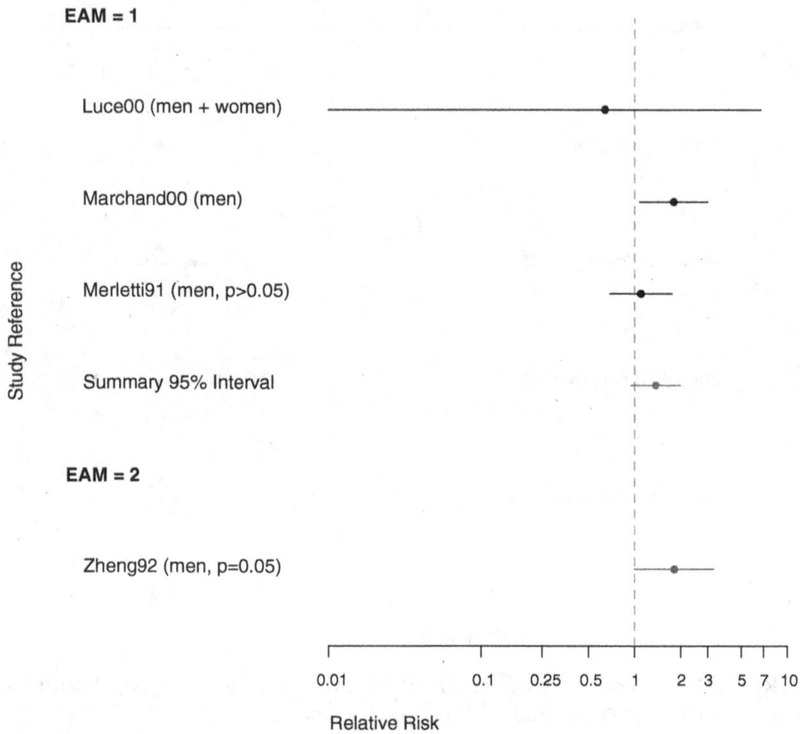

FIGURE 7.5 Case-control studies: RR of pharyngeal cancer in people with "any" exposure to asbestos compared with people with none, stratified on quality of exposure assessment (top, EAM = 1: higher-quality exposure assessment; bottom, EAM = 2: lower-quality exposure assessment).

data were looked at in a stratified fashion (Table 7.2), there was some suggestion that smoking modified the risk of hypopharyngeal cancer associated with asbestos exposure, which was comparable with their findings on the association of smoking and asbestos exposure with laryngeal cancer (Table 8.2).

In a European multicenter study of laryngeal and hypopharyngeal cancer, Berrino et al. (2003) found similar results when comparing the asbestos exposure of 100 men diagnosed with hypopharyngeal cancer before age 55 with 819 controls. The odds ratios (ORs) for those with either possible or probable exposure to asbestos were both 1.8, adjusted for alcohol consumption and smoking; there was no examination of effect modification. When these 100 cases of hypopharyngeal cancer were analyzed in combination with 215 cases of laryngeal cancer (see Table E.2), the OR increased slightly with duration of exposure. Merletti et al. (1991) found an RR of

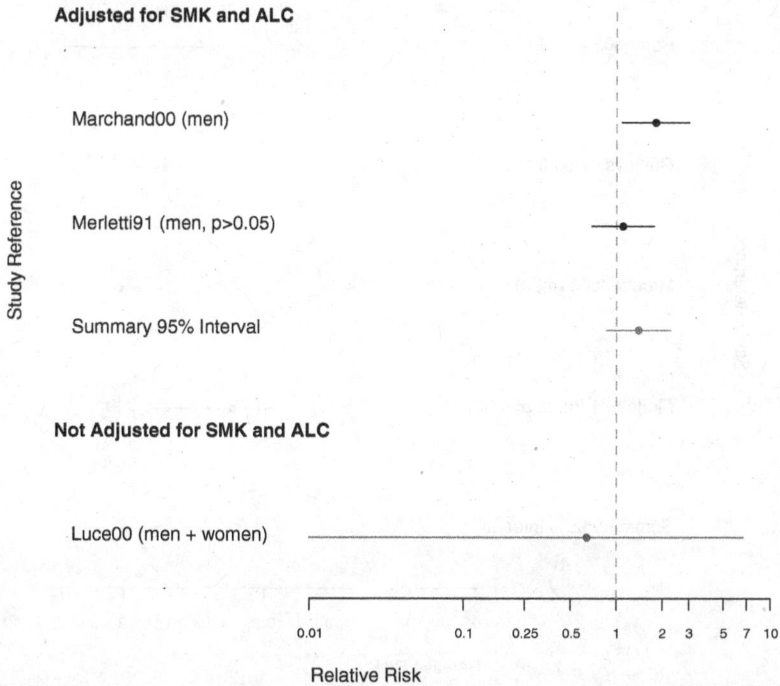

FIGURE 7.6 Case-control studies: RR of pharyngeal cancer in people with "any" exposure to asbestos compared with people with none, in studies with higher-quality exposure assessment, stratified on quality of confounder assessment (top: adjusted; bottom: unadjusted).

1.1 in a population-based case-control study of 86 men with cancer of the oral cavity or oropharynx, of whom 45 had definitely been exposed to asbestos. In a study of 138 Swedish men with pharyngeal cancer, Gustavsson et al. (1998) found no suggestion of an association of this cancer with asbestos exposure.

The other two case-control studies failed to adjust for confounding. Zheng et al. (1992) conducted a population-based case-control study in Shanghai, China, using 204 incident cases of pharyngeal cancer and 414 controls, with the primary purpose of investigating the role of diet in pharyngeal-cancer causation; more asbestos exposure was seen in the cases than the controls, and the crude RR was 1.7. In a case-control study of only 5 cases of hypopharyngeal cancer among residents of New Caledonia, Luce et al. (2000) found no indication of increased risk of pharyngeal cancer with exposure to tremolite asbestos in whitewash.

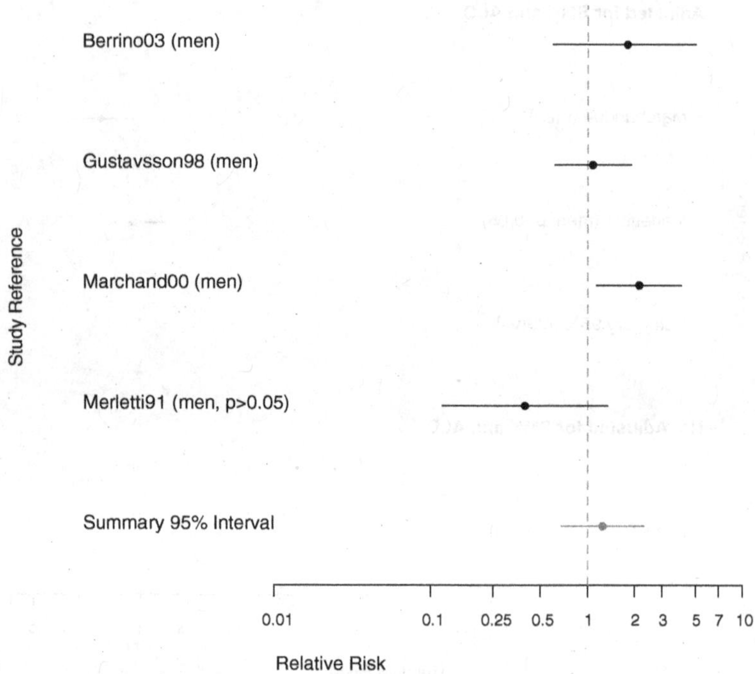

FIGURE 7.7 Case-control studies: RR of pharyngeal cancer among people in the most extreme exposure category compared with those with none. (If multiple exposure gradients were presented in study, highest and lowest estimates for the most extreme categories were plotted.)

TABLE 7.2 Effect Modification for Pharyngeal Cancer Associated with Asbestos Exposure and Smoking

Study	Smoking History (pack-years)	RRs with 95% CIs for Asbestos Exposure: None or Low (cumulative)	RRs with 95% CIs for Asbestos Exposure: Intermediate or High (cumulative)
Marchand et al. (2000)	<30	1.0	1.2 (0.6-2.3)
(adjusted for age and for alcohol consumption)	30+	4.0 (2.2-7.2)	6.2 (3.4-11.4)

EVIDENCE INTEGRATION AND CONCLUSION

Evidence Considered

The committee reviewed 16 cohort populations and six case-control studies of pharyngeal cancer, of which four included high-quality exposure assessment or adjustment for possible confounding by smoking and alcohol consumption. The committee noted that epidemiologic evidence on pharyngeal cancer was based on a more heterogeneous grouping of subsites than was the evidence on cancer at the other selected sites considered in this review. No increase in pharyngeal tumors has been observed in animals exposed chronically to asbestos by inhalation (Hesterberg et al. 1993, 1994; McConnell 2005; McConnell et al. 1994a,b, 1999).

Consistency

Overall, the cohort studies were rather consistent; the plots present a pattern of modestly positive associations which is similar, to but fainter than, that seen for laryngeal cancer (see Chapter 8). Few RRs were less than 1.0. The few case-control studies were inconsistent and showed some suggestion of effect modification by smoking.

Although the information from the case-control studies was sparse, the aggregated risk estimate for any asbestos exposure was modest and similar to that for the more numerous cohort studies. For both types of study, the limited data on extreme exposures tended toward lower risks than the aggregate risk for any exposure, suggesting the lack of a dose-response relationship.

Strength of Association

The summary RR for the cohort studies was almost exactly midway between 1.0 and 2.0, but there were too few studies with quantitative measures of exposure to examine exposure-response trends.

Coherence

Squamous-cell carcinomas arising from the oropharynx and hypopharynx are similar to squamous-cell carcinomas of the lung and larynx in their histogenesis; however, they arise from oral and pharyngeal epithelium, which differs from the respiratory epithelium from which lung and laryngeal cancers arise. The major risk factors for pharyngeal cancer are tobacco-smoking, tobacco-chewing, and use of snuff alone or in combination with alcohol consumption. The combination of asbestos exposure and tobacco-smoking is an established risk factor for lung cancer, but for pharyngeal cancer only a single case-control study has addressed asbestos exposure as a cofactor with tobacco use.

There are no published reports of recovery of asbestos fibers or asbestos bodies from the pharynx; the absence of such data neither supports nor refutes the possibility that fibers accumulate at this site.

Conclusion

Several cohort studies suggest an association between pharyngeal cancer and asbestos. The contrast with the abundance and consistency of data available on the larynx, the absence of information on a dose-response relationship, and the lack of supportive data from animal studies reduce the overall degree of evidence for causality. Nonetheless, several of the positive cohort studies and at least one case-control study support the determination that the evidence is **suggestive but not sufficient** to infer a causal relationship between asbestos exposure and pharyngeal cancer.

REFERENCES

Battista G, Belli S, Comba P, Fiumalbi C, Grignoli M, Loi F, Orsi D, Paredes I. 1999. Mortality due to asbestos-related causes among railway carriage construction and repair workers. *Occupation Medicine (London)* 49(8): 536-539.

Berrino F, Richiardi L, Boffetta P, Esteve J, Belletti I, Raymond L, Troschel L, Pisani P, Zubiri L, Ascunce N, Guberan E, Tuyns A, Terracini B, Merletti F. 2003. Occupation and larynx and hypopharynx cancer: A job-exposure matrix approach in an international case-control study in France, Italy, Spain and Switzerland. *Cancer Causes and Control* 14(3): 213-223.

Berry G, Newhouse ML, Wagner JC. 2000. Mortality from all cancers of asbestos factory workers in east London 1933-80. *Occupational and Environmental Medicine* 57(11): 782-785.

Enterline PE, Hartley J, Henderson V. 1987. Asbestos and cancer: A cohort followed up to death. *British Journal of Industrial Medicine* 44(6): 396-401.

Giaroli C, Belli S, Bruno C, Candela S, Grignoli M, Minisci S, Poletti R, Ricco G, Vecchi G, Venturi G, Ziccardi A, Combra P. 1994. Mortality study of asbestos cement workers. *International Archives of Occupational and Environmental Health* 66(1): 7-11.

Gustavsson P, Jakobsson R, Johansson H, Lewin F, Norell S, Rutkvist LE. 1998. Occupational exposures and squamous cell carcinoma of the oral cavity, pharynx, larynx, and oesophagus: A case-control study in Sweden. *Occupational and Environmental Medicine* 55(6): 393-400.

Hesterberg TW, Miller WC, Mast R, McConnell EE, Bernstein DM, Anderson R. 1994. Relationship between lung biopersistence and biological effects of man-made vitreous fibers after chronic inhalation in rats. *Environmental Health Perspectives* 102 (Supplement 5): 133-137.

Hesterberg TW, Miller WC, McConnell EE, Chevalier J, Hadley JG, Bernstein DM, Thevenaz P, Anderson R. 1993. Chronic inhalation toxicity of size-separated glass fibers in Fischer 344 rats. *Fundamental and Applied Toxicology* 20(4): 464-476.

Hughes JM, Weill H, Hammad YY. 1987. Mortality of workers employed in two asbestos cement manufacturing plants. *British Journal of Industrial Medicine* 44(3): 161-174.

IARC (International Agency for Research on Cancer). 1995. *Wood Dust and Formaldehyde.* IARC Monograph on the Evaluation of Carcinogenic Risks to Humans. Volume 84. Lyon, France: World Health Organization. Pp. 282-294.

Jemal A, Siegel R, Ward E, Murray T, Xu J, Smigal C, Thun M. 2006. Cancer statistics, 2006. *CA: A Cancer Journal for Clinicians* 56: 106-130.

Lefebvre JL, Chevalier D, Luboinski B, Kirkpatrick A, Collette L, Sahmoud T. 1996. Larynx preservation in pyriform sinus cancer: Preliminary results of a European Organization for Research and Treatment of Cancer phase III trial. *Journal of the National Cancer Institute* 88(13): 890-899.

Levin J, McLarty J, Hurst GA, Smith A, Frank AL. 1998. Tyler asbestos workers: Mortality experience in a cohort exposed to amosite. *Occupational and Environmental Medicine* 55(3): 155-160.

Luce D, Bugel I, Goldberg P, Goldberg M, Salomon C, Billon-Galland MA, Nicolau J, Quenel P, Fevotte J, Brochard P. 2000. Environmental exposure to tremolite and respiratory cancer in New Caledonia: A case-control study. *American Journal of Epidemiology* 151(3): 259-265.

Marchand JL, Luce D, Leclerc A, Goldberg P, Orlowski E, Bugel I, Brugere J. 2000. Laryngeal and hypopharyngeal cancer and occupational exposure to asbestos and man-made vitreous fibers: Results of a case-control study. *American Journal of Industrial Medicine* 37(6): 581-589.

McConnell EE. 2005 (October 27). *Personal Communication to Mary Paxton for the Committee on Asbestos: Selected Health Effects.* Available in IOM Public Access Files.

McConnell E, Kamstrup O, Musselman R, Hesterberg T, Chevalier J, Miller W, Thevenaz P. 1994a. Chronic inhalation study of size-separated rock and slag wool insulation fibers in Fischer 344/N rats. *Inhalation Toxicology* 6(6): 571-614.

McConnell E, Mast R, Hesterberg T, Chevalier J, Kotin P, Bernstein D, Thevenaz P, Glass L, Anderson R. 1994b. Chronic inhalation toxicity of a kaolin-based refactory cermaic fiber in Syrian golden hamsters. *Inhalation Toxicology* 6(6): 503-532.

McConnell EE, Axten C, Hesterberg TW, Chevalier J, Miller WC, Everitt J, Oberdorster G, Chase GR, Thevenaz P, Kotin P. 1999. Studies on the inhalation toxicology of two fiberglasses and amosite asbestos in the Syrian golden hamster: Part II. Results of chronic exposure. *Inhalation Toxicology* 11(9): 785-835.

Merletti F, Boffetta P, Ferro G, Pisani P, Terracini B. 1991. Occupation and cancer of the oral cavity or oropharynx in Turin, Italy. *Scandinavian Journal of Work, Environment and Health* 17(4): 248-254.

Meurman LO, Pukkala E, Hakama M. 1994. Incidence of cancer among anthophyllite asbestos miners in Finland. *Occupational and Environmental Medicine* 51(6): 421-425.

Miller BA, Kolonel LN, Bernstein L, Young JL Jr, Swanson GM, West D, Key CR, Liff JM, Glover, Alexander GA (eds). 1996. *Racial/Ethnic Patterns of Cancer in the United States 1988-1992.* (NIH publication no. 96-4104). Bethesda, Maryland: National Cancer Institute.

Mueller N. 1995. Overview: Viral agents and cancer. *Environmental Health Perspectives* 103 (Supplement 8): 259-261.

Parnes SM. 1990. Asbestos and cancer of the larynx: Is there a relationship? *Laryngoscope* 100(3): 254-261.

Pfister DG, Hu KS, Lefebvre JL. 2004. Cancer of the hypopharynx and cervical esophagus. In: *Head and Neck Cancer: A Multidisciplinary Approach.* 2nd edition. Baltimore, MD: Lippincott Williams and Wilkins. Pp. 404-454.

Piolatto G, Negri E, La Vecchia C, Pira E, Decarli A, Peto J. 1990. An update of cancer mortality among chrysotile asbestos miners in Balangero, northern Italy. *British Journal of Industrial Medicine* 47(12): 810-814.

Pira E, Pelucchi C, Buffoni L, Palmas A, Turbiglio M, Negri E, Piolatto PG, La Vecchia C. 2005. Cancer mortality in a cohort of asbestos textile workers. *British Journal of Cancer* 92(3): 580-586.

Puntoni R, Merlo F, Borsa L, Reggiardo G, Garrone E, Ceppi M. 2001. A historical cohort mortality study among shipyard workers in Genoa, Italy. *American Journal of Industrial Medicine* 40(4): 363-370.

Raffn E, Lynge E, Juel K, Korsgaard B. 1989. Incidence of cancer and mortality among employees in the asbestos cement industry in Denmark. *British Journal of Industrial Medicine* 46(2): 90-96.

Reid A, Ambrosini G, de Klerk N, Fritschi L, Musk B. 2004. Aerodigestive and gastrointestinal tract cancers and exposure to crocidolite (blue asbestos): Incidence and mortality among former crocidolite workers. *International Journal of Cancer* 111(5): 757-761.

Selikoff IJ, Seidman H. 1991. Asbestos-associated deaths among insulation workers in the United States and Canada, 1967-1987. *Annals of the New York Academy of Sciences* 643: 1-14.

Sluis-Cremer GK, Liddell FD, Logan WP, Bezuidenhout BN. 1992. The mortality of amphibole miners in South Africa, 1946-80. *British Journal of Industrial Medicine* 49(8): 566-575.

Zheng W, Blot WJ, Shu XO, Diamond EL, Gao YT, Ji BT, Fraumeni JF Jr. 1992. Risk factors for oral and pharyngeal cancer in Shanghai, with emphasis on diet. *Cancer Epidemiology, Biomarkers and Prevention* 1(6): 441-448.

8

Laryngeal Cancer and Asbestos

NATURE OF THIS CANCER TYPE

The larynx, commonly known as the voice box or Adam's apple, is above the trachea and below the pharynx (Figures 7.1 and 8.1). It includes three anatomic subsites: the *glottis*, including the vocal fold or vocal cords, depicted near the middle of Figure 8.1; the *supraglottis*, which encompasses all tissues above the vocal folds and below the pharynx and includes the epiglottis, a fold that closes the larynx during swallowing to prevent food inhalation; and the *subglottis*, or area below the vocal fold.

The American Cancer Society (Jemal et al. 2006) has estimated that about 9,510 new cases of and 3,740 deaths from cancer of the larynx (ICD-9 161; ICD-O C32.0-C32.9) will occur in 2006. Laryngeal cancer ranks 16th in incidence and mortality among men in the United States, and 28th and 25th in incidence and mortality, respectively, among women. Both incidence and mortality are more than 4 times higher in men than women and are higher among blacks than whites, especially in men. The risk of developing laryngeal cancer increases with age. However, the incidence of laryngeal cancer, adjusted for age, has decreased by an average of 2.6% per year since 1988.

Most cancers of the larynx are squamous-cell carcinomas that arise from the thin, flat cells (squamous cells) that line the upper airway. Those tumors, like squamous-cell carcinomas of the oral cavity and pharynx, develop gradually as normal cells develop into clones of progressively abnormal cells. As the clones accumulate genetic damage, some may undergo malignant transformation, first into carcinoma in situ, and later into inva-

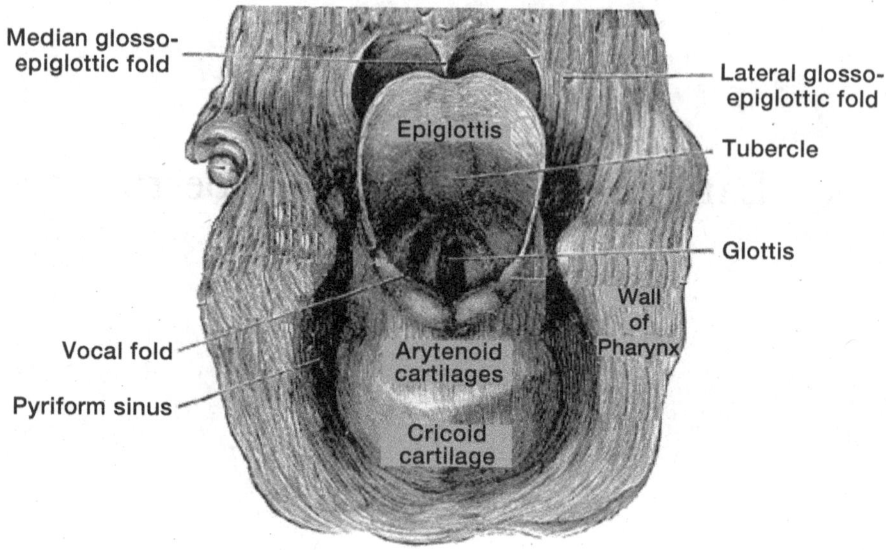

FIGURE 8.1 Larynx viewed from behind.
SOURCE: Modified from *Grey's Anatomy of the Human Body*. Available at http://www.bartleby.com/107/236.html.

sive cancer. Premalignant lesions often regress after the discontinuation of tobacco use and alcohol consumption.

The most important risk factors for laryngeal cancer are tobacco-smoking (all forms) (IARC 2004) and heavy consumption of alcohol, especially when drinking and smoking occur in combination (IARC 1988). Cancer of the larynx is rare in lifelong nonsmokers, even though nonsmoking drinkers have been reported to have increased risk (Burch et al. 1981, Elwood et al. 1984). Risk increases with the number of cigarettes smoked per day and duration of smoking. The independent effect of tobacco on laryngeal cancer is greater than that of alcohol consumption. The effects of occupation on the risk of laryngeal cancer have been difficult to study, because of the powerful relationship of this cancer with tobacco use and alcohol consumption, and the little information on alcohol consumption and tobacco use in many occupational studies. Exposure to strong sulfuric acid mist is an established cause of laryngeal cancer (IARC 1987). Other factors that may increase risk, but on which current data are limited, include exposure to mustard gas (HHS 2004), steam and fumes from isopropyl alcohol (IARC 1987), metalworking fluids (Eisen et al. 1994, Zeka et al. 2004), and chronic infection with human papilloma virus (Rees et al. 2004).

The combination of tobacco-smoking and heavy drinking causes a much larger increase in laryngeal cancer risk than would be expected from the sum of the relative risk (RR) estimates associated with the separate exposures. For example, a study of laryngeal cancer published in 1976 (Wynder and Hoffmann 1976) found that, compared with men who neither smoked nor drank, those who reported both smoking (35 or more cigarettes per day) and drinking (seven or more alcoholic drinks per day) had an RR of 22.1 (95% confidence interval [CI] 7.8-62.1). Smoking alone was associated with an RR of 7.0 (95% CI 2.5-19.4), whereas the RR of this level of alcohol consumption alone could not be calculated because of the absence of cases. That study, conducted during the period when many studied occupational populations were experiencing exposure to asbestos, illustrates the strength of the association of laryngeal cancer with smoking and drinking.

EPIDEMIOLOGIC EVIDENCE CONSIDERED

The association between asbestos exposure and cancer of the larynx has been examined in many cohort and case-control studies. As discussed previously, the major strengths of the occupational cohort studies are that the magnitudes and durations of asbestos exposure tend to be substantially higher and the exposure information better documented than in case-control studies of the general population. Most of the cohort studies address death from laryngeal cancer—an imperfect surrogate of incidence because survival of laryngeal cancer is high. The case-control studies are also important with respect to laryngeal cancer because their analyses are based on incident cases rather than deaths; the number of cases is larger, thus providing greater statistical power; and some of the case-control studies collect information that can be used to adjust for or stratify on tobacco or alcohol use.

Cohort Studies

The cohorts that presented usable information about the risk of laryngeal cancer and their design properties are described in Table B.1, and the details of their results concerning cancer at this site are abstracted in Table D.2. The results of the cohort and case-control studies are summarized in Table 8.1, and Figures 8.2 and 8.3 are plots of RRs for overall exposure and for exposure-response gradients from the cohort studies reviewed.

The committee identified and included in its analyses 35 cohort populations from 29 published papers that examined the RR of a diagnosis of or death from laryngeal cancer among among people with any occupational exposure to asbestos compared with people in the general population with-

TABLE 8.1 Summary of Epidemiologic Findings Regarding Cancer of the Larynx

Study Type	Figure	Comparison	Study Populations Included	No. Study Populations	Summary RR (95% CI)	Between-Study SD
Cohort	8.2	Any vs none	All	35	1.40 (1.19-1.64)	—
	8.3	High vs none[a]	Lower bound[b]	11	2.02 (1.64-2.47)	—
			Upper bound[b]	11	2.57 (1.47-4.49)	—
Case-control	8.4	Any vs none	All	15	1.43 (1.15-1.78)	0.27
	8.5	Any vs none	EAM = 1	10	1.21 (1.04-1.40)	0.02
			EAM = 2	5	2.56 (1.20-5.43)	0.65
	8.6	Any vs none	EAM = 1 Adjusted[c]	7	1.18 (1.01-1.37)	0.00
			EAM = 1 Unadjusted[c]	3	1.58 (0.86-2.91)	0.27
	8.7	High vs none[a]	EAM = 1 Lower bound[b]	7	1.38 (1.02-1.86)	0.27
			EAM = 1 Upper bound[b]	7	1.53 (1.21-1.93)	0.07

NOTE: CI = Confidence interval; EAM = exposure-assessment method; high quality, EAM = 1; lower quality, EAM = 2; RR = relative risk; SD = standard deviation.

[a]Used studies that reported dose-response relationship (RR on an exposure gradient).
[b]Some studies reported dose-response relationship on multiple gradient metrics. In computing the summary RR, "lower bound" calculation used the smallest "high vs none" RR, and "upper bound" calculation used largest "high vs none" RR.
[c]Adjusted: RR was adjusted for both smoking and alcohol use.

out such exposure (Table D.2 and Figure 8.2). Other reports were not included in the analysis, because they were superseded by later reports based on longer follow-up of the same cohort (e.g., Clemmensen and Hjalgrim-Jensen 1981; McDonald et al. 1986, 1993; Rubino et al. 1979), were not primarily asbestos cohorts (e.g., Magnani et al. 1986, Imbernon et al. 1995),

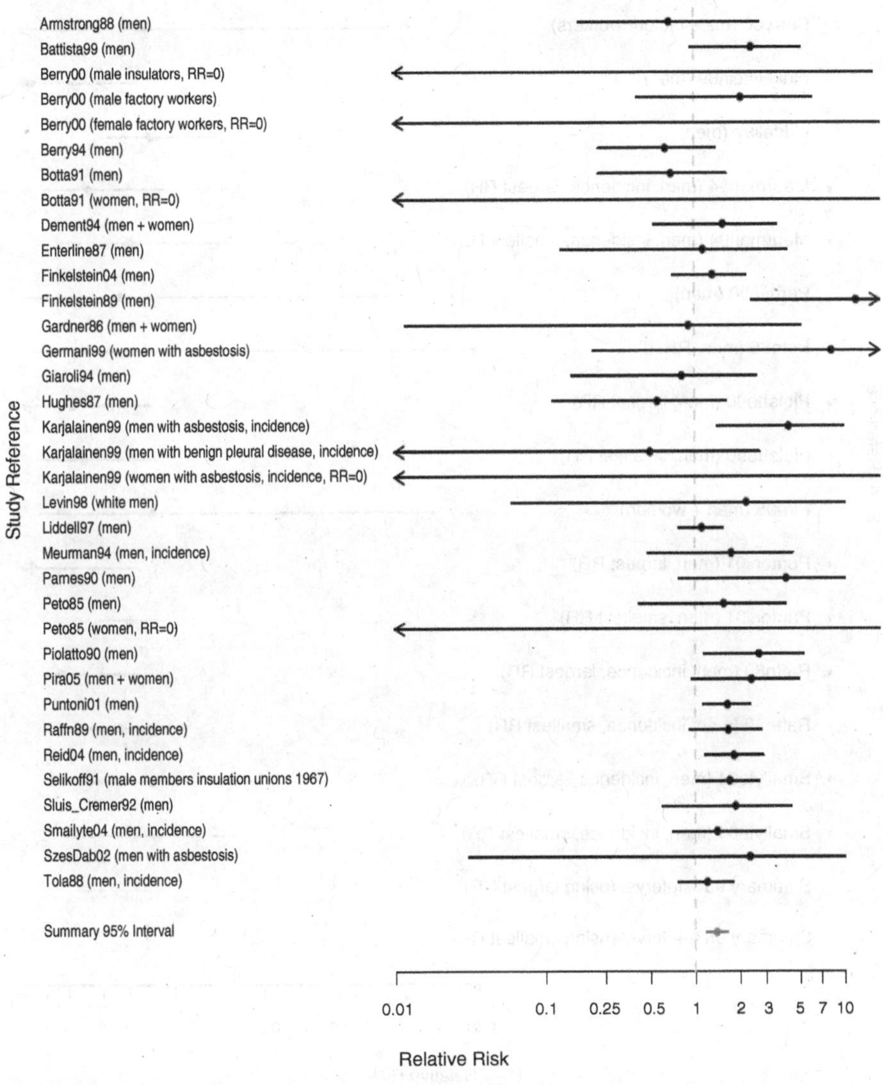

FIGURE 8.2 Cohort studies: RR of laryngeal cancer in people with "any" exposure to asbestos compared with people who report none.

did not specify the standardized mortality ratio or expected number of cases of laryngeal cancer (e.g., Djerassi et al. 1979; McDonald et al. 1983, 1984; Zhu and Wang 1993), or did not report the larynx as a separate cancer site (e.g., Seidman et al. 1986, Selikoff et al. 1979).

Figure 8.2 shows the RR estimates and 95% CI estimates in 34 cohort

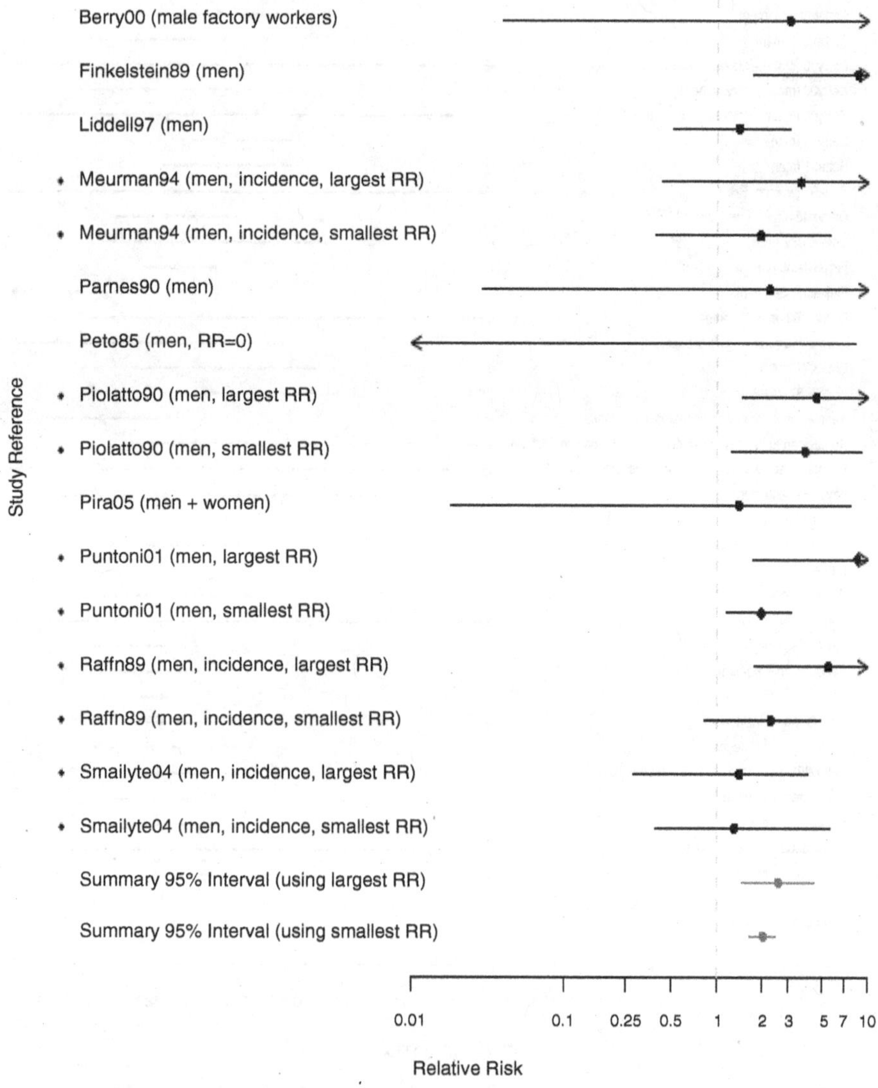

FIGURE 8.3 Cohort studies: RRs of laryngeal cancer among people in most extreme exposure category compared with those with no exposure (♦ = more than one exposure gradient reported in citation, so the plot contains both highest and lowest estimates of risk at most extreme category over all gradients).

study populations that reported "any" occupational exposure to asbestos, compared with unexposed subjects. The cohorts were drawn from a wide array of industries, including mining, textiles, and insulation. Five of the studies (Karjalainen et al. 1999, Meurman et al. 1994, Raffn et al. 1989, Reid et al. 2004, Smailyte et al. 2004) compared the incidence of laryngeal cancer in exposed and unexposed subjects; the remainder assessed mortality. The number of cases or deaths in the reports ranged from 1 (Gardner and Powell 1986, Germani et al. 1999, Szeszenia-Dabrowska et al. 2002) to 36 (Liddell et al. 1997). The RR estimates exceeded 1.0 in all cohorts with 10 or more cases of or deaths from laryngeal cancer (Finkelstein and Verma 2004, Liddell et al. 1997, Puntoni et al. 2001, Raffn et al. 1989, Reid et al. 2004, Selikoff and Hammond 1978, Selikoff and Seidman 1991, Tola et al. 1988) and in the largest study of patients with asbestosis (Karjalainen et al. 1999). Some of the heterogeneity seen in Figure 8.2 reflects the statistical imprecision of subgroup analyses, especially for women. The combined RR associated with any occupational exposure to asbestos (Figure 8.2) was 1.40 (95% CI 1.19-1.64).

Further analyses examined whether the association between asbestos exposure and laryngeal cancer was stronger among the most highly exposed subjects in a subset of 11 cohorts in which this information was available. The analysis was done in several ways to take account of the multiple indexes used by many of the studies to define the intensity or duration of exposure (duration of employment, cumulative exposure, peak exposure, probability of exposure, and so on). We plotted the highest and lowest RRs for subjects who were in one of the "most exposed" categories by any definition. Figure 8.3 presents the plots for the 11 cohorts in which this information was available. In each of the individual cohorts, the RR estimates exceeded 1.0. The aggregate RR estimate in the most highly exposed subjects was 2.57 (95% CI 1.47-4.49) for the strongest association reported and 2.02 (95% CI 1.64-2.47) for the weakest association reported; both are higher than the combined estimate associated with any exposure to asbestos 1.40 (95% CI 1.19-1.64).

Our last approach in assessing the cohort studies of asbestos exposure in relation to laryngeal-cancer risk was to examine the association in cohorts with extremely high exposure to asbestos, such as the patients with asbestosis studied by Karjalainen et al. (1999). The standardized incidence ratios (SIRs) of mesothelioma (RR = 32, 95% CI 14.4-60.0) and of lung cancer (RR = 6.7, 95%CI 5.6-7.9) were significantly increased in this cohort, compared with the incidence in the general population of Finland. The SIR of laryngeal cancer was also increased (RR = 4.2, 95% CI 1.4-9.8) in men but not women.

In summary, the larger cohort studies consistently show increased risk of laryngeal cancer in asbestos-exposed workers employed in a wide array of industries and in a large cohort of workers with asbestosis. There is some evidence of a dose-response relationship in the meta-analyses.

Case-Control Studies

The case-control studies of laryngeal cancer that were retained for thorough evaluation after exclusion of studies that did not assess exposure to asbestos or did not meet other exclusion criteria are listed in Table 6.5 according to quality of their exposure assessment. The details of the design aspects of those studies are presented in Table C.1 and their detailed results are abstracted in Table E.2. The findings of the studies are summarized in Table 8.1 and in the plots presented in Figures 8.4-8.7.

The committee identified 18 published case-control studies that provide data on the association between risk of laryngeal cancer and exposure to asbestos or any employment in an occupation or industry where asbestos exposure was known to occur. The studies involved from 20 cases (Luce et al. 2000) to 940 cases (Elci et al. 2002). Seven of the studies had 200 or more subjects (Berrino et al. 2003, Deitz et al. 2002, Elci et al. 2002, Marchand et al. 2000, Olsen and Sabroe 1984, Wortley et al. 1992, Zheng et al. 1992), while seven more included at least 100 (Ahrens et al. 1991, Brown et al. 1988, Burch et al. 1981, De Stefani et al. 1998, Gustavsson et al. 1998, Muscat and Wynder 1992, Stell and McGill 1973). Over 97% of cases in these studies were male. The male predominance reflects the facts that about 80% of laryngeal cancers occur in men and that occupational exposures to asbestos typically occur in trades where nearly all workers have been men.

Figure 8.4 provides the RR or odds ratio estimates associated with reporting "any" exposure to asbestos in 15 studies that compared subjects with any occupational exposure to those with no exposure to asbestos. Three case-control studies are excluded from this analysis (Berrino et al. 2000, Gustavsson et al. 1998, Wortley et al. 1992), because they present results for larynx only in relation to dose. Only one (Luce et al. 2000) of the 15 studies included in Figure 8.5 has an RR estimate below 1.0. The meta-analysis, combining 15 studies, found an RR of 1.43 (95% CI 1.15-1.78) associated with "any" exposure to asbestos.

To assess whether the association between asbestos exposure and risk of laryngeal cancer was stronger in studies with higher exposure information, the committee separated the studies into those with better measures of exposure and those with more limited data, as shown in Figure 8.5. The RR from the combined analysis of 10 studies with higher-quality exposure information was 1.21 (95% CI 1.04-1.40). Among the studies considered to have more limited information on asbestos exposure were two (Shettigara and Morgan 1975, Stell and McGill 1973) in which the association with

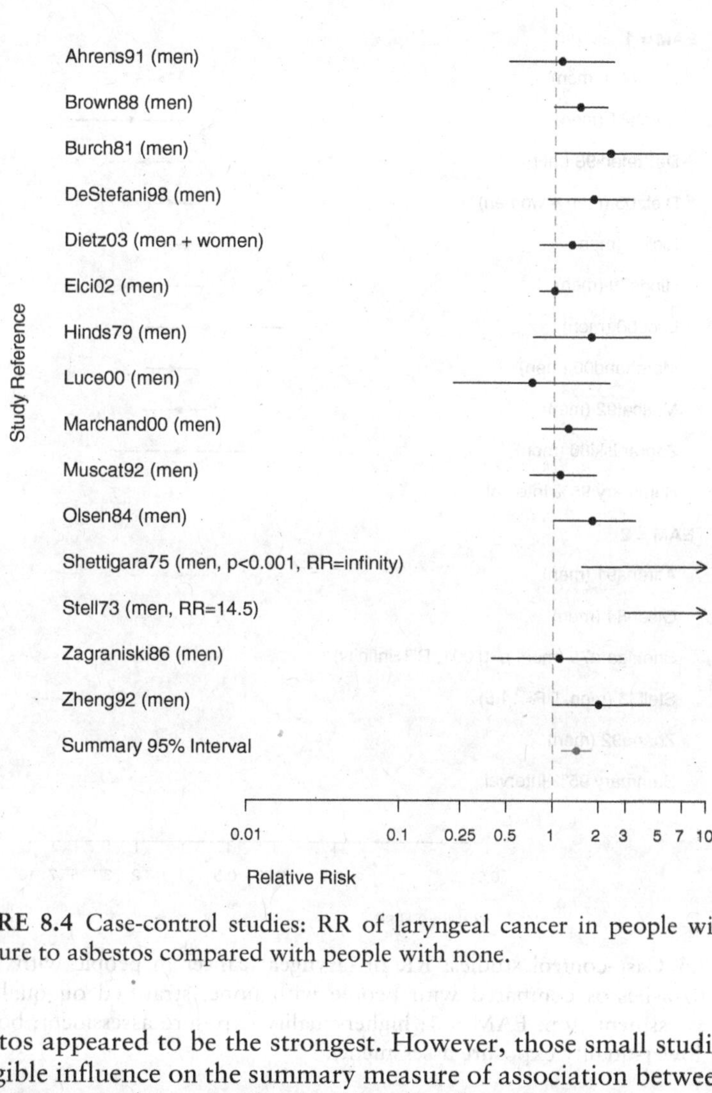

FIGURE 8.4 Case-control studies: RR of laryngeal cancer in people with "any" exposure to asbestos compared with people with none.

asbestos appeared to be the strongest. However, those small studies had a negligible influence on the summary measure of association between asbestos exposure and increased risk of laryngeal cancer. The association persisted with or without the inclusion of studies with weaker exposure data.

Most of the case-control studies made some attempt to control for tobacco and alcohol consumption in examining the association between asbestos exposure and laryngeal cancer. Two of the studies whose results are presented in Figure 8.6 with adjustment for those risk factors also gave unadjusted estimates in the citation. In Dietz et al. (2004), the association between asbestos exposure and laryngeal cancer was weakened by controlling for other covariates; but in Brown et al. (1988), controlling for tobacco

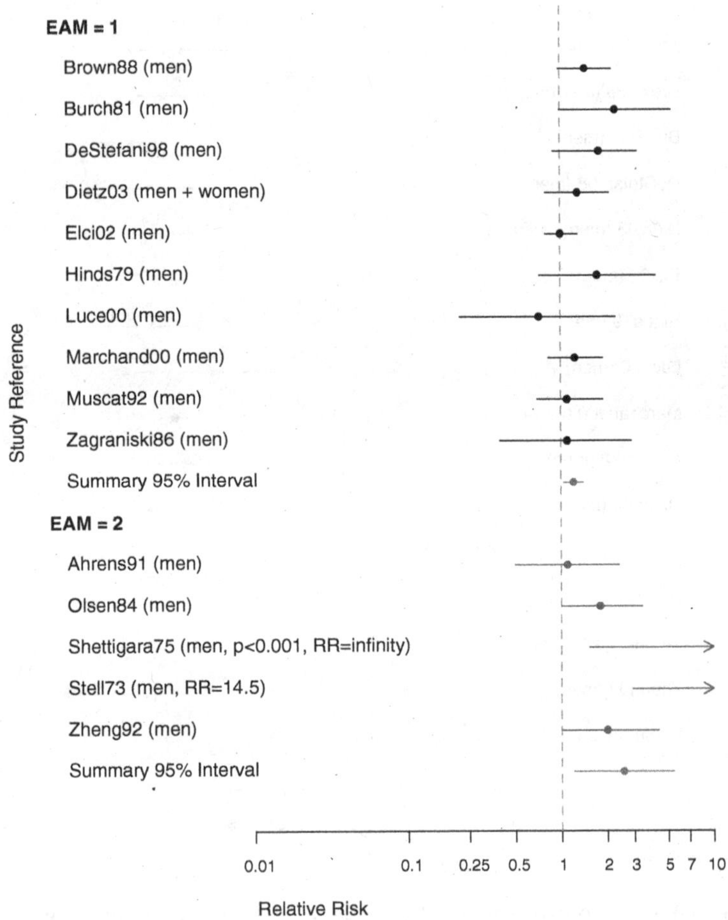

FIGURE 8.5 Case-control studies: RR of laryngeal cancer in people with "any" exposure to asbestos compared with people with none, stratified on quality of exposure assessment (top, EAM = 1: higher-quality exposure assessment; bottom, EAM = 2: lower-quality exposure assessment).

use and alcohol consumption made little difference. Overall, with adjustment for the other two prominent risk factors for laryngeal cancer, an association with asbestos exposure appears to persist (RR = 1.18, 95% CI 1.01-1.37). Given the propensity that has been demonstrated for smoking to act as an effect modifier in lung cancer rather than merely as a simple additive factor, however, it may be more appropriate to consider stratified analyses than adjusted multivariate findings.

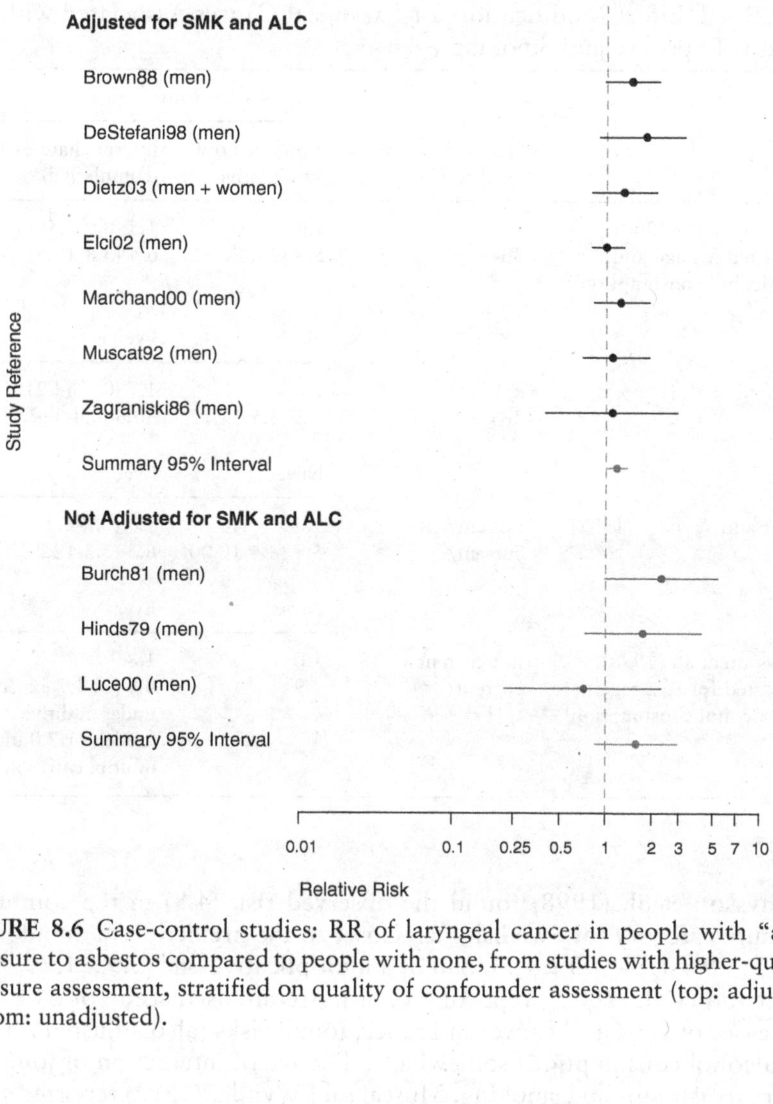

FIGURE 8.6 Case-control studies: RR of laryngeal cancer in people with "any" exposure to asbestos compared to people with none, from studies with higher-quality exposure assessment, stratified on quality of confounder assessment (top: adjusted; bottom: unadjusted).

Five of the case-control studies presented results stratified by tobacco or alcohol consumption and allowed limited consideration of whether asbestos exposure might modify the laryngeal carcinogenicity of tobacco or alcohol exposure (Burch et al. 1981, De Stefani et al. 1998, Gustavsson et al. 1998, Marchand et al. 2000, Muscat and Wynder 1992). The information presented in Burch et al. (1981) did not conform to a tabular presentation, but the results from the others are abstracted in Table 8.2.

TABLE 8.2 Effect Modification for Laryngeal Cancer Associated with Asbestos Exposure and Smoking

Study	Smoking History (pack-years)	Asbestos Exposure: None or Low (cumulative)	Asbestos Exposure: Intermediate or High (cumulative)
Marchand et al. (2000) (adjusted for age and for alcohol consumption)	<30	1.0	1.5 (0.9-2.5)
	30+	5.3 (3.2-8.8)	6.5 (3.8-10.8)
		Never	Ever
De Stefani et al. (1998)	≤ 35	1.0	1.7 (0.2-14.2)
	36+	6.2 (3.5-11.1)	30.6 (8.4-112.1)
		Never	Ever
Muscat and Wynder (1992)	not current	1.0	1.3 (0.7-2.4)
	current	5.8 (3.4-10.00	6.3 (3.3-12.2)
		Never	Ever
Gustavsson et al. (1998) (adjusted for age, region, and alcohol consumption)	not current	1.0	1.8
	current	3.9	4.8 [vs 4.7 expected under additive model; or 7.0 under multiplicative model]

Gustavsson et al. (1998) found the observed risk (4.8) in the combined exposure category for Swedish men closer to the prediction of an additive model (3.9 + 1.7 – 1.0 = 4.7) than of a multiplicative one (3.9 × 1.7 = 7.0). Marchand et al. (2000), reporting on a hospital-based study of 315 incident cases of laryngeal cancer in France, found risks (also adjusted for age and alcohol consumption) somewhat indicative of interaction of joint exposure to asbestos and smoking. Muscat and Wynder (1992) reported similar results in a hospital-based study of 194 white males in the United States. De Stefani et al. (1998), however, found a much stronger association with having "ever" been exposed to asbestos among Uruguayan heavy smokers than in asbestos-exposed men who had not smoked as much. A limitation of all of those studies is that, although the risk was higher among men who were exposed than those who were not unexposed to asbestos, the data were not stratified into narrowly defined combinations of asbestos exposure, tobacco-smoking, and alcohol consumption.

As in the analyses of cohort studies, the committee examined the risks in the extreme categories of exposure-related gradients (longest duration, highest probability of exposure, cumulative exposure, and so on) in the case-control studies. As depicted in Figure 8.7, the aggregate results for the weakest (RR = 1.38, 95% CI 1.02-1.86) and the strongest (RR = 1.53, 95% CI 1.21-1.93) reported associations for extreme exposure groups were both higher than the aggregated estimate for subjects with any exposure to asbestos in the studies with more reliable exposure assessment (top of Figure 8.5), and this a suggests of dose-response relationship.

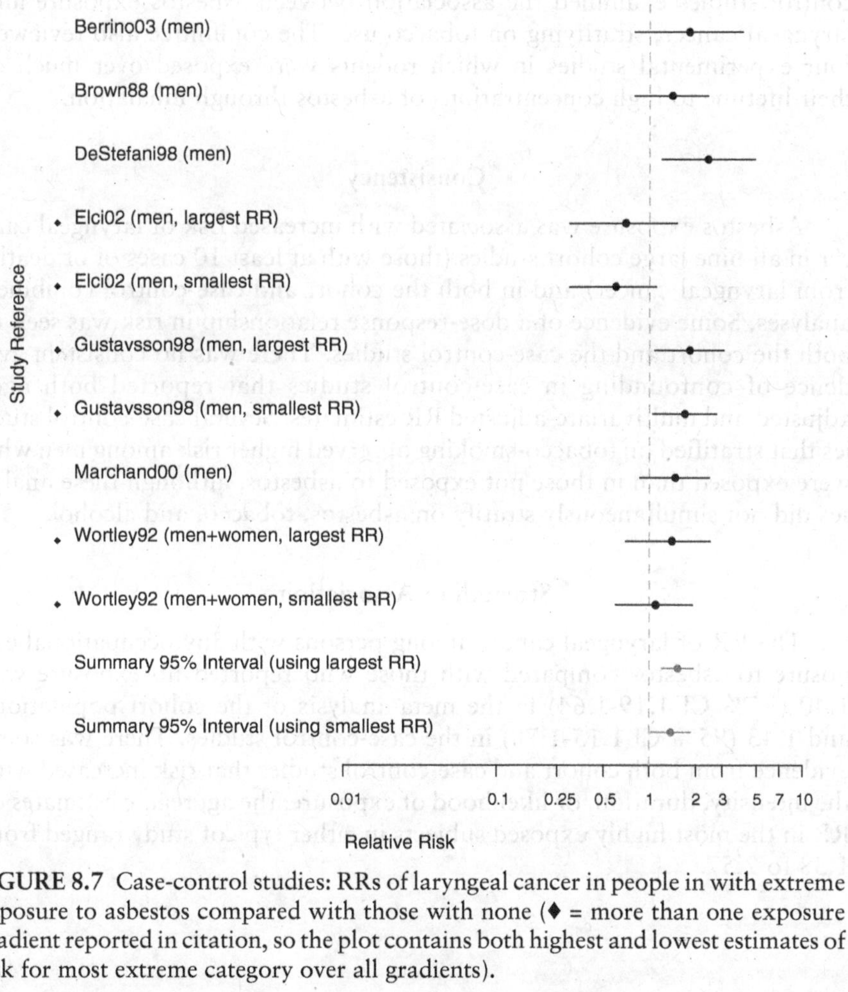

FIGURE 8.7 Case-control studies: RRs of laryngeal cancer in people in with extreme exposure to asbestos compared with those with none (♦ = more than one exposure gradient reported in citation, so the plot contains both highest and lowest estimates of risk for most extreme category over all gradients).

EVIDENCE INTERGRATION AND CONCLUSION

Evidence Considered

The evidence base included a larger number of epidemiologic studies of asbestos exposure and laryngeal cancer, particularly of the case-control design, than were available for other cancer sites. The committee reviewed the results on 35 cohort populations and 18 case-control studies. Subjects in the studies had been exposed to asbestos in a wide array of industries and occupations in North America, South America, Europe, and Japan. Many of the case-control studies collected some data with which to control for confounding by tobacco-smoking and alcohol consumption. Several case-control studies examined the association between asbestos exposure and laryngeal cancer, stratifying on tobacco use. The committee also reviewed four experimental studies in which rodents were exposed over much of their lifetime to high concentrations of asbestos through inhalation.

Consistency

Asbestos exposure was associated with increased risk of laryngeal cancer in all nine large cohort studies (those with at least 10 cases of or deaths from laryngeal cancer) and in both the cohort and case-control combined analyses. Some evidence of a dose-response relationship in risk was seen in both the cohort and the case-control studies. There was no consistent evidence of confounding in case-control studies that reported both age-adjusted and multivariate-adjusted RR estimates. Several case-control studies that stratified on tobacco-smoking observed higher risk among men who were exposed than in those not exposed to asbestos, although these analyses did not simultaneously stratify on asbestos, tobacco, and alcohol.

Strength of Association

The RR of laryngeal cancer among persons with any occupational exposure to asbestos compared with those who reported no exposure was 1.40 (95% CI 1.19-1.64) in the meta-analysis of the cohort populations and 1.43 (95% CI 1.15-1.78) in the case-control studies. There was some evidence from both cohort and case-control studies that risk increased with the intensity, duration, or likelihood of exposure; the aggregate estimates of RR in the most highly exposed subjects in either type of study ranged from 1.38 to 2.57.

Coherence

Several factors contribute to the biologic plausibility that asbestos may cause cancer of the larynx. The larynx, like the lung, is anatomically in the direct path of inhaled asbestos fibers. Inflammation or damage of the vocal folds could disrupt laminar airflow and predispose to the deposition and accumulation of asbestos fibers in the larynx. Squamous-cell carcinomas of the lung and larynx have histologic and clinical similarities. Cancers at both sites arise from the respiratory epithelium in regions of squamous metaplasia and dysplasia. Tobacco-smoking is the most important risk factor for both sites. Asbestos exposure is an established cause of lung cancer. On the basis of theoretical considerations, tobacco-smoking, alone or in combination with alcohol consumption, may predispose to the accumulation of asbestos fibers in the epithelial lining of the larynx. Aerodynamic turbulence at bifurcations of the large conducting airways is known to contribute to the deposition of long asbestos fibers in the lung (Asgharian and Yu 1988). Bronchogenic carcinomas commonly arise in those areas (Schlesinger and Lippmann 1978). The accumulation of asbestos fibers, together with smoking and/or drinking, could produce chronic irritation or inflammation and thus accelerates the progression of neoplasia.

The committee identified and considered several limitations in the evidence related to biologic plausibility. Foremost were the absence of clinical data documenting that asbestos fibers accumulate and persist in the larynx and the lack of experimental support from animal studies. The presence or absence of asbestos fibers in laryngeal tissue from occupationally exposed people has been investigated in only a few studies, in which contamination from other tissues is always a concern; Roggli et al. (1980) reported asbestos bodies and Kambic et al. (1989) reported fibers in this anatomic area. Studies in rats and Syrian hamsters found that asbestos inhalation, at levels sufficient to cause mesothelioma in both species and lung cancer in rats, did not induce chronic inflammation or increase cancer of the larynx (Hesterberg et al. 1993, 1994; McConnell 2005; McConnell et al. 1994a,b, 1999). These rodent models do not, however, reflect exposure to cofactors, such as tobacco-smoking and alcohol consumption, which may affect fiber deposition and/or persistence that may exacerbate local tissue injury and inflammation.

Conclusion

Considering all lines of evidence, the committee placed greater weight on the consistency of the epidemiologic studies and the biologic plausibility of the hypothesis than on the lack of confirmatory evidence from animal studies or documentation of fiber deposition in the larynx. The committee concluded that the evidence is *sufficient* to infer a causal relationship between asbestos exposure and laryngeal cancer.

REFERENCES

Ahrens W, Jockel K, Patzak W, Elsner G. 1991. Alcohol, smoking, and occupational factors in cancer of the larynx: A case-control study. *American Journal of Industrial Medicine* 20(4): 477-493.

Armstrong BK, de Klerk NH, Musk AW, Hobbs MS. 1988. Mortality in miners and millers of crocidolite in Western Australia. *British Journal of Industrial Medicine* 45(1): 5-13.

Asgharian B, Yu C. 1988. Deposition of inhaled fibrous particles in the human lung. *Journal of Aerosol Medicine* 1: 37-50.

Battista G, Belli S, Comba P, Fiumalbi C, Grignoli M, Loi F, Orsi D, Paredes I. 1999. Mortality due to asbestos-related causes among railway carriage construction and repair workers. *Occupation Medicine (London)* 49(8): 536-539.

Berrino F, Richiardi L, Boffetta P, Esteve J, Belletti I, Raymond L, Troschel L, Pisani P, Zubiri L, Ascunce N, Guberan E, Tuyns A, Terracini B, Merletti F. 2003. Occupation and larynx and hypopharynx cancer: A job-exposure matrix approach in an international case-control study in France, Italy, Spain and Switzerland. *Cancer Causes and Control* 14(3): 213-223.

Berry G. 1994. Mortality and cancer incidence of workers exposed to chrysotile asbestos in the friction-products industry. *Annals of Occupational Hygiene* 38(4): 539-546.

Berry G, Newhouse ML, Wagner JC. 2000. Mortality from all cancers of asbestos factory workers in east London 1933-1980. *Occupational and Environmental Medicine* 57(11): 782-785.

Botta M, Magnani C, Terracini B, Bertolone GP, Castagneto B, Cocito V, DeGiovanni D, Paglieri P. 1991. Mortality from respiratory and digestive cancers among asbestos cement workers in Italy. *Cancer Detection and Prevention* 15(6): 445-447.

Brown LM, Mason TJ, Pickle LW, Stewart PA, Buffler PA, Burau K, Ziegler RG, Fraumeni JF Jr. 1988. Occupational risk factors for laryngeal cancer on the Texas Gulf Coast. *Cancer Research* 48(7): 1960-1964.

Burch JD, Howe GR, Miller AB, Semenciw R. 1981. Tobacco, alcohol, asbestos, and nickel in the etiology of cancer of the larynx: A case-control study. *Journal of the National Cancer Institute* 67(6): 1219-1224.

Clemmensen J, Hjalgrim-Jensen S. 1981. Cancer incidence among 5686 asbestos-cement workers followed from 1943 through 1976. *Ecotoxicology Environment Safety* 5(1): 15-23.

De Stefani E, Boffetta P, Oreggia F, Ronco A, Kogevinas M, Mendilaharsu M. 1998. Occupation and the risk of laryngeal cancer in Uruguay. *American Journal of Industrial Medicine* 33(6): 537-542.

Dement JM, Brown DP, Okun A. 1994. Follow-up study of chrysotile asbestos textile workers: Cohort mortality and case-control analyses. *American Journal of Industrial Medicine* 26(4): 431-447.

Dietz A, Ramroth H, Urban T, Ahrens W, Becher H. 2004. Exposure to cement dust, related occupational groups and laryngeal cancer risk: Results of a population based case-control study. *International Journal of Cancer* 108(6): 907-911.

Djerassi L, Kaufmann G, Bar-Nets M. 1979. Malignant disease and environmental control in an asbestos cement plant. *Annals of the New York Academy of Sciences* 330: 243-253.

Eisen EA, Tolbert PE, Hallock MF, Monson RR, Smith TJ, Woskie SR.1994. Mortality studies of machining fluid exposure in the automobile industry: III. A case-control study of larynx cancer. *American Journal of Industrial Medicine* 26(2): 185-202.

Elci OC, Akpinar-Elci M, Blair A, Dosemeci M. 2002. Occupational dust exposure and the risk of laryngeal cancer in Turkey. *Scandinavian Journal of Work, Environment and Health* 28(4): 278-284.

Elwood JM, Pearson JC, Skippen DH, Jackson SM. 1984. Alcohol, smoking, social and occupational factors in the aetiology of cancer of the oral cavity, pharynx and larynx. *International Journal of Cancer* 34(5): 603-612.

Enterline PE, Hartley J, Henderson V. 1987. Asbestos and cancer: A cohort followed up to death. *British Journal of Industrial Medicine* 44(6): 396-401.

Finkelstein MM. 1989. Mortality rates among employees potentially exposed to chrysotile asbestos at two automotive parts factories. *Canadian Medical Association Journal* 141(2): 125-130.

Finkelstein MM, Verma DK. 2004. A cohort study of mortality among Ontario pipe trades workers. *Occupational and Environmental Medicine* 61(9): 736-742.

Gardner MJ, Powell CA. 1986. Mortality of asbestos cement workers using almost exclusively chrysotile fibre. *Journal of the Society of Occupational Medicine* 36(4): 124-126.

Germani D, Belli S, Bruno C, Grignoli M, Nesti M, Pirastu R, Comba P. 1999. Cohort mortality study of women compensated for asbestosis in Italy. *American Journal of Industrial Medicine* 36(1): 129-134.

Giaroli C, Belli S, Bruno C, Candela S, Grignoli M, Minisci S, Poletti R, Ricco G, Vecchi G, Venturi G, Ziccardi A, Combra P. 1994. Mortality study of asbestos cement workers. *International Archives of Occupational and Environmental Health* 66(1): 7-11.

Gustavsson P, Jakobsson R, Johansson H, Lewin F, Norell S, Rutkvist LE. 1998. Occupational exposures and squamous cell carcinoma of the oral cavity, pharynx, larynx, and oesophagus: A case-control study in Sweden. *Occupational and Environmental Medicine* 55(6): 393-400.

Hesterberg TW, Miller WC, Mast R, McConnell EE, Bernstein DM, Anderson R. 1994. Relationship between lung biopersistence and biological effects of man-made vitreous fibers after chronic inhalation in rats. *Environmental Health Perspectives* 102 (Supplement 5): 133-137.

Hesterberg TW, Miller WC, McConnell EE, Chevalier J, Hadley JG, Bernstein DM, Thevenaz P, Anderson R. 1993. Chronic inhalation toxicity of size-separated glass fibers in Fischer 344 rats. *Fundamental and Applied Toxicology* 20(4): 464-476.

HHS (US Department of Health and Human Services). 2004. *11th Report on Carcinogens.* Washington, DC: National Toxicology Program.

Hinds MW, Thomas DB, O'Reilly HP. 1979. Asbestos, dental X-rays, tobacco, and alcohol in the epidemiology of laryngeal cancer. *Cancer* 44(3): 1114-1120.

Hughes JM, Weill H, Hammad YY. 1987. Mortality of workers employed in two asbestos cement manufacturing plants. *British Journal of Industrial Medicine* 44(3): 161-174.

IARC (International Agency for Research on Cancer). 1987. *Overall Evaluations of Carcinogenity: An Updating of IARC Monographs Volume 1 to 42.* IARC Monographs on the Evaluation of Carcinogenic Risks of Chemicals to Man. Supplement 7. Lyon, France: World Health Organization.

IARC. 1988. *Alcohol Drinking.* IARC Monographs on the Evaluation of Carcinogenic Risks to Human. Volume 44. Lyon, France: World Health Organization.

IARC. 2004. *Tobacco Smoke and Involuntary Smoking.* IARC Monographs on the Evaluation of Carcinogenic Risks to Human. Volume 83. Lyon, France: World Health Organization.

Imbernon E, Goldberg M, Bonenfant S, Chevalier A, Guenel P, Vatre R, Dehaye J. 1995. Occupational respiratory cancer and exposure to asbestos: A case-control study in a cohort of workers in the electricity and gas industry. *American Journal of Industrial Medicine* 28(3): 339-352.

Jemal A, Siegel R, Ward E, Murray T, Xu J, Smigal C, Thun M. 2006. Cancer statistics, 2006. *CA: A Cancer Journal for Clinicians* 56: 106-130.

Kambic V, Radsel Z, Gale N. 1989. Alterations in the laryngeal mucosa after exposure to asbestos. *British Journal of Industrial Medicine* 46(10): 717-723.

Karjalainen A, Pukkala E, Kauppinen T, Partanen T. 1999. Incidence of cancer among Finnish patients with asbestos-related pulmonary or pleural fibrosis. *Cancer Causes and Control* 10(1): 51-57.

Levin J, McLarty J, Hurst GA, Smith A, Frank AL. 1998. Tyler asbestos workers: Mortality experience in a cohort exposed to amosite. *Occupational and Environmental Medicine* 55(3): 155-160.

Liddell FD, McDonald AD, McDonald JC. 1997. The 1891-1920 birth cohort of Quebec chrysotile miners and millers: Development from 1904 and mortality to 1992. *Annals of Occupational Hygiene* 41(1): 13-36.

Luce D, Bugel I, Goldberg P, Goldberg M, Salomon C, Billon-Galland MA, Nicolau J, Quenel P, Fevotte J, Brochard P. 2000. Environmental exposure to tremolite and respiratory cancer in New Caledonia: A case-control study. *American Journal of Epidemiology* 151(3): 259-265.

Magnani C, Nardini I, Governa M, Serio A. 1986. [A cohort study of the personnel assigned to a state railroad repair shop]. *Medicina del Lavoro* 77(2): 154-161.

Marchand JL, Luce D, Leclerc A, Goldberg P, Orlowski E, Bugel I, Brugere J. 2000. Laryngeal and hypopharyngeal cancer and occupational exposure to asbestos and man-made vitreous fibers: Results of a case-control study. *American Journal of Industrial Medicine* 37(6): 581-589.

McConnell EE. 2005 (October 27). *Personal Communication to Mary Paxton for the Committee on Asbestos: Selected Health Effects.* Available in IOM Public Access Files.

McConnell E, Kamstrup O, Musselman R, Hesterberg T, Chevalier J, Miller W, Thevenaz P. 1994a. Chronic inhalation study of size-separated rock and slag wool insulation fibers in Fischer 344/N rats. *Inhalation Toxicology* 6(6): 571-614.

McConnell E, Mast R, Hesterberg T, Chevalier J, Kotin P, Bernstein D, Thevenaz P, Glass L, Anderson R. 1994b. Chronic inhalation toxicity of a kaolin-based refactory cermaic fiber in Syrian golden hamsters. *Inhalation Toxicology* 6(6): 503-532.

McConnell EE, Axten C, Hesterberg TW, Chevalier J, Miller WC, Everitt J, Oberdorster G, Chase GR, Thevenaz P, Kotin P. 1999. Studies on the inhalation toxicology of two fiberglasses and amosite asbestos in the Syrian golden hamster: Part II. Results of chronic exposure. *Inhalation Toxicology* 11(9): 785-835.

McDonald AD, Fry JS, Woolley AJ, McDonald JC. 1984. Dust exposure and mortality in an American chrysotile asbestos friction products plant. *British Journal of Industrial Medicine* 41(2): 151-157.

McDonald JC, Liddell FD. 1979. Mortality in Canadian miners and millers exposed to chrysotile. *Annals of the New York Academy of Sciences* 330: 1-9.

McDonald JC, McDonald AD. 1997. Chrysotile, tremolite and carcinogenicity. *Annals of Occupational Hygiene* 41(6): 699-705.

McDonald JC, McDonald AD, Gibbs GW, Siemiatycki J, Rossiter CE. 1971. Mortality in the chrysotile asbestos mines and mills of Quebec. *Archives of Environmental Health* 22(6): 677-686.

McDonald JC, Liddell FD, Gibbs GW, Eyssen GE, McDonald AD. 1980. Dust exposure and mortality in chrysotile mining, 1910-75. *British Journal of Industrial Medicine* 37(1): 11-24.

McDonald AD, Fry JS, Woolley AJ, McDonald J. 1983. Dust exposure and mortality in an American chrysotile textile plant. *British Journal of Industrial Medicine* 40(4): 361-367.

McDonald JC, McDonald AD, Armstrong B, Sebastien P. 1986. Cohort study of mortality of vermiculite miners exposed to tremolite. *British Journal of Industrial Medicine* 43(7): 436-444.

McDonald JC, Liddell FD, Dufresne A, McDonald AD. 1993. The 1891-1920 birth cohort of Quebec chrysotile miners and millers: Mortality 1976-88. *British Journal of Industrial Medicine* 50(12): 1073-1081.

Meurman LO, Pukkala E, Hakama M. 1994. Incidence of cancer among anthophyllite asbestos miners in Finland. *Occupational and Environmental Medicine* 51(6): 421-425.

Muscat J, Wynder E. 1992. Tobacco, alcohol, asbestos, and occupational risk factors for laryngeal cancer. *Cancer* 69(9): 2244-2251.

Olsen J, Sabroe S. 1984. Occupational causes of laryngeal cancer. *Journal of Epidemiology and Community Health* 38: 117-121.

Parnes SM. 1990. Asbestos and cancer of the larynx: Is there a relationship? *Laryngoscope* 100(3): 254-261.

Peto J, Doll R, Hermon C, Binns W, Clayton R, Goffe T. 1985. Relationship of mortality to measures of environmental asbestos pollution in an asbestos textile factory. *Annals of Occupational Hygiene* 29(3): 305-355.

Piolatto G, Negri E, La Vecchia C, Pira E, Decarli A, Peto J. 1990. An update of cancer mortality among chrysotile asbestos miners in Balangero, northern Italy. *British Journal of Industrial Medicine* 47(12): 810-814.

Pira E, Pelucchi C, Buffoni L, Palmas A, Turbiglio M, Negri E, Piolatto PG, La Vecchia C. 2005. Cancer mortality in a cohort of asbestos textile workers. *British Journal of Cancer* 92(3): 580-586.

Puntoni R, Merlo F, Borsa L, Reggiardo G, Garrone E, Ceppi M. 2001. A historical cohort mortality study among shipyard workers in Genoa, Italy. *American Journal of Industrial Medicine* 40(4): 363-370.

Raffn E, Lynge E, Juel K, Korsgaard B. 1989. Incidence of cancer and mortality among employees in the asbestos cement industry in Denmark. *British Journal of Industrial Medicine* 46(2): 90-96.

Rees L, Birchall M, Bailey M, Thomas S. 2004. A systematic review of case-control studies of human papillomavirus infection in laryngeal squamous cell carcinoma. *Clinical Otolaryngology and Allied Sciences* 29(4): 301-306.

Reid A, Ambrosini G, de Klerk N, Fritschi L, Musk B. 2004. Aerodigestive and gastrointestinal tract cancers and exposure to crocidolite (blue asbestos): Incidence and mortality among former crocidolite workers. *International Journal of Cancer* 111(5): 757-761.

Roggli VL, Greenberg SD, McLarty JL, Hurst GA, Spivey CG, Heiger LR. 1980. Asbestos body content of the larnyx in asbestos workers: A study of five cases. *Archives of Otolaryngology* 106(9): 533-535.

Rubino GF, Piolatto G, Newhouse ML, Scansetti G, Aresini GA, Murray R. 1979. Mortality of chrysotile asbestos workers at the Balangero Mine, northern Italy. *British Journal of Industrial Medicine* 36(3): 187-194.

Schlesinger RB, Lippmann M. 1978. Selective particle deposition and bronchogenic carcinoma. *Environmental Research* 15(3): 424-431.

Seidman H, Selikoff IJ, Gelb SK. 1986. Mortality experience of amosite asbestos factory workers: Dose-response relationships 5 to 40 years after onset of short-term work exposure. *American Journal of Industrial Medicine* 10(5-6): 479-514.

Selikoff IJ, Hammond EC. 1978. Asbestos-associated disease in United States shipyards. *CA: A Cancer Journal for Clinicians* 28(2): 87-99.

Selikoff IJ, Seidman H. 1991. Evaluation of selection bias in a cross-sectional survey. *American Journal of Industrial Medicine* 20(5): 615-627.

Selikoff IJ, Hammond EC, Seidman H. 1979. Mortality experience of insulation workers in the United States and Canada, 1943-1976. *Annals of the New York Academy of Sciences* 330: 91-116.

Shettigara PT, Morgan RW. 1975. Asbestos, smoking, and laryngeal carcinoma. *Archives of Environmental Health* 30(10): 517-519.

Sluis-Cremer GK, Liddell FD, Logan WP, Bezuidenhout BN. 1992. The mortality of amphibole miners in South Africa, 1946-80. *British Journal of Industrial Medicine* 49(8): 566-575.

Smailyte G, Kurtinaitis J, Andersen A. 2004. Cancer mortality and morbidity among Lithuanian asbestos-cement producing workers. *Scandinavian Journal of Work, Environment and Health* 30(1): 64-70.

Stell P, McGill T. 1973. Asbestos and laryngeal carcinoma. *Lancet* 2(7826): 416-417.

Szeszenia-Dabrowska N, Urszula W, Szymczak W, Strzelecka A. 2002. Mortality study of workers compensated for asbestosis in Poland, 1970-1997. *International Journal Occupational Medicine and Environmental Health* 15(3): 267-278.

Tola S, Kalliomaki PL, Pukkala E, Asp S, Korkala ML. 1988. Incidence of cancer among welders, platers, machinists, and pipe fitters in shipyards and machine shops. *British Journal of Industrial Medicine* 45(4): 209-218.

Wortley P, Vaughan TL, Davis S, Morgan MS, Thomas DB. 1992. A case-control study of occupational risk factors for laryngeal cancer. *British Journal of Industrial Medicine* 49(12): 837-844.

Wynder EL, Hoffmann D. 1976. Tobacco and tobacco smoke. *Seminars in Oncology* 3(1): 5-15.

Zagraniski RT, Kelsey JL, Walter SD. 1986. Occupational risk factors for laryngeal carcinoma: Connecticut, 1975-1980. *American Journal of Epidemiology* 124(1): 67-76.

Zeka A, Eisen EA, Kriebel D, Gore R, Wegman DH. 2004. Risk of upper aerodigestive tract cancers in a case-cohort study of autoworkers exposed to metalworking fluids. *Occupational and Environmental Medicine* 61(5): 426-431.

Zheng W, Blot WJ, Shu XO, Gao YT, Ji BT, Ziegler RG, Fraumeni JF Jr. 1992. Diet and other risk factors for laryngeal cancer in Shanghai, China. *American Journal of Epidemiology* 136(2): 178-191.

Zhu H, Wang Z. 1993. Study of occupational lung cancer in asbestos factories in China. *British Journal of Industrial Medicine* 50(11): 1039-1042.

9

Esophageal Cancer and Asbestos

NATURE OF THIS CANCER TYPE

The esophagus is a muscular tube that carries food and liquid from the mouth to the stomach (Figures 7.1 and 9.1).

The American Cancer Society (Jemal et al. 2006) has estimated that 14,550 new cases of and 13,770 deaths from esophageal cancer (ICD-9 150; ICD-O-3 C15.0-15.9) will occur in the United States in 2006. Esophageal cancer ranks 19th in numbers of cases of cancer in the United States and sixth in developing countries (Kleihues and Stewart 2003).

The incidence is nearly 4 times higher in men than in women in the United States and slightly higher among blacks than among whites. The incidence has increased among men by an average of 1.7% per year since 1975, although the predominant histologic type and location of cancers in the esophagus have changed since the 1970s in most economically developed countries. Historically, the most common form of esophageal cancer worldwide was squamous-cell carcinoma, which occurred largely in the upper two-thirds of the esophagus (Blot 1994). Since the 1970s, the incidence of adenocarcinoma of the lower one-third of the esophagus and the junction with the stomach has increased by a factor of more than 5 among white and black men in the United States, whereas the incidence of squamous-cell carcinoma has decreased moderately. Rates of adenocarcinoma are also rising in women but are much lower than in men. Adenocarcinoma now makes up more than half of the esophageal cancers in white males, whereas squamous-cell carcinoma remains the predominant histologic type among black people and in high-incidence populations worldwide (Blot and McLaughlin 1999).

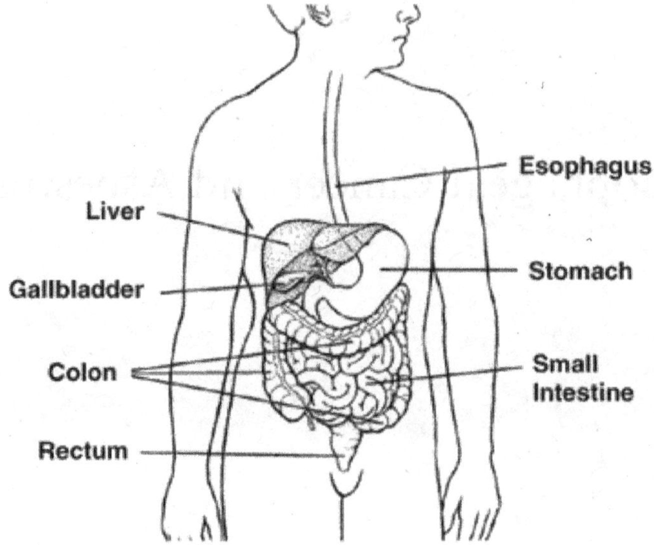

FIGURE 9.1 Anatomy of the esophagus, colon, rectum, and other digestive organs. SOURCE: Copyright 2005 American Cancer Society, Inc. Reprinted with permission from www.cancer.org.

The incidence of carcinoma of the esophagus varies widely among countries. In regions extending from Iran through the steppes of Central Asia, Mongolia, and the northern portion of China, cancer frequencies are 10-100 times higher than in the countries at lowest risk. Squamous-cell carcinoma still predominates in the areas of high endemic risk, whereas adenocarcinoma now makes up about 50% of all cases in the low-risk areas of the United States, Europe, South Africa, Southeast Asia, and Japan.

The known risk factors differ somewhat for the two major histologic types of esophageal cancer. Known risk factors for squamous-cell carcinoma include all forms of tobacco-smoking (cigarettes, cigars, pipes, and bidis), use of chewing tobacco or snuff, and excessive consumption of alcohol. The combination of tobacco use and alcohol consumption potentiates the risk of either factor alone. Factors known to increase the risk of adenocarcinoma include chronic esophageal reflux (regurgitation of stomach acid and bile through the lower esophageal sphincter into the lower esophagus), obesity (which contributes to reflux), smoking, and achalasia (a type of esophageal dysfunction).

Adenocarcinoma of the esophagus develops from Barrett's esophagus, a premalignant condition in which normal squamous epithelium of the lower esophagus is replaced with metaplastic columnar epithelium. The main cause of Barrett's esophagus is thought to be chronic gastroesophageal reflux. People with Barrett's esophagus are at increased risk for developing cancer of the esophagus and should be followed closely by their doctors. Even though they are at greater than average risk, most people with Barrett's esophagus do not develop cancer of the esophagus.

EPIDEMIOLOGIC EVIDENCE CONSIDERED

Cohort Studies

The cohorts that presented usable information on the risk of esophageal cancer were indicated in Table 6.1. Their histories and design properties are described in Table B.1, and the details of their results concerning cancer at this site are abstracted in Table D.3. The results of both the cohort and case-control studies are summarized in Table 9.1, and Figures 9.2 and 9.3 are plots of relative risks (RRs) for overall exposure and for exposure-response gradients from the cohort studies reviewed.

TABLE 9.1 Summary of Epidemiologic Findings Regarding Cancer of Esophagus

Study Type	Figure	Comparison	Study Populations Included	No. Study Populations	Summary RR (95% CI)	Between-Study SD
Cohort	9.2	Any vs none	All	25	0.99 (0.79-1.27)	
	9.3	High vs none[a]	Lower bound[b]	7	1.35 (0.81-2.27)	
			Upper bound[b]	7	1.43 (0.79-2.58)	—
Case-control	—	Any vs none	All	2	1.47 (0.87-2.47)	0.00
	—	Any vs none	EAM = 1	1		
			EAM = 2	1		
	—	High vs none[a]	EAM = 1	2	1.04 (0.50-1.80)	0.00

NOTE: CI = Confidence interval; EAM = exposure-assessment method; high quality, EAM = 1; lower quality, EAM = 2; RR = relative risk; SD = standard deviation.

[a]Used studies that reported dose-response relationship (RR on an exposure gradient).

[b]For studies that reported dose-response relationship on multiple gradient metrics, smallest "high vs none" RR was used to compute lower bound, and largest "high vs none" RR was used in computing the upper bound.

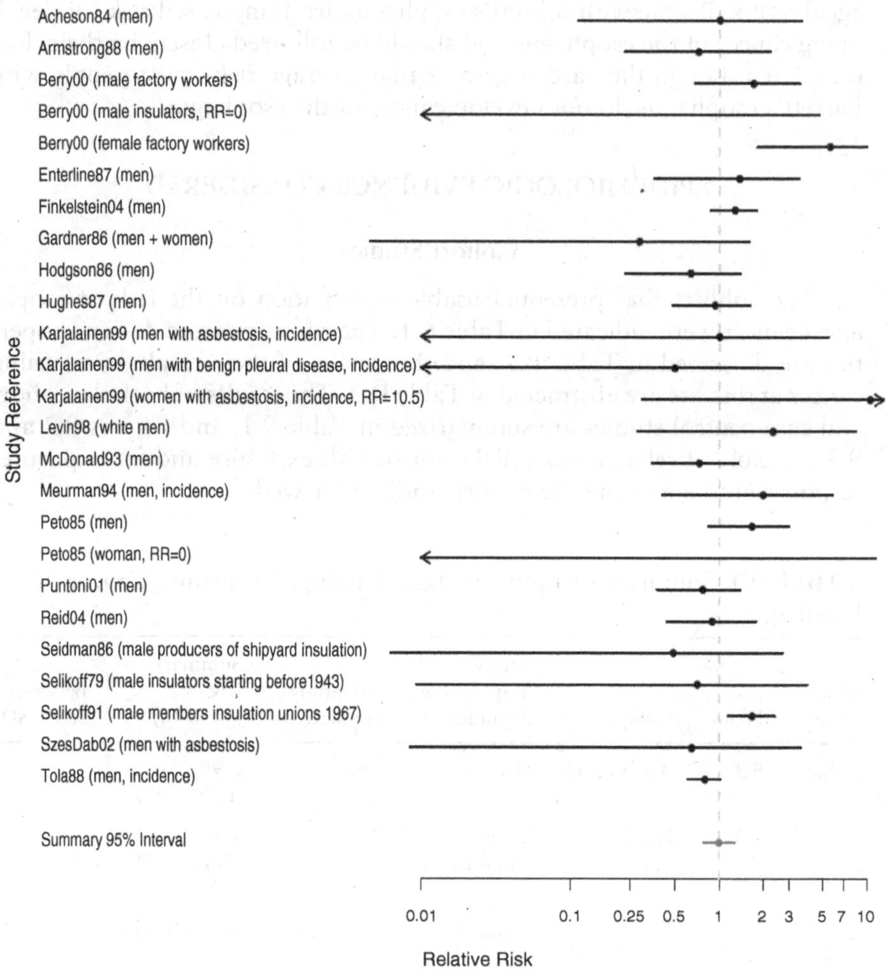

FIGURE 9.2 Cohort studies: RR of esophageal cancer in people with "any" exposure to asbestos compared with people who report no exposure.

Few studies presented data explicitly on esophageal cancer, because of its rarity. Therefore, observed numbers, and hence statistical precision, were low. Only UK asbestos-factory workers (Berry et al. 2000) and North American insulation workers (Selikoff and Seidman 1991) showed strong evidence of increased risk with any asbestos exposure. A suggestion that risk might be dose-dependent was seen among Finnish anthophyllite miners (Meurman et al. 1994) and UK textile workers (Peto et al. 1985). The

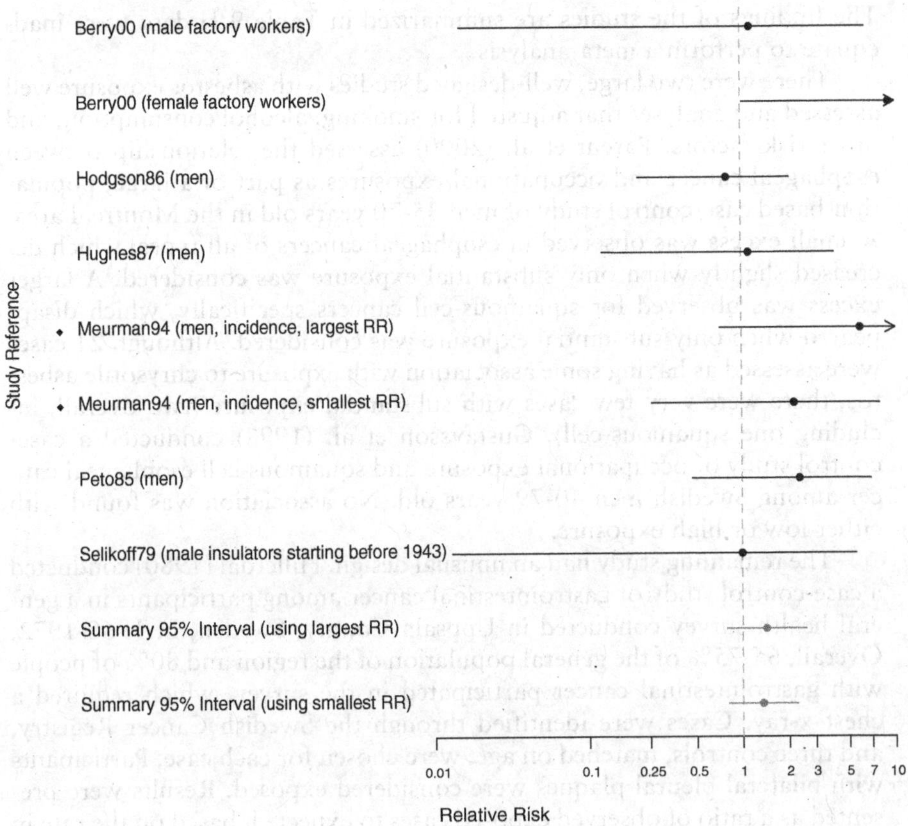

FIGURE 9.3 Cohort studies: RRs of esophageal cancer among people in extreme exposure category compared with those with none (♦ = more than one exposure gradient reported in citation, so the plot contains both highest and lowest estimates of risk for extreme category over all gradients).

aggregate estimated risk for all 25 cohort populations with information on esophageal cancer risk following any exposure to asbestos was neutral (RR = 0.99, 95% CI 0.79-1.27).

Case-Control Studies

The three case-control studies retained for thorough evaluation after excluding studies that did not assess exposure to asbestos or did not meet other exclusion criteria are listed Table 6.5 according to quality of their exposure assessment. The details of the design aspects of these studies are presented in Table C.1 and their detailed results are abstracted in Table E.3.

The findings of the studies are summarized in Table 9.1; data were inadequate to perform a meta-analysis.

There were two large, well-designed studies with asbestos exposure well assessed and analyses that adjusted for smoking, alcohol consumption, and other risk factors. Parent et al. (2000) assessed the relationship between esophageal cancer and occupational exposures as part of a large, population-based case-control study of men 35-70 years old in the Montreal area. A small excess was observed in esophageal cancers of all types, which decreased slightly when only substantial exposure was considered. A larger excess was observed for squamous-cell cancers specifically, which disappeared when only substantial exposure was considered. Although 21 cases were assessed as having some association with exposure to chrysotile asbestos, there were very few cases with substantial exposure (two overall, including one squamous-cell). Gustavsson et al. (1998) conducted a case-control study of occupational exposure and squamous-cell esophageal cancer among Swedish men 40-79 years old. No association was found with either low or high exposure.

The remaining study had an unusual design. Hillerdal (1980) conducted a case-control study of gastrointestinal cancer among participants in a general health survey conducted in Uppsala County, Sweden, in 1968-1972. Overall, 65-75% of the general population of the region and 80% of people with gastrointestinal cancer participated in the survey, which required a chest x-ray. Cases were identified through the Swedish Cancer Registry, and three controls, matched on age, were chosen for each case. Participants with bilateral pleural plaques were considered exposed. Results were presented as a ratio of observed exposed cases to expected, based on the rate in controls. One of the 21 people with esophageal cancer cases had pleural plaques vs 0.35 expected.

EVIDENCE INTEGRATION AND CONCLUSION

Evidence Considered

Both case-control and cohort studies of esophageal cancer were reviewed. Only three case-control studies met the criteria for inclusion, and so there were too few for a useful quantitative meta-analysis. There were relevant results from 25 cohort populations, although the number of cases was often small. The mortality studies did not distinguish between histologic subtypes, so associations could have been obscured. In assessing biologic plausibility, the cell type, potential dose at the target tissues, results, and possible mechanisms were considered. Findings related to the response to asbestos by esophageal tissues were evaluated from several well conducted chronic rodent studies, four with inhalation exposure and six with dietary administration.

Consistency

The three case-control studies did not have consistent results, and the number of exposed cases was generally small. Two incorporated adjustment for tobacco and alcohol consumption; one of these observed an excess risk of squamous-cell cancer without evidence of a dose-response relationship, and the other found no evidence of an excess. A third, older study found an excess based on a single case, which was difficult to interpret.

Because of the relative rarity of esophageal cancer, few cohort studies presented data explicitly on this endpoint; and when they did, the statistical precision was routinely low. The results of the 20 citations that presented information on esophageal cancer in 25 cohort populations were mixed. Berry et al. (2000) and Selikoff and Seidman (1991) saw strong evidence of increased risk with any exposure, while Meurman et al. (1994) and Peto et al. (1985) found some evidence of a dose-response relationship. Findings from the remaining studies either were close to null, presented mixed or inconsistent results, or indicated lower than expected risks.

Strength of Association

There were too few case-control studies for a meaningful combined analysis. Several cohort studies did observe a dose-response relationship based on relatively small numbers; but when all 25 cohort populations were considered in the meta-analysis, no increase in RR was observed. Some studies did observe excess risks, but overall there was little consistency in the epidemiologic data.

Coherence

The most common histologic type of cancer arising in the upper two-thirds of the esophagus is squamous-cell carcinoma. That is probably the most common histologic type encountered in the epidemiologic studies of workers in the 1970s and earlier. The major risk factors are tobacco-smoking and tobacco-chewing, snuff use, and alcohol consumption. Since the 1970s, the major histologic type of esophageal cancer has been adenocarcinoma arising in the lower one-third of this anatomic region. Major risk factors for this type of esophageal cancer are reflux, obesity, achalasia, and tobacco-smoking. Although the combination of asbestos exposure and tobacco-smoking is an established risk factor for lung cancer, there is no epidemiologic or experimental evidence addressing whether asbestos is a cofactor with tobacco use or alcohol consumption in the development of esophageal cancer.

Asbestos bodies have been identified in the esophagus (Kobayashi et al. 1987), but contamination during collection or processing of tissue samples is a possibility, as discussed in Chapter 4.

No increase in esophageal tumors has been observed in animals exposed chronically to asbestos either by inhalation (Hesterberg et al. 1993, 1994; McConnell 2005; McConnell et al. 1994a,b, 1999) or by oral feeding (HHS 1983, 1985, 1988, 1990a,b,c). There is no other experimental evidence that asbestos fibers act as a direct or indirect carcinogen specifically in the esophagus.

Conclusion

Some studies have found an association between asbestos exposure and esophageal cancer, but the overall results of epidemiologic studies are mixed. In addition, what little evidence there is from animal experiments about asbestos's carcinogenic potential specifically on esophageal tissues does not support biological activity at this site. On the basis of those observations, the committee concluded that the evidence is *inadequate* to infer the presence or absence of a causal relationship between asbestos exposure and esophageal cancer.

REFERENCES

Acheson ED, Gardner MJ, Winter PD, Bennett C. 1984. Cancer in a factory using amosite asbestos. *International Journal of Epidemiology* 13(1): 3-10.

Armstrong BK, de Klerk NH, Musk AW, Hobbs MS. 1988. Mortality in miners and millers of crocidolite in Western Australia. *British Journal of Industrial Medicine* 45(1): 5-13.

Berry G, Newhouse ML, Wagner JC. 2000. Mortality from all cancers of asbestos factory workers in east London 1933-1980. *Occupational and Environmental Medicine* 57(11): 782-785.

Blot WJ. 1994. Esophageal cancer trends and risk factors. *Seminars in Oncology* 21(4): 403-410.

Blot WJ, McLaughlin JK. 1999. The changing epidemiology of esophageal cancer. *Seminars in Oncology* 26 (5 Supplement 15): 2-8.

Enterline PE, Hartley J, Henderson V. 1987. Asbestos and cancer: A cohort followed up to death. *British Journal of Industrial Medicine* 44(6): 396-401.

Finkelstein MM, Verma DK. 2004. A cohort study of mortality among Ontario pipe trades workers. *Occupational and Environmental Medicine* 61(9): 736-742.

Gardner MJ, Winter PD, Pannett B, Powell CA. 1986. Follow up study of workers manufacturing chrysotile asbestos cement products. *British Journal of Industrial Medicine* 43(11): 726-732.

Gustavsson P, Jakobsson R, Johansson H, Lewin F, Norell S, Rutkvist LE. 1998. Occupational exposures and squamous cell carcinoma of the oral cavity, pharynx, larynx, and oesophagus: A case-control study in Sweden. *Occupational and Environmental Medicine* 55(6): 393-400.

Hesterberg TW, Miller WC, McConnell EE, Chevalier J, Hadley JG, Bernstein DM, Thevenaz P, Anderson R. 1993. Chronic inhalation toxicity of size-separated glass fibers in Fischer 344 rats. *Fundamental and Applied Toxicology* 20(4): 464-476.

Hesterberg TW, Miller WC, Mast R, McConnell EE, Bernstein DM, Anderson R. 1994. Relationship between lung biopersistence and biological effects of man-made vitreous fibers after chronic inhalation in rats. *Environmental Health Perspectives* 102 (Supplement 5): 133-137.

HHS (US Department of Health and Human Services). 1983. *Lifetime Carcinogenesis Studies of Amosite Asbestos (CAS NO. 12172-73-5) in Syrian Golden Hamsters (Feed Studies).* NTP TR 249. Research Triangle Park, NC: National Toxicology Program.

HHS. 1985. *Toxicology and Carcinogenesis Studies of Chrysotile Asbestos (CAS No. 12001-29-5) in F344/N Rats (Feed Studies).* NTP TR 295. Research Triangle Park, NC: National Toxicology Program.

HHS. 1988. *Toxicology and Carcinogenesis Studies of Crocidolite Asbestos (CAS No. 12001-28-4) in F344/N Rats (Feed Studies).* NTP TR 280. Research Triangle Park, NC: National Toxicology Program.

HHS. 1990a. *Lifetime Carcinogenesis Studies of Chrysotile Asbestos (CAS No. 12001-29-5) in Syrian Golden Hamsters (Feed Studies).* NTP TR 246. Research Triangle Park, North Carolina: National Toxicology Program.

HHS. 1990b. *Toxicology and Carcinogenesis Studies of Amosite Asbestos (CAS No. 12172-73-5) in F344/N Rats (Feed Studies).* NTP TR 279. Research Triangle Park, NC: National Toxicology Program.

HHS. 1990c. *Toxicology and Carcinogenesis Studies of Tremolite (CAS No. 14567-73-8) in F344/N Rats (Feed Studies).* NTP TR 277. Research Triangle Park, NC: National Toxicology Program.Hillerdal G. 1980. Gastrointestinal carcinoma and occurrence of pleural plaques on pulmonary X-ray. *Journal of Occupational Medicine* 22(12): 806-809.

Hodgson JT, Jones RD. 1986. Mortality of asbestos workers in England and Wales 1971-81. *British Journal of Industrial Medicine* 43(3): 158-164.

Hughes JM, Weill H, Hammad YY. 1987. Mortality of workers employed in two asbestos cement manufacturing plants. *British Journal of Industrial Medicine* 44(3): 161-174.

Jemal A, Siegel R, Ward E, Murray T, Xu J, Smigal C, Thun M. 2006. Cancer statistics, 2006. *CA: A Cancer Journal for Clinicians* 56: 106-130.

Karjalainen A, Pukkala E, Kauppinen T, Partanen T. 1999. Incidence of cancer among Finnish patients with asbestos-related pulmonary or pleural fibrosis. *Cancer Causes and Control* 10(1): 51-57.

Kleihues P, Stewart BW, eds. 2003. *World Cancer Report.* Lyon, France: International Agency for Research on Cancer.

Kobayashi H, Ming ZW, Watanabe H, Ohnishi Y. 1987. A quantitative study on the distribution of asbestos bodies in extrapulmonary organs. *ACTA Pathologica Japonica* 37(3): 375-383.

Levin J, McLarty J, Hurst GA, Smith A, Frank AL. 1998. Tyler asbestos workers: Mortality experience in a cohort exposed to amosite. *Occupational and Environmental Medicine* 55(3): 155-160.

McConnell EE. 2005 (October 27). *Personal Communication to Mary Paxton for the Committee on Asbestos: Selected Health Effects.* Available in IOM Public Access Files.

McConnell E, Kamstrup O, Musselman R, Hesterberg T, Chevalier J, Miller W, Thevenaz P. 1994a. Chronic inhalation study of size-separated rock and slag wool insulation fibers in Fischer 344/N rats. *Inhalation Toxicology* 6(6): 571-614.

McConnell E, Mast R, Hesterberg T, Chevalier J, Kotin P, Bernstein D, Thevenaz P, Glass L, Anderson R. 1994b. Chronic inhalation toxicity of a kaolin-based refactory cermaic fiber in Syrian golden hamsters. *Inhalation Toxicology* 6(6): 503-532.

McConnell EE, Axten C, Hesterberg TW, Chevalier J, Miller WC, Everitt J, Oberdorster G, Chase GR, Thevenaz P, Kotin P. 1999. Studies on the inhalation toxicology of two fiberglasses and amosite asbestos in the Syrian golden hamster: Part II. Results of chronic exposure. *Inhalation Toxicology* 11(9): 785-835.

McDonald JC, Liddell FD, Dufresne A, McDonald AD. 1993. The 1891-1920 birth cohort of Quebec chrysotile miners and millers: Mortality 1976-88. *British Journal of Industrial Medicine* 50(12): 1073-1081.

Meurman LO, Pukkala E, Hakama M. 1994. Incidence of cancer among anthophyllite asbestos miners in Finland. *Occupational and Environmental Medicine* 51(6): 421-425.

Parent ME, Siemiatycki J, Fritschi L. 2000. Workplace exposures and oesophageal cancer. *Occupational and Environmental Medicine* 57(5): 325-334.

Peto J, Doll R, Hermon C, Binns W, Clayton R, Goffe T. 1985. Relationship of mortality to measures of environmental asbestos pollution in an asbestos textile factory. *Annals of Occupational Hygiene* 29(3): 305-355.

Puntoni R, Merlo F, Borsa L, Reggiardo G, Garrone E, Ceppi M. 2001. A historical cohort mortality study among shipyard workers in Genoa, Italy. *American Journal of Industrial Medicine* 40(4): 363-370.

Reid A, Ambrosini G, de Klerk N, Fritschi L, Musk B. 2004. Aerodigestive and gastrointestinal tract cancers and exposure to crocidolite (blue asbestos): Incidence and mortality among former crocidolite workers. *International Journal of Cancer* 111(5): 757-761.

Seidman H, Selikoff IJ, Gelb SK. 1986. Mortality experience of amosite asbestos factory workers: Dose-response relationships 5 to 40 years after onset of short-term work exposure. *American Journal of Industrial Medicine* 10(5-6): 479-514.

Selikoff IJ, Seidman H. 1991. Asbestos-associated deaths among insulation workers in the United States and Canada, 1967-1987. *Annals of the New York Academy of Sciences* 643: 1-14.

Selikoff IJ, Hammond EC, Seidman H. 1979. Mortality experience of insulation workers in the United States and Canada, 1943-1976. *Annals of the New York Academy of Sciences* 330: 91-116.

Szeszenia-Dabrowska N, Urszula W, Szymczak W, Strzelecka A. 2002. Mortality study of workers compensated for asbestosis in Poland, 1970-1997. *International Journal of Occupational Medicine and Environmental Health* 15(3): 267-278.

Tola S, Kalliomaki PL, Pukkala E, Asp S, Korkala ML. 1988. Incidence of cancer among welders, platers, machinists, and pipe fitters in shipyards and machine shops. *British Journal of Industrial Medicine* 45(4): 209-218.

10

Stomach Cancer and Asbestos

NATURE OF THIS CANCER TYPE

Despite a major decline in the incidence of stomach cancer (ICD-9 151; ICD-O-3 C16.0-16.9; see Figure 9.1) worldwide, and particularly in industrialized countries over the last century, it remains the second most common fatal cancer worldwide. An estimated 22,280 new cases and 11,430 deaths are projected to occur in the United States in 2006 (Jemal et al. 2006). The incidence of stomach cancer is about twice as high among men as among women, and is higher among nonwhites than among whites. In the United States, the incidence per 100,000 people varies markedly by race and ethnicity: the incidence in Asian and Pacific islanders is 23.0 and 12.8 in males and females, respectively; in blacks, 19.9 and 9.9; in Hispanics, 18.1 and 10.0; in American Indians and Alaska natives, 14.4 and 8.3; and in white non-Hispanics, 10.0 and 4.3. The age-standardized death rate from stomach cancer has declined on average by 2.5-3.0% per year since 1975.

The known risk factors for stomach cancer depend on the location of the tumor. Obesity is the principal known risk factor for cancers that develop in the upper portion (cardia) of the stomach in the United States. In contrast, severe nutritional deficiency is responsible for the high endemic incidence of that type of stomach cancer in some regions of China. Chronic infection with the bacterium *Helicobacter pylori* (*H. pylori*) in combination with tobacco-smoking is the main cause of cancer of the body (fundus) of the stomach and of the gastric antrum. Chronic infection with *H. pylori* causes chronic gastritis and loss of the acid-producing potential of the stomach.

About 90-95% of stomach cancers are adenocarcinomas, although other, less common tumors do occur. Most adenocarcinomas are thought to develop slowly—over many years. Premalignant lesions and early-stage cancers generally begin in the mucosa or inner lining of the stomach. The cells become progressively abnormal as they accumulate genetic damage. With malignant transformation, the cancers develop the capacity to invade the submucosa and muscle wall of the stomach, to extend from there into the subserosa and the outermost serosa that wrap the stomach, or to metastasize to other organs, such as the liver, lungs, and bones. Some types of lymphoma, a cancer of the immune system, also occur in the wall of the stomach; they account for about 4% of stomach cancers. Included among the other tumors are the slow-growing (indolent) lymphoma of mucosa-associated lymphoid tissue (MALT) and carcinoid, a hormone-producing tumor of the stomach and other organs.

In the United States, the median survival of persons with stomach cancer is less than 1 year after diagnosis, although the 5-year survival rate has increased slightly from 15.1% for patients diagnosed in 1974-1976 to 23.2% for those diagnosed in 1995-2001.

EPIDEMIOLOGIC EVIDENCE CONSIDERED

The committee deemed 36 papers on occupational cohorts and five population-based case-control studies to be informative for assessing the association of asbestos and stomach cancer. In that several citations on the cohorts reported separate findings for subgroups (by sex or by separate factory workforces), a total of 42 cohorts were included in this review.

Cohort Studies

The cohorts that presented usable information on the risk of stomach cancer were indicated in Table 6.1. Their histories and design properties are described in Table B.1, and the details of their results concerning cancer at this site are abstracted in Table D.4. The results of the cohort and case-control studies are summarized in Table 10.1, and Figures 10.1 and 10.2 are plots of RRs for overall exposures and for exposure-response gradients from the cohort studies reviewed.

Most of the occupational cohort studies were conducted in predominantly white populations in North America, Europe, and Australia. Two studies in China (Pang et al. 1997, Zhu and Wang 1993) were also included in the review. The reported associations between stomach cancer and occupational asbestos exposure in cohort studies were based on somewhat larger numbers of cases than those related to esophageal cancer, but statistical power in individual studies was generally low

TABLE 10.1 Summary of Epidemiologic Findings Regarding Cancer of the Stomach

Study Type	Figure	Comparison	Study Populations Included	No. Study Populations	Summary RR (95% CI)	Between-Study SD
Cohort	10.1	Any vs none	All	42	1.17 (1.07-1.28)	
	10.2	High vs none[a]	Lower bound[b]	12[c]	1.31 (0.97-1.76)	
			Upper bound[b]	13	1.33 (0.98-1.79)	—
Case-control	10.3	Any vs none	All	5	1.11 (0.76-1.64)	0.32
	10.4	Any vs none	EAM = 1	3	0.91 (0.45-1.84)	0.48
			EAM = 2	2	1.43 (0.70-2.93)	0.42
	10.5	High vs none[a]	EAM = 1	5	1.42 (0.92-2.20)	0.00

NOTE: CI = Confidence interval; EAM = exposure-assessment method; high quality, EAM = 1; lower quality, EAM = 2; RR = relative risk; SD = standard deviation.

[a]Included studies that reported dose-response relationship (RR on an exposure gradient).
[b]For studies that reported dose-response relationship on multiple gradient metrics, the smallest "high vs none" RR was used to compute the lower bound, and the largest "high vs none" RR was used in computing the upper bound.
[c]This calculation omitted de Klerk et al. (1989), which reported RR = 0, but gave no information on the expected number of cases.

because stomach cancer is a rare outcome in whites. Mortality was the outcome in most of the cohort studies reviewed. Insofar as stomach cancer generally has a high case-fatality rate, mortality is a relatively accurate measure of disease incidence.

All the cohort studies lacked data on stomach-cancer subsites and on potential confounding factors, such as *H. pylori* infection or diet. Confounding by factors related to socioeconomic status, which may be associated with these and other stomach-cancer risk factors, may have occurred in the comparisons of overall risks between occupational cohorts and the general population (such as standardized mortality ratios). However, the extent of potential confounding in the comparisons can only be speculated. Internal comparisons of exposure-response gradients within cohorts were unlikely to have been confounded appreciably, because important potential

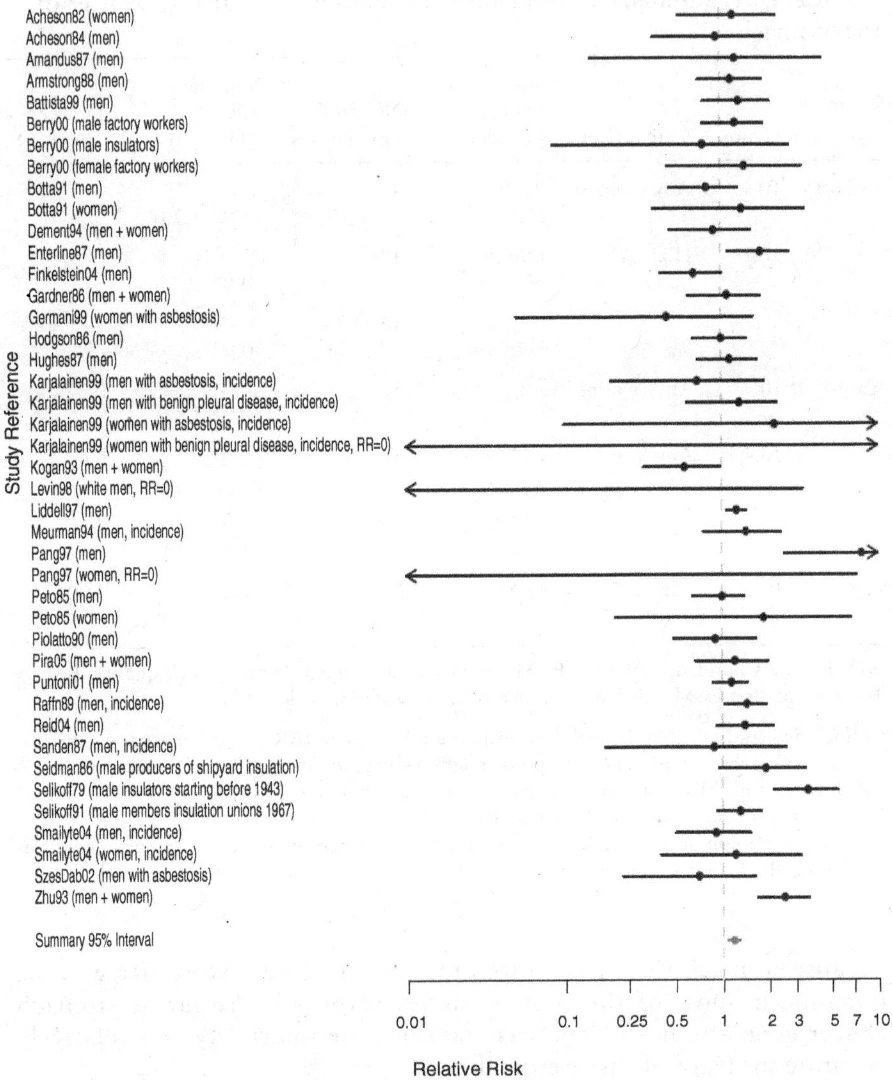

FIGURE 10.1 Cohort studies: RR of stomach cancer in people with "any" exposure to asbestos compared with people who report none.

confounders were probably, at most, weakly correlated with cumulative asbestos exposure.

The majority of overall cohort RR estimates exceeded the null value (1.0), indicating excesses, although estimates varied considerably in strength. The largest overall cohort RRs were seen among the earliest New

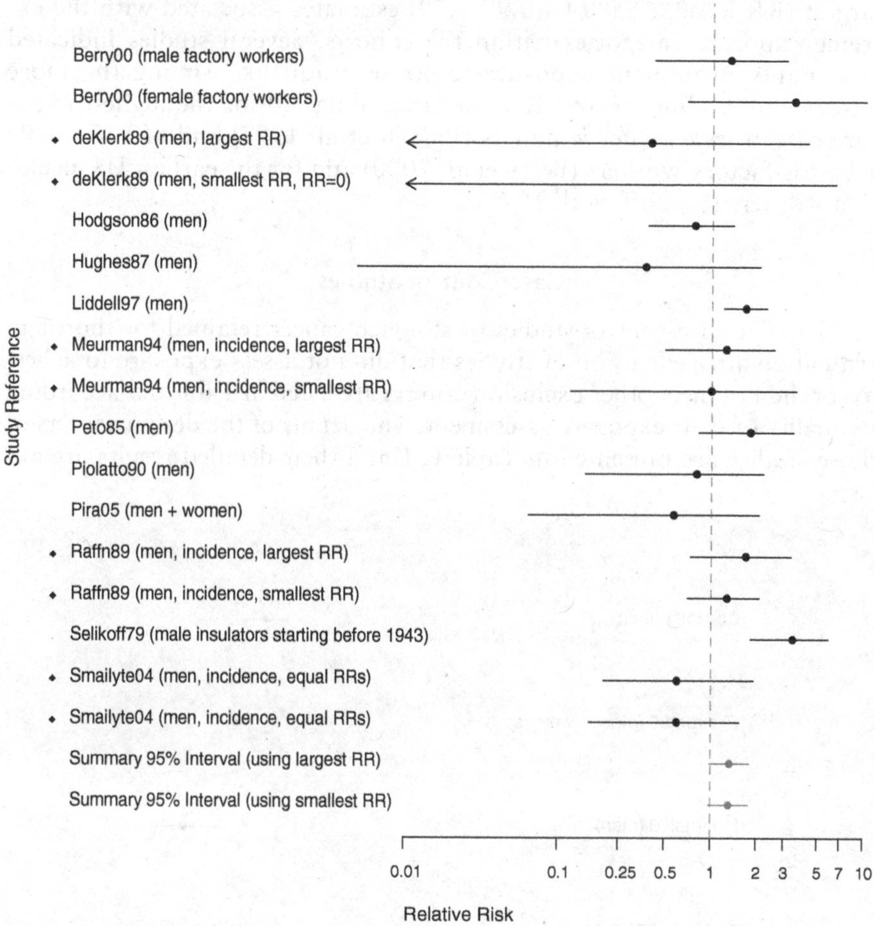

FIGURE 10.2 Cohort studies: RRs of stomach cancer among people in most extreme exposure category compared to those with none (♦ = more than one exposure gradient reported in citation, so the plot contains both highest and lowest estimates of risk for most extreme category over all gradients).

York-New Jersey insulation workers whose RR was 3.52 (Selikoff et al. 1979) and among two sets of workers in Chinese asbestos factories whose RRs were 4.4 and 2.4, respectively (Pang et al. 1997, Zhu and Wang 1993). The majority of studies reported small to modest overall cohort wide excesses (RR < 1.5). The combined RR was 1.17 (95% CI 1.07-1.28) (Table 10.1).

With respect to dose-response gradients, the summary estimates were stable whether based on the smallest (RR = 1.31, 95% CI 0.97-1.76) or largest (RR = 1.33, 95% CI 0.97-1.79) estimates associated with the extreme exposure categories within the cohorts. Several studies indicated reasonably prominent exposure-response gradients. Among the more noteworthy findings were RR values exceeding 3.0 for the highest exposure categories of Quebec miners (Liddell et al. 1997) and of UK female asbestos-factory workers (Berry et al. 2000) and for the earliest US insulation workers (Selikoff et al. 1979).

Case-Control Studies

The five case-control studies of stomach cancer retained for thorough evaluation after exclusion of studies that did not assess exposure to asbestos or did not meet other exclusion criteria are listed in Table 6.5 according to quality of their exposure assessment. The details of the design aspects of those studies are presented in Table C.1 and their detailed results are ab-

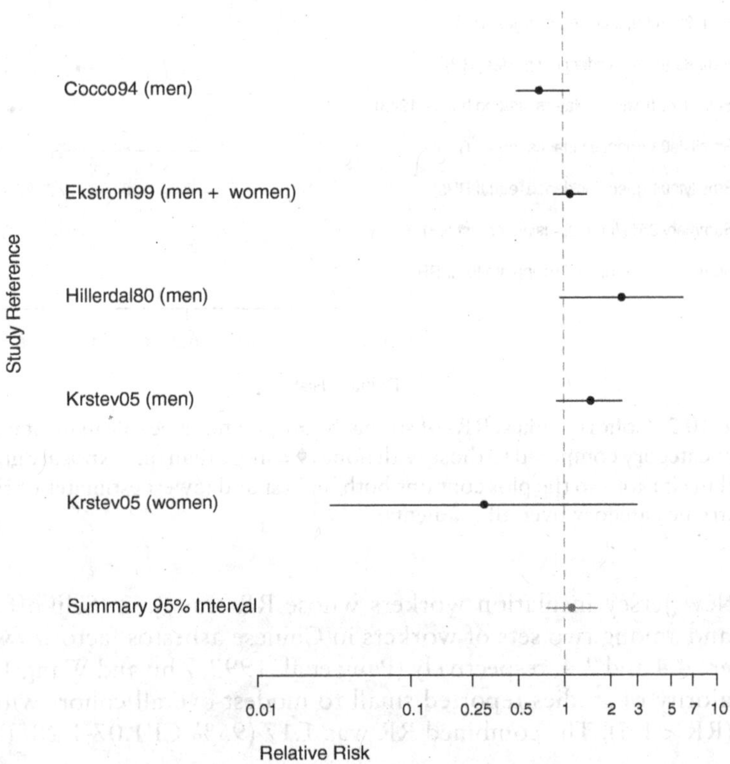

FIGURE 10.3 Case-control studies: RR of stomach cancer in people with "any" exposure to asbestos compared with people with none.

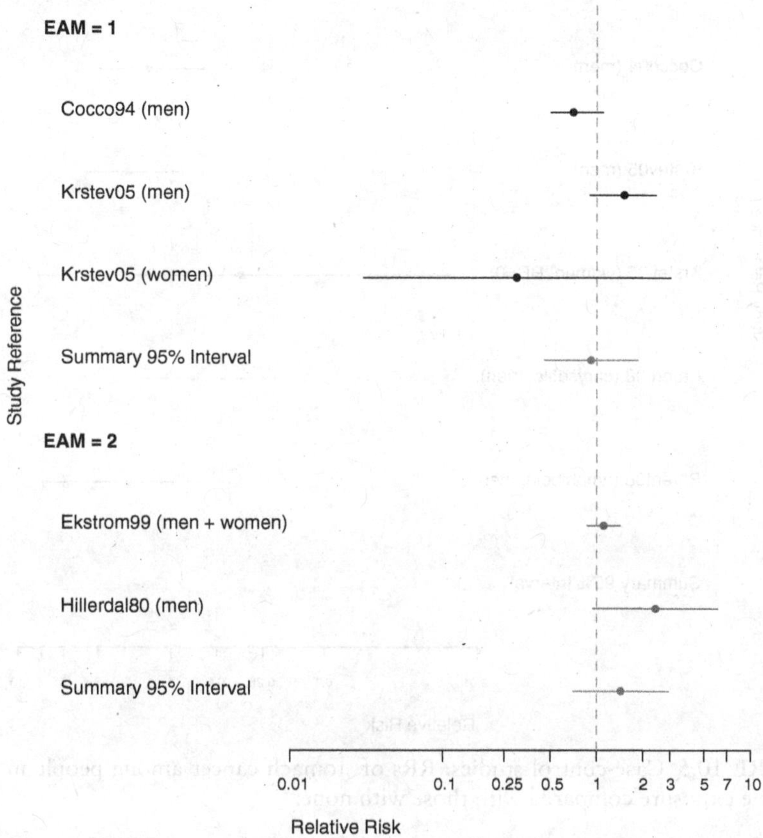

FIGURE 10.4 Case-control studies: RR of stomach cancer in people with "any" exposure to asbestos compared with people with none, stratified on quality of exposure assessment (top, EAM = 1: higher-quality exposure assessment; bottom, EAM = 2: lower-quality exposure assessment).

stracted in Table E.4. The findings of the studies are summarized in Table 10.1 and in the plots presented in Figures 10.3-10.5. Four of the case-control studies gathered data on potential confounders and adjusted risk estimates for asbestos exposure accordingly.

The findings for the case-control study populations with results reported for any asbestos exposure were mixed (Figure 10.3). Two found evidence of an increased stomach-cancer risk, two reported mostly null associations, and one suggested a deficit of stomach-cancer risk among women exposed to asbestos. The combined RR across these five was 1.11 (95% CI 0.76-1.64). That small overall RR increase was based largely on the two studies

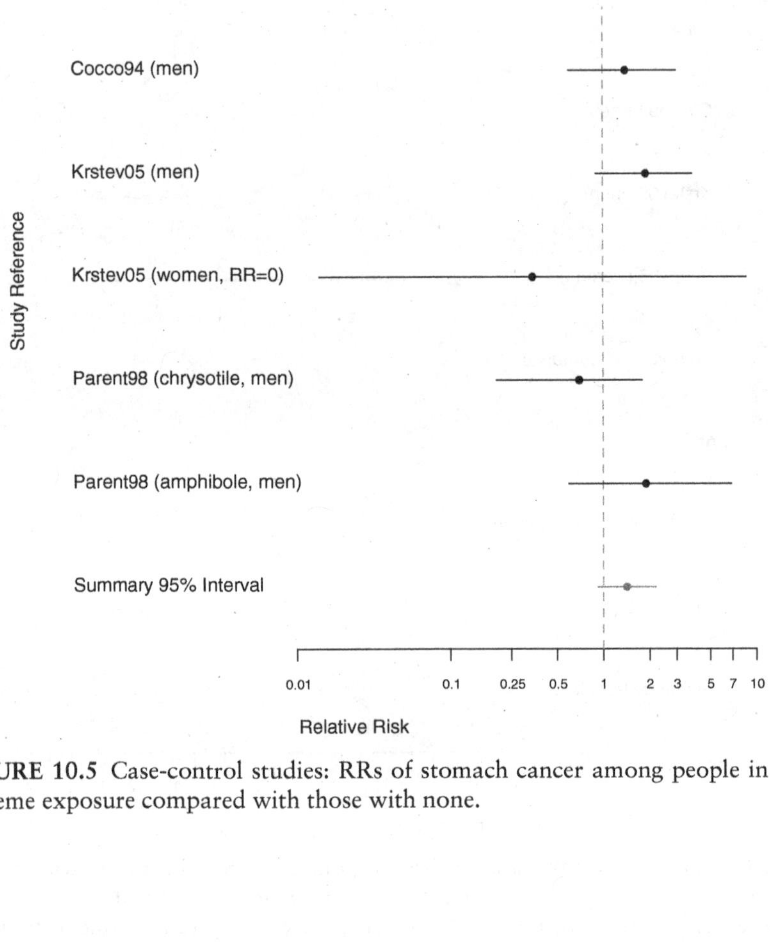

FIGURE 10.5 Case-control studies: RRs of stomach cancer among people in with extreme exposure compared with those with none.

with lower-quality exposure assessment (see Figure 10.4), whose aggregate RR estimate was 1.43 (95% CI 0.70-2.93), whereas the combined RR estimate for the three findings with better exposure assessments was 0.91 (95% CI 0.45-1.84). The strongest association (RR=2.40) was reported by a study in which asbestos exposure was inferred indirectly from the presence of pleural plaques rather than being based on quantitative estimates of cumulative exposure or duration (Hillerdal 1980).

The summary odds ratio (OR) increased when only extreme exposure was considered (OR = 1.42, 95% CI 0.92-2.20), but evidence suggesting a dose-response relationship was also inconsistent (Figure 10.5). The largest study (Cocco et al. 2004) gave a suggestion of greater risk with longer exposure, but the other two citations (Krstev et al. 2005, Parent et al. 1998) both had one study group showing somewhat greater risk with more exposure and another group showing the reverse.

EVIDENCE INTERGRATION AND CONCLUSION

Evidence Considered

The committee's final review covered 34 occupational-cohort studies, including a total of 42 cohorts, and five population-based case-control studies that provided data on stomach-cancer risk. The studies were conducted primarily among whites in North America, Europe, and Australia. Some of the studies reviewed information on exposure that enabled dose-response evaluation. In addition, the committee considered studies in which animals were exposed chronically to asbestos either by inhalation (Hesterberg et al. 1993, 1994; McConnell 2005; McConnell et al. 1994a,b, 1999) or by oral feeding (HHS 1983, 1985, 1988, 1990a,b,c); none reported increased incidence of stomach tumors.

Consistency

The occupational-cohort studies generally, although not uniformly, suggested a slightly increased risk of stomach cancer relative to the general population. There were also several instances in which reasonably strong dose-response gradients were observed in the occupational cohort studies. In contrast, the results from case-control studies were inconsistent, with no clear pattern emerging from the estimated risks of stomach cancer associated with asbestos exposure.

Strength of Association

Considering only the cohort studies, the committee noted that observed risk increases were weak to modest. There was also evidence from several studies supportive of relatively strong dose-response relationships. However, the few weak suggestions of dose-response gradients seen among the cohorts did little to augment the overall strength of evidence of a causal association. The case-control studies were far less informative than the cohort studies in their characterization of either overall associations or dose-response relationships between asbestos and stomach cancer.

Coherence

Asbestos bodies have been identified in human stomach tissue and at other sites in the gastrointestinal tract (Auerbach et al. 1980, Kobayashi et al. 1987). It is plausible that asbestos fibers could accumulate at sites of mucosal injury and ulceration in the stomach, but the extent to which this occurs in exposed persons has not been investigated. As is the case for finding asbestos bodies at other sites, contamination during collection or processing of tissue samples is a possibility, as discussed in Chapter 4. The potential role of asbestos fibers as a cofactor with established risk factors (such as *H. pylori*) has not been investigated experimentally or epidemiologically.

Stomach cancer has received far less attention than mesothelioma or lung cancer in toxicologic research on asbestos. The very limited available literature on the topic provides no experimental evidence that asbestos fibers act as a direct or indirect carcinogen in the stomach.

Conclusion

Several considerations led the committee to its conclusion regarding causality for this site. The occupational-cohort studies were the most informative source of evidence. They revealed a generally consistent pattern of fairly modest risk increases. There was also some evidence, albeit inconsistent, of dose-dependence. Considerations of biological plausibility did not strengthen the case for causation. In particular, the extent of asbestos-fiber deposition and retention in human stomach mucosa is not known. Moreover, the limited available evidence from experimental research does not indicate that asbestos is carcinogenic to the stomach.

The committee concluded that evidence is *suggestive but not sufficient* to infer a causal relationship between asbestos exposure and stomach cancer.

REFERENCES

Acheson ED, Gardner MJ, Pippard EC, Grime LP. 1982. Mortality of two groups of women who manufactured gas masks from chrysotile and crocidolite asbestos: A 40-year follow-up. *British Journal of Industrial Medicine* 39(4): 344-348.

Acheson ED, Gardner MJ, Winter PD, Bennett C. 1984. Cancer in a factory using amosite asbestos. *International Journal of Epidemiology* 13(1): 3-10.

Amandus HE, Wheeler R, Jankovic J, Tucker J. 1987. The morbidity and mortality of vermiculite miners and millers exposed to tremolite-actinolite: Part I. Exposure estimates. *American Journal of Industrial Medicine* 11(1): 1-14.

Armstrong BK, de Klerk NH, Musk AW, Hobbs MS. 1988. Mortality in miners and millers of crocidolite in Western Australia. *British Journal of Industrial Medicine* 45(1): 5-13.

Auerbach O, Conston AS, Garfinkel L, Parks VR, Kaslow HD, Hammond EC. 1980. Presence of asbestos bodies in organs other than the lung. *Chest* 77(2): 133-137.

Battista G, Belli S, Comba P, Fiumalbi C, Grignoli M, Loi F, Orsi D, Paredes I. 1999. Mortality due to asbestos-related causes among railway carriage construction and repair workers. *Occupation Medicine (London)* 49(8): 536-539.

Berry G, Newhouse ML, Wagner JC. 2000. Mortality from all cancers of asbestos factory workers in east London 1933-80. *Occupational and Environmental Medicine* 57(11): 782-785.

Botta M, Magnani C, Terracini B, Bertolone GP, Castagneto B, Cocito V, DeGiovanni D, Paglieri P. 1991. Mortality from respiratory and digestive cancers among asbestos cement workers in Italy. *Cancer Detection and Prevention* 15(6): 445-447.

Cocco P, Palli D, Buiatti E, Cipriani F, DeCarli A, Manca P, Ward MH, Blot WJ, Fraumeni JF Jr. 1994. Occupational exposures as risk factors for gastric cancer in Italy. *Cancer Causes and Control* 5(3): 241-248.

de Klerk NH, Armstrong BK, Musk AW, Hobbs MS. 1989. Cancer mortality in relation to measures of occupational exposure to crocidolite at Wittenoom Gorge in Western Australia. *British Journal of Industrial Medicine* 46(8): 529-536.

Dement JM, Brown DP, Okun A. 1994. Follow-up study of chrysotile asbestos textile workers: Cohort mortality and case-control analyses. *American Journal of Industrial Medicine* 26(4): 431-447.

Ekstrom AM, Eriksson M, Hansson LE, Lindgren A, Signorello LB, Nyren O, Hardell L. 1999. Occupational exposures and risk of gastric cancer in a population-based case-control study. *Cancer Research* 59(23): 5932-5937.

Enterline PE, Hartley J, Henderson V. 1987. Asbestos and cancer: A cohort followed up to death. *British Journal of Industrial Medicine* 44(6): 396-401.

Finkelstein MM, Verma DK. 2004. A cohort study of mortality among Ontario pipe trades workers. *Occupational and Environmental Medicine* 61(9): 736-742.

Gardner MJ, Winter PD, Pannett B, Powell CA. 1986. Follow up study of workers manufacturing chrysotile asbestos cement products. *British Journal of Industrial Medicine* 43(11): 726-732.

Germani D, Belli S, Bruno C, Grignoli M, Dstat MN, Pirastu R, Comba P. 1999. Cohort mortality study of women compensated for asbestosis in Italy. *American Journal Industrial Medicine* 36(1): 129-134.

Hesterberg TW, Miller WC, McConnell EE, Chevalier J, Hadley JG, Bernstein DM, Thevenaz P, Anderson R. 1993. Chronic inhalation toxicity of size-separated glass fibers in Fischer 344 rats. *Fundamental and Applied Toxicology* 20(4): 464-476.

Hesterberg TW, Miller WC, Mast R, McConnell EE, Bernstein DM, Anderson R. 1994. Relationship between lung biopersistence and biological effects of man-made vitreous fibers after chronic inhalation in rats. *Environmental Health Perspectives* 102 (Supplement 5): 133-137.

HHS (US Department of Health and Human Services). 1983. *Lifetime Carcinogenesis Studies of Amosite Asbestos (CAS NO. 12172-73-5) in Syrian Golden Hamsters (Feed Studies).* NTP TR 249. Research Triangle Park, NC: National Toxicology Program.

HHS. 1985. *Toxicology and Carcinogenesis Studies of Chrysotile Asbestos (CAS No. 12001-29-5) in F344/N Rats (Feed Studies).* NTP TR 295. Research Triangle Park, NC: National Toxicology Program.

HHS. 1988. *Toxicology and Carcinogenesis Studies of Crocidolite Asbestos (CAS No. 12001-28-4) in F344/N Rats (Feed Studies).* NTP TR 280. Research Triangle Park, NC: National Toxicology Program.

HHS. 1990a. *Lifetime Carcinogenesis Studies of Chrysotile Asbestos (CAS No. 12001-29-5) in Syrian Golden Hamsters (Feed Studies).* NTP TR 246. Research Triangle Park, North Carolina: National Toxicology Program.

HHS. 1990b. *Toxicology and Carcinogenesis Studies of Amosite Asbestos (CAS No. 12172-73-5) in F344/N Rats (Feed Studies).* NTP TR 279. Research Triangle Park, NC: National Toxicology Program.

HHS. 1990c. *Toxicology and Carcinogenesis Studies of Tremolite (CAS No. 14567-73-8) in F344/N Rats (Feed Studies).* NTP TR 277. Research Triangle Park, NC: National Toxicology Program.

Hillerdal G. 1980. Gastrointestinal carcinoma and occurrence of pleural plaques on pulmonary X-ray. *Journal of Occupational Medicine* 22(12): 806-809.

Hodgson JT, Jones RD. 1986. Mortality of asbestos workers in England and Wales 1971-81. *British Journal of Industrial Medicine* 43(3): 158-164.

Hughes JM, Weill H, Hammad YY. 1987. Mortality of workers employed in two asbestos cement manufacturing plants. *British Journal of Industrial Medicine* 44(3): 161-174.

Jemal A, Siegel R, Ward E, Murray T, Xu J, Smigal C, Thun M. 2006. Cancer statistics, 2006. *CA: A Cancer Journal for Clinicians* 56: 106-130.

Karjalainen A, Pukkala E, Kauppinen T, Partanen T. 1999. Incidence of cancer among Finnish patients with asbestos-related pulmonary or pleural fibrosis. *Cancer Causes and Control* 10(1): 51-57.

Kobayashi H, Ming ZW, Watanabe H, Ohnishi Y. 1987. A quantitative study on the distribution of asbestos bodies in extrapulmonary organs. *ACTA Pathologica Japonica* 37(3): 375-383.

Kogan PM, Yatsenko AS, Tregubov ES, Gurvich EB, Kuzina LE. 1993. Evaluation of carcinogenic risk in friction product workers. *Medicina del Lavoro* 84(4): 290-296.

Krstev S, Dosemeci M, Lissowska J, Chow WH, Zatonski W, Ward MH. 2005. Occupation and risk of stomach cancer in Poland. *Occupational and Environmental Medicine* 62(5): 318-324.

Levin J, McLarty J, Hurst GA, Smith A, Frank AL. 1998. Tyler asbestos workers: Mortality experience in a cohort exposed to amosite. *Occupational and Environmental Medicine* 55(3): 155-160.

Liddell FD, McDonald AD, McDonald JC. 1997. The 1891-1920 birth cohort of Quebec chrysotile miners and millers: Development from 1904 and mortality to 1992. *Annals of Occupational Hygiene* 41(1): 13-36.

McConnell EE. 2005 (October 27). *Personal Communication to Mary Paxton for the Committee on Asbestos: Selected Health Effects.* Available in IOM Public Access Files.

McConnell E, Kamstrup O, Musselman R, Hesterberg T, Chevalier J, Miller W, Thevenaz P. 1994a. Chronic inhalation study of size-separated rock and slag wool insulation fibers in Fischer 344/N rats. *Inhalation Toxicology* 6(6): 571-614.

McConnell E, Mast R, Hesterberg T, Chevalier J, Kotin P, Bernstein D, Thevenaz P, Glass L, Anderson R. 1994b. Chronic inhalation toxicity of a kaolin-based refactory cermaic fiber in Syrian golden hamsters. *Inhalation Toxicology* 6(6): 503-532.

McConnell EE, Axten C, Hesterberg TW, Chevalier J, Miller WC, Everitt J, Oberdorster G, Chase GR, Thevenaz P, Kotin P. 1999. Studies on the inhalation toxicology of two fiberglasses and amosite asbestos in the Syrian golden hamster: Part II. Results of chronic exposure. *Inhalation Toxicology* 11(9): 785-835.

Meurman LO, Pukkala E, Hakama M. 1994. Incidence of cancer among anthophyllite asbestos miners in Finland. *Occupational and Environmental Medicine* 51(6): 421-425.

Pang ZC, Zhang Z, Wang Y, Zhang H. 1997. Mortality from a Chinese asbestos plant: Overall cancer mortality. *American Journal of Industrial Medicine* 32(5): 442-444.

Parent ME, Siemiatycki J, Fritschi L. 1998. Occupational exposures and gastric cancer. *Epidemiology* 9(1): 48-55.

Peto J, Doll R, Hermon C, Binns W, Clayton R, Goffe T. 1985. Relationship of mortality to measures of environmental asbestos pollution in an asbestos textile factory. *Annals of Occupational Hygiene* 29(3): 305-355.

Piolatto G, Negri E, La Vecchia C, Pira E, Decarli A, Peto J. 1990. An update of cancer mortality among chrysotile asbestos miners in Balangero, northern Italy. *British Journal of Industrial Medicine* 47(12): 810-814.

Pira E, Pelucchi C, Buffoni L, Palmas A, Turbiglio M, Negri E, Piolatto PG, La Vecchia C. 2005. Cancer mortality in a cohort of asbestos textile workers. *British Journal of Cancer* 92(3): 580-586.

Puntoni R, Merlo F, Borsa L, Reggiardo G, Garrone E, Ceppi M. 2001. A historical cohort mortality study among shipyard workers in Genoa, Italy. *American Journal of Industrial Medicine* 40(4): 363-370.

Raffn E, Lynge E, Juel K, Korsgaard B. 1989. Incidence of cancer and mortality among employees in the asbestos cement industry in Denmark. *British Journal of Industrial Medicine* 46(2): 90-96.

Reid A, Ambrosini G, de Klerk N, Fritschi L, Musk B. 2004. Aerodigestive and gastrointestinal tract cancers and exposure to crocidolite (blue asbestos): Incidence and mortality among former crocidolite workers. *International Journal of Cancer* 111(5): 757-761.

Sanden A, Jarvholm B. 1987. Cancer morbidity in Swedish shipyard workers 1978-1983. *International Archives of Occupational and Environmental Health* 59(5): 455-462.

Seidman H, Selikoff IJ, Gelb SK. 1986. Mortality experience of amosite asbestos factory workers: Dose-response relationships 5 to 40 years after onset of short-term work exposure. *American Journal of Industrial Medicine* 10(5-6): 479-514.

Selikoff IJ, Seidman H. 1991. Asbestos-associated deaths among insulation workers in the United States and Canada, 1967-1987. *Annals of the New York Academy of Sciences* 643: 1-14.

Selikoff IJ, Hammond EC, Seidman H. 1979. Mortality experience of insulation workers in the United States and Canada, 1943-1976. *Annals of the New York Academy of Sciences* 330: 91-116.

Smailyte G, Kurtinaitis J, Andersen A. 2004. Cancer mortality and morbidity among Lithuanian asbestos-cement producing workers. *Scandinavian Journal of Work, Environment and Health* 30(1): 64-70.

Szeszenia-Dabrowska N, Urszula W, Szymczak W, Strzelecka A. 2002. Mortality study of workers compensated for asbestosis in Poland, 1970-1997. *International Journal of Occupation Medicine and Environmental Health* 15(3): 267-278.

Zhu H, Wang Z. 1993. Study of occupational lung cancer in asbestos factories in China. *British Journal of Industrial Medicine* 50(11): 1039-1042.

11

Colorectal Cancer and Asbestos

NATURE OF THIS CANCER TYPE

Together, cancers of the colon and rectum (ICD-9 153-154; ICD-O-3 C18.0-C20.9; see Figure 9.1) are the third-most common cancer and cause of cancer death among men and women in the United States. The American Cancer Society (Jemal et al. 2006) has projected that 148,610 new cases (106,680 colon and 41,930 rectum) and 55,170 deaths will occur in the United States in 2006. Colon and rectum cancers together account for about 10% of all cancer deaths. The incidence of cancers of the colon and rectum combined decreased by an average of 2.2% per year from 1998 to 2002, presumably in part because of increased screening and removal of adenomatous polyps that might otherwise progress to cancer. The age-standardized death rate from colorectal cancer decreased by an average of 1.8% per year from 1984 to 2002. The decreasing mortality reflects both the decrease in incidence and improvements in treatment and survival.

The risk of colon and rectum cancer increases with age; more than 90% of cases are diagnosed in people over 50 years old. Other risk factors for colon cancer are obesity (especially in men), physical inactivity, heavy consumption of alcohol and of red or processed meat, a history of inflammatory bowel disease, and a family history of colon or rectum cancer, especially in persons under 40 years old. Tobacco-smoking is an established risk factor for ademomatous polyps, the main precursor of colon cancer. Studies suggest that treatment with nonsteroidal anti-inflammatory drugs (NSAIDs), such as aspirin, and estrogen alone or in sequential use with progestin hormone therapy may reduce colorectal-cancer risk. However, no medical organizations recommend treatment with NSAIDs or postmenopausal estrogen and progestin hormone replacement to prevent cancer because of potential side effects of NSAIDs and hormones. Women who take hormone-replacement therapy may be more likely to have colorectal cancer diagnosed at a more advanced stage.

The 1- and 5-year survival rates for persons with colorectal cancer are 83% and 63%, respectively. Survival continues to decline beyond 5 years to 57% at 10 years after diagnosis. When colorectal cancers are detected at an early, localized stage, the 5-year survival rate is 90%; however, only 39% of colorectal cancers are diagnosed at this stage, mostly because of low rates of screening. After the cancer has spread regionally to involve adjacent organs or lymph nodes, the 5-year survival rate drops to 67%. The 5-year survival rate for persons with distant metastases is 10%.

EPIDEMIOLOGIC EVIDENCE CONSIDERED

Results varied from study to study (for both cohort and case-control designs) in whether they were presented as colorectal or for colon and for rectum separately. In reviewing the available data on cancers of the colon and rectum in association with exposure to asbestos, the committee conducted three preliminary meta-analyses on the information presented separately for colon, for rectum, and for colorectal cancer as already combined by the original researchers. The plots and summary tables for those runs are presented in Appendix F. For the 15 cohort populations with individual results for colon and for rectum there did not appear to be any systematic difference, and their aggregate results were similar to those for the studies that had precombined their observations into a colorectal category. The results when the case-control results were considered in this fashion were so sparse that strong contrasts could not be drawn, but no major difference was apparent.

Condensing these three datasets into a single analysis would provide a better chance of amassing adequate information to reach a conclusion, and did not seem contraindicated by the screening runs. Furthermore, the legislation driving the committee's charge specified colorectal cancer as a single endpoint. Age and sex are the primary known risk factors for rectal cancer, while colon cancer also appears more clearly associated with family history, physical inactivity, and several other factors such as body mass index and dietary and alcohol intake (Wei et al. 2004). Less ability to detect risk factors may itself be a function of limited statistical power arising from the fact that rectal cancer comprises only about 30% of tumors of the large intestine. Because these subsites are not clearly or consistently distinguished from each other on death certificates, colon and rectum cancer are frequently combined in analyses based on mortality, as was the case of a majority of the cohort studies in this review. Taking account of all these factors, the committee decided to group separate results for colon and rectum within individual cohort studies and to discuss all the findings as colorectal.

In only two cohort studies were separate results for colon not accompanied by separate results for rectum. Only statistics on colon cancer were available for the women reported in Karjalainen et al. (1999), and subsequent tables revealed that the three colorectal cancers among all men reported by Sanden and Jarvholm (1987) were all rectal cancers in people with more than 20 years since first exposure. Otherwise, reported expectations permitted accurate combination to derive relative risks (RRs) for colorectal cancers within all the cohort populations. The 11 case-control citations were somewhat more problematic, because when colon- or rectum-specific results were given combined RRs could not be calculated from information present in the papers; the outcomes that each actually reported are indicated in the plots below.

Cohort Studies

The cohorts that presented usable information on the risk of colorectal cancer were indicated in Table 6.1. Their histories and design properties are described in Table B.1, and the details of their results concerning cancer at this site are abstracted in Table D.5. The results of both the cohort and the case-control studies are summarized in Table 11.1, and Figures 11.1 and 11.2 are plots of RRs for overall exposure and for exposure-response gradients from the cohort studies reviewed. Colorectal cancer occurred with far greater frequency than either esophageal or stomach cancer in the cohorts studied, and this enabled more statistically precise risk estimation. Thirty-two citations on cohort studies presented results on the association between asbestos exposure and colorectal cancer for a total of 41 distinct subpopulations.

The cohort studies were limited in that they were largely restricted to mortality, which may not give a complete account of occurrence of colorectal cancer. Also, data on known risks (such as family history of colorectal cancer and/or diet) were not available in any of the cohort studies; because such non-occupational risk factors are not likely to have been associated with asbestos exposure, however, they probably do not represent important confounders.

The Finnish women with asbestos-related diseases (Karjalainen et al. 1999), for whom only colon cancer was reported, had the highest RRs. The largest excesses of colorectal cancer were observed among the earliest North American insulation workers (Selikoff et al. 1979) and British male insulation workers (Berry et al. 2000). In contrast, numerous reports were consistent with no association and several were consistent with a negative asso-

TABLE 11.1 Summary of Epidemiologic Findings Regarding Cancer of the Colon or Rectum

Study Type	Figure	Comparison	Study Populations Included	No. Study Populations	Summary RR (95% CI)	Between-Study SD
Cohort	11.1	Any vs none	All	41	1.15 (1.01-1.31)	
	11.2	High vs none[a]	Lower bound[b]	13	1.24 (0.91-1.69)	—
			Upper bound[b]	13	1.38 (1.14-1.67)	—
Case-control	11.3	Any vs none	All	13	1.16 (0.90-1.49)	0.32
	11.4	Any vs none	EAM = 1	8	0.98 (0.75-1.29)	.29
			EAM = 2	5	2.00 (1.28-3.14)	.00
	11.5	High vs none[a]	EAM = 1 Lower bound[b]	7	1.02 (0.57-1.82)	.51
			EAM = 1 Upper bound[b]	7	1.14 (0.70-1.89)	.45

NOTE: CI = Confidence interval; EAM = exposure-assessment method; high quality, EAM = 1; lower quality, EAM = 2; RR = relative risk; SD = standard deviation.

[a]Used studies that reported dose-response relationship (RR on an exposure gradient).

[b]For studies that reported dose-response relationship on multiple gradient metrics, the smallest "high vs none" RR was used to compute the lower bound, and the largest "high vs none" RR was used to compute the upper bound.

ciation. Overall, the cohort studies (Figure 11.2) showed a small and marginally significant association between asbestos exposure and colorectal cancer (RR = 1.15, 95% CI 1.02-1.31).

The summary estimate derived by aggregating the highest of the reported extreme-exposure RR was 1.38 (95% CI 1.14-1.67), whereas the estimate of association from combining the lowest of the reported RR for the extreme category of an exposure gradient was 1.24 (95% CI 0.91-1.67) (Figure 11.2). Although those summary risk estimates for extreme exposures are greater than the summary for any exposure (1.15 from Figure 11.1), the difference is small.

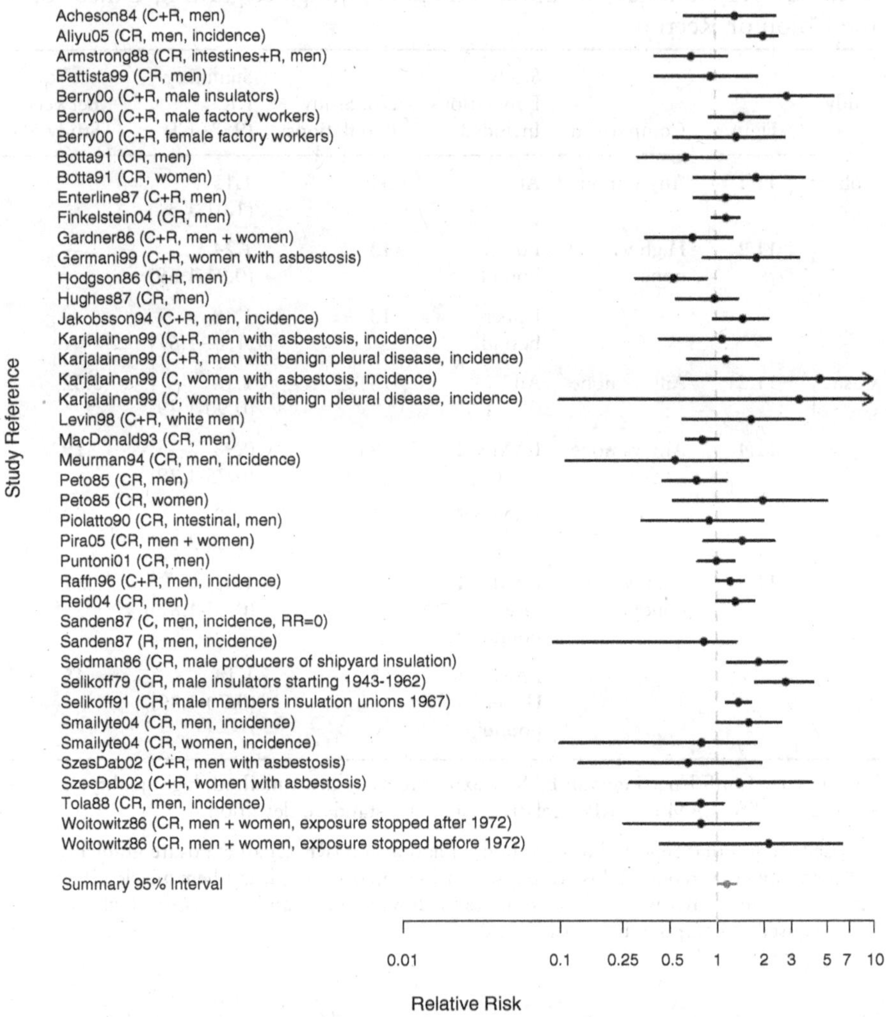

FIGURE 11.1 Cohort studies: RR of colorectal cancer in people with "any" exposure to asbestos compared with people who report none.

Case-Control Studies

The case-control studies retained for thorough evaluation after exclusion of studies that did not assess exposure to asbestos or did not meet other exclusion criteria are listed in Table 6.5 according to quality of their exposure assessment. The details of the design aspects of those studies are presented in Table C.1 and their detailed results are abstracted in Table E.5.

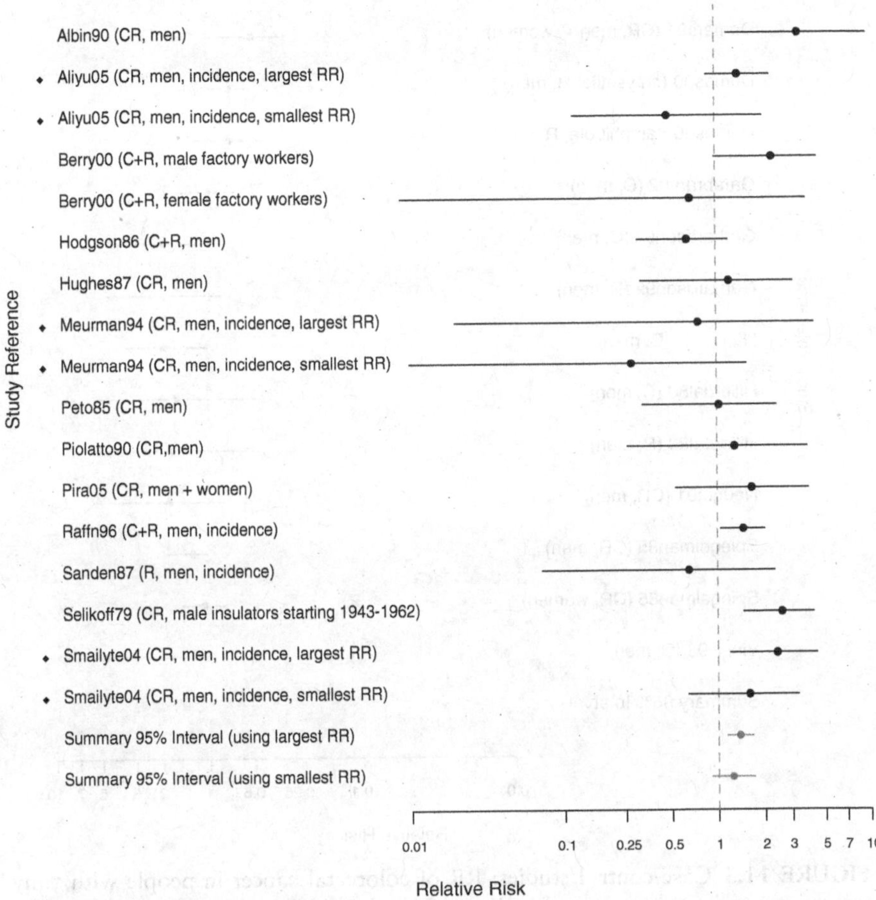

FIGURE 11.2 Cohort studies: RRs of colorectal cancer among people in most extreme exposure category compared to those with none (♦ = more than one exposure gradient reported in citation, so the plot contains both highest and lowest estimates of risk for most extreme category over all gradients).

Of the 11 citations, one (Dumas et al. 2000) reported only on rectal cancer, and five investigated only colon cancer (Fredriksson et al. 1989, Garabrant et al. 1992, Goldberg et al. 2001, Hardell 1981, Vineis et al. 1993). Separate results for colon and rectal cancers could not be readily merged into a colorectal grouping as was done for the cohorts, but the results have been considered together in this review. The findings of all 11 studies are summarized in Table 11.1 and in the plots presented in Figures 11.3-11.5, where the citation labels indicate whether the RR pertains to colon (C), rectum (R), or both (CR). The committee did not seek adjustment for confounders

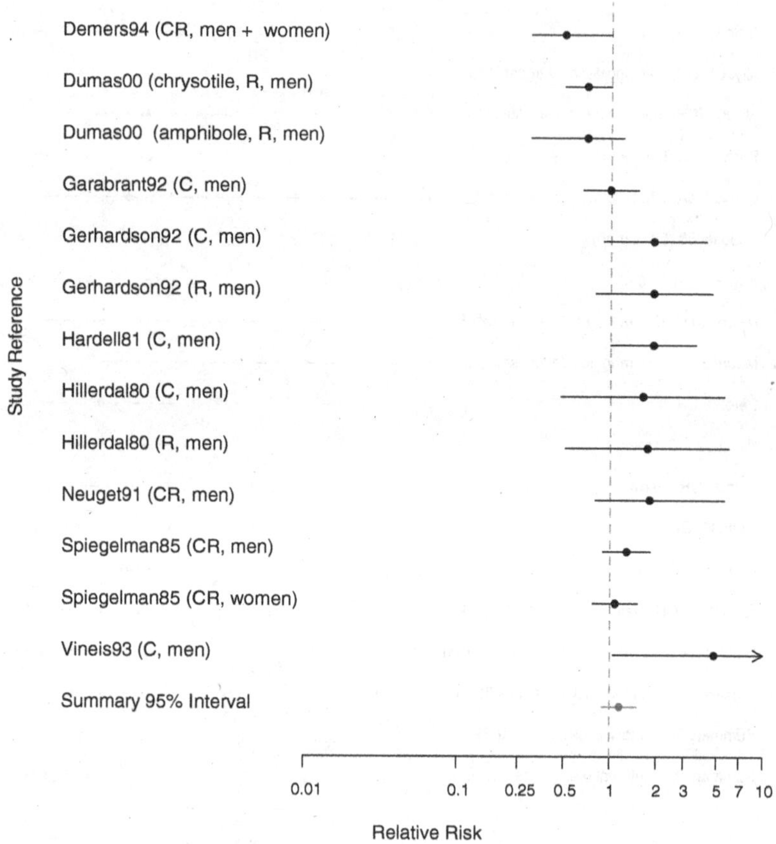

FIGURE 11.3 Case-control studies: RR of colorectal cancer in people with "any" exposure to asbestos compared with people with none.

other than sex and age for this cancer type, so a plot stratified on adjustment was not generated.

Thirteen results for any exposure were reviewed; eight point estimates exceeded 1.0, two were almost exactly 1.0, and three point estimates were less than 1.0 (Figure 11.3). When they were combined, the average estimate of association was 1.16 (95% CI 0.90-1.49).

We next considered separately high-quality and lower-quality studies (Figure 11.4). In the colorectal case-control studies with higher-quality assessment of asbestos exposure, the summary estimate of association was essentially null (95% CI 0.75-1.29); in the lower-quality studies, the summary estimate of association was significantly positive (RR = 2.00, 95% CI 1.28-3.14). That pattern suggests that lower-quality studies—those with

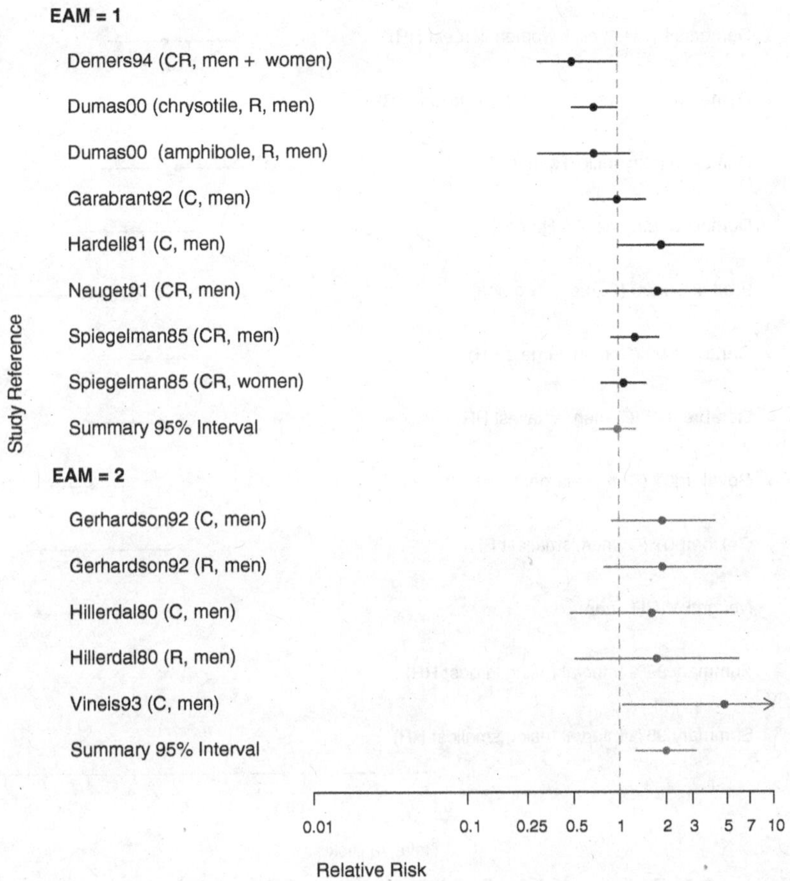

FIGURE 11.4 Case-control studies: RR of colorectal cancer in people with "any" exposure to asbestos compared with people with none, stratified on quality of exposure assessment (top, EAM = 1: higher-quality exposure assessment; bottom, EAM = 2: lower-quality exposure assessment).

less rigorous classification of exposure and typically without adjustment for confounding—were more likely to show associations between asbestos exposure and colorectal cancer.

The case-control studies evaluating gradients of exposure (Figure 11.5) did not find stronger associations between the highest exposure and colorectal cancer (RR = 1.02, 95% CI 0.57-1.82 for lowest estimates; and RR = 1.14, 95% CI 0.70-1.89 for highest estimates). That is, among groups with colorectal cancer those with high exposure did not, in aggregate, have a greater risk of cancer than those with simply any exposure.

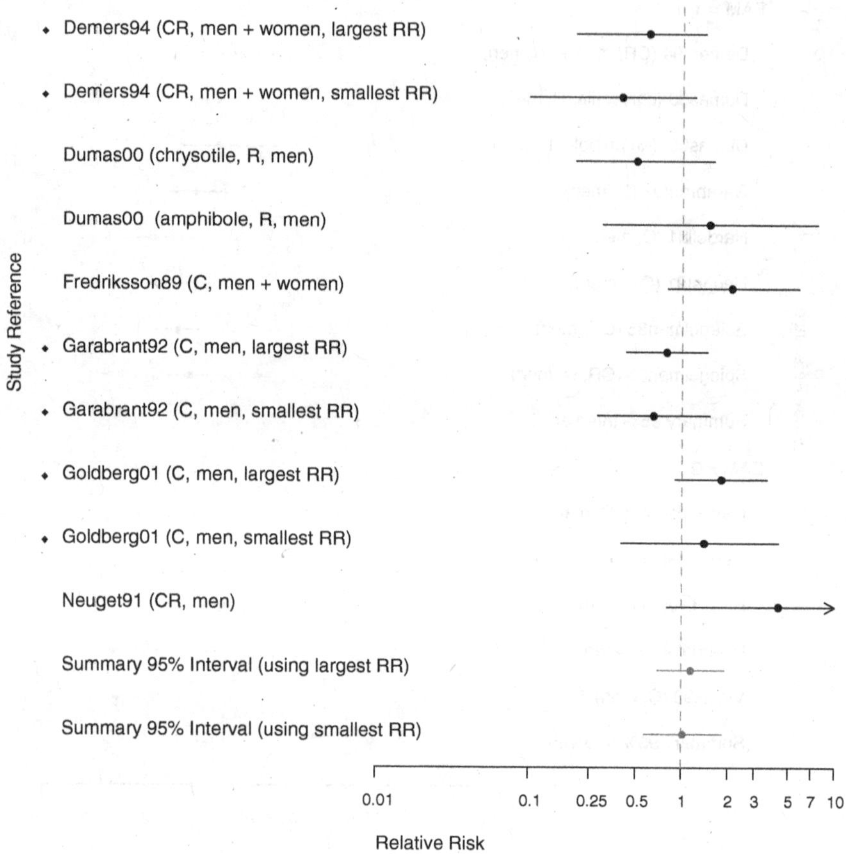

FIGURE 11.5 Case-control studies: RRs of colorectal cancer among people in most extreme exposure category compared to those with none (♦ = more than one exposure gradient reported in citation, so the plot contains both highest and lowest estimates of risk for most extreme category over all gradients).

EVIDENCE INTEGRATION AND CONCLUSION

Evidence Considered

Thirty-two citations containing relevant information on 41 occupational cohort populations and 11 case-control studies of colorectal cancer contributed epidemiologic data. Findings related to the response to asbestos by tissues in the colon and rectum were evaluated from several well conducted chronic rodent studies, four with inhalation exposure and six with dietary administration.

Consistency

The occupational-cohort studies suggested fairly consistently, although not uniformly, that the risk of colorectal cancer was higher in exposed people than in the general population. In contrast, the case-control studies lacked consistency: estimated effects of asbestos exposure range from apparently protective to seemingly harmful, whereas the one study with the most detailed asbestos-exposure assessment and analysis (Garabrant et al. 1992) had essentially null findings.

Strength of Associations

For the case-control studies, the summary estimate of association was close to null and not statistically significant. Moreover, evidence of a dose-response relationship in the case-control studies was lacking. The overall observed risk estimate from cohort studies was modestly above 1.0 and statistically significant with some—albeit modest—evidence of a dose-response relationship.

Coherence

Colorectal tumors are most commonly adenocarcinomas that arise in polyps. Multiple risk factors are associated with colon cancer, including age, familial predisposition, obesity, physical inactivity, and inflammatory bowel disease. The potential role of asbestos fibers as a cofactor has not been investigated in epidemiologic or experimental studies.

Asbestos bodies and asbestos fibers have been identified in the colon. Ehrlich et al. (1991) recovered both from the biopsy samples from a third of a small group of asbestos workers with colon cancer, but none from the colons of patients without a history of asbestos exposure. Auerbach et al. (1980) recovered asbestos bodies from colon tissue, as did Kobayashi et al. (1987), who reported recovering them from both the large and small intestine. In patients with inflammatory bowel disease and colon tumors, it is uncertain whether fibers accumulate secondarily at sites of mucosal injury or ulceration associated with inflammation or in an expanding tumor. As is the case for finding asbestos bodies at other sites, contamination during collection or processing of tissue samples is a possibility, as discussed in Chapter 4.

One animal study (Amacher et al. 1974) showed that even a single dose of chrysotile fed to rats, if large enough, consistently caused a transient increase in DNA synthesis in the colon weeks later suggesting gastrointestinal absorption had occurred at some unspecified site, but overall animal models have failed to produce colon or colorectal cancer. Thorough examination of rats and Syrian hamsters exposed to asbestos by inhalation at levels sufficient to cause mesothelioma in both species and lung cancer in rats did not find colorectal malignancies (Hesterberg et al. 1993, 1994; McConnell 2005; McConnell et al. 1994a,b, 1999). One (HHS 1985) of six lifetime, high-dose asbestos feeding studies in rodents (HHS 1983, 1985, 1988, 1990a,b,c) did, however, produced benign adenomatous colon polyps in rats after chrysotile exposure. Benign adematous colon polyps are a precursor of the most common type of colon cancer in humans. No polyps were produced by chronic asbestos feeding in hamsters.

Conclusion

The committee judged that some aspects of the evidence were supportive of a causal association: a positive but small aggregate association with a narrow confidence band arising from the many cohort findings possible biologic plausibility suggested by the presence of asbestos bodies and fibers in the colons of asbestos workers and the experimental induction of colon polyps, albeit benign, in rats. The overall lack of consistency or of the suggestion of an association among the case-control studies (even those of the highest quality) and the absence of convincing dose-response relationships in either type of study design, however, weigh against causality.

Thus, the committee determined that the evidence is *suggestive but not sufficient* to infer a causal relationship between asbestos exposure and colorectal cancer.

REFERENCES

Acheson ED, Gardner MJ, Winter PD, Bennett C. 1984. Cancer in a factory using amosite asbestos. *International Journal of Epidemiology* 13(1): 3-10.

Albin M, Jakobsson K, Attewell R, Johansson L, Welinder H. 1990. Mortality and cancer morbidity in cohorts of asbestos cement workers and referents. *British Journal of Industrial Medicine* 47(9): 602-610.

Aliyu OA, Cullen MR, Barnett MJ, Balmes JR, Cartmel B, Redlich CA, Brodkin CA, Barnhart S, Rosenstock L, Israel L, Goodman GE, Thornquist MD, Omenn GS. 2005. Evidence for excess colorectal cancer incidence among asbestos-exposed men in the Beta-Carotene and Retinol Efficacy Trial. *American Journal of Epidemiology* 162(9): 868-878.

Amacher DE, Alarif A, Epstein SS. 1974. Effects of ingested chrysotile on DNA synthesis in the gastrointestinal tract and liver of the rat. *Environmental Health Perspectives* 9: 319-324.

Armstrong BK, de Klerk NH, Musk AW, Hobbs MS. 1988. Mortality in miners and millers of crocidolite in Western Australia. *British Journal of Industrial Medicine* 45(1): 5-13.

Auerbach O, Conston AS, Garfinkel L, Parks VR, Kaslow HD, Hammond EC. 1980. Presence of asbestos bodies in organs other than the lung. *Chest* 77(2): 133-137.

Battista G, Belli S, Comba P, Fiumalbi C, Grignoli M, Loi F, Orsi D, Paredes I. 1999. Mortality due to asbestos-related causes among railway carriage construction and repair workers. *Occupation Medicine (London)* 49(8): 536-539.

Berry G, Newhouse ML, Wagner JC. 2000. Mortality from all cancers of asbestos factory workers in east London 1933-80. *Occupational and Environmental Medicine* 57(11): 782-785.

Botta M, Magnani C, Terracini B, Bertolone GP, Castagneto B, Cocito V, DeGiovanni D, Paglieri P. 1991. Mortality from respiratory and digestive cancers among asbestos cement workers in Italy. *Cancer Detection and Prevention* 15(6): 445-447.

Demers RY, Burns PB, Swanson GM. 1994. Construction occupations, asbestos exposure, and cancer of the colon and rectum. *Journal of Occupational Medicine* 36(9): 1027-1031.

Dumas S, Parent ME, Siemiatycki J, Brisson J. 2000. Rectal cancer and occupational risk factors: A hypothesis-generating, exposure-based case-control study. *International Journal of Cancer* 87(6): 874-879.

Ehrlich A, Gordon RE, Dikman SH. 1991. Carcinoma of the colon in asbestos-exposed workers: Analysis of asbestos content in colon tissue. *American Journal of Industrial Medicine* 19(5): 629-636.

Enterline PE, Hartley J, Henderson V. 1987. Asbestos and cancer: A cohort followed up to death. *British Journal of Industrial Medicine* 44(6): 396-401.

Finkelstein MM, Verma DK. 2004. A cohort study of mortality among Ontario pipe trades workers. *Occupational and Environmental Medicine* 61(9): 736-742.

Fredriksson M, Bengtsson NO, Hardell L, Axelson O. 1989. Colon cancer, physical activity, and occupational exposures: A case-control study. *Cancer* 63(9): 1838-1842.

Garabrant DH, Peters RK, Homa DM. 1992. Asbestos and colon cancer: Lack of association in a large case-control study. *American Journal of Epidemiology* 135(8): 843-853.

Gardner MJ, Powell CA. 1986. Mortality of asbestos cement workers using almost exclusively chrysotile fibre. *Journal of the Society of Occupational Medicine* 36(4): 124-126.

Gerhardsson de Verdier M, Plato N, Steineck G, Peters JM.1992. Occupational exposures and cancer of the colon and rectum. *American Journal of Industrial Medicine* 22(3): 291-303.

Germani D, Belli S, Bruno C, Grignoli M, Nesti M, Pirastu R, Comba P. 1999. Cohort mortality study of women compensated for asbestosis in Italy. *American Journal of Industrial Medicine* 36(1): 129-134.

Goldberg MS, Parent ME, Siemiatycki J, Desy M, Nadon L, Richardson L, Lakhani R, Latreille B, Valois MF. 2001. A case-control study of the relationship between the risk of colon cancer in men and exposures to occupational agents. *American Journal of Industrial Medicine* 39(6): 531-546.

Hardell L. 1981. Relation of soft-tissue sarcoma, malignant lymphoma and colon cancer to phenoxy acids, chlorophenols and other agents. *Scandinavian Journal of Work, Environment and Health* 7(2): 119-130.

Hesterberg TW, Miller WC, McConnell EE, Chevalier J, Hadley JG, Bernstein DM, Thevenaz P, Anderson R. 1993. Chronic inhalation toxicity of size-separated glass fibers in Fischer 344 rats. *Fundamental and Applied Toxicology* 20(4): 464-476.

Hesterberg TW, Miller WC, Mast R, McConnell EE, Bernstein DM, Anderson R. 1994. Relationship between lung biopersistence and biological effects of man-made vitreous fibers after chronic inhalation in rats. *Environmental Health Perspectives* 102 (Supplement 5): 133-137.

HHS (US Department of Health and Human Services). 1983. *Lifetime Carcinogenesis Studies of Amosite Asbestos (CAS NO. 12172-73-5) in Syrian Golden Hamsters (Feed Studies).* NTP TR 249. Research Triangle Park, NC: National Toxicology Program.

HHS. 1985. *Toxicology and Carcinogenesis Studies of Chrysotile Asbestos (CAS No. 12001-29-5) in F344/N Rats (Feed Studies).* NTP TR 295. Research Triangle Park, NC: National Toxicology Program.

HHS. 1988. *Toxicology and Carcinogenesis Studies of Crocidolite Asbestos (CAS No. 12001-28-4) in F344/N Rats (Feed Studies).* NTP TR 280. Research Triangle Park, NC: National Toxicology Program.

HHS. 1990a. *Lifetime Carcinogenesis Studies of Chrysotile Asbestos (CAS No. 12001-29-5) in Syrian Golden Hamsters (Feed Studies)*. NTP TR 246. Research Triangle Park, North Carolina: National Toxicology Program.

HHS. 1990b. *Toxicology and Carcinogenesis Studies of Amosite Asbestos (CAS No. 12172-73-5) in F344/N Rats (Feed Studies)*. NTP TR 279. Research Triangle Park, NC: National Toxicology Program.

HHS. 1990c. *Toxicology and Carcinogenesis Studies of Tremolite (CAS No. 14567-73-8) in F344/N Rats (Feed Studies)*. NTP TR 277. Research Triangle Park, NC: National Toxicology Program.Hillerdal G. 1980. Gastrointestinal carcinoma and occurrence of pleural plaques on pulmonary X-ray. *Journal of Occupational Medicine* 22(12): 806-809.

Hodgson J, Jones R. 1986. Mortality of asbestos workers in England and Wales 1971-1981. *British Journal of Industrial Medicine* 43(3): 158-164.

Hughes JM, Weill H, Hammad YY. 1987. Mortality of workers employed in two asbestos cement manufacturing plants. *British Journal of Industrial Medicine* 44(3): 161-174.

Jakobsson K, Albin M, Hagmar L. 1994. Asbestos, cement, and cancer in the right part of the colon. *Occupational and Environmental Medicine* 51(2): 95-101.

Jemal A, Siegel R, Ward E, Murray T, Xu J, Smigal C, Thun M. 2006. Cancer statistics, 2006. *CA: A Cancer Journal for Clinicians* 56: 106-130.

Karjalainen A, Pukkala E, Kauppinen T, Partanen T. 1999. Incidence of cancer among Finnish patients with asbestos-related pulmonary or pleural fibrosis. *Cancer Causes and Control* 10(1): 51-57.

Kobayashi H, Ming ZW, Watanabe H, Ohnishi Y. 1987. A quantitative study on the distribution of asbestos bodies in extrapulmonary organs. *ACTA Pathologica Japonica* 37(3): 375-383.

Levin J, McLarty J, Hurst GA, Smith A, Frank AL. 1998. Tyler asbestos workers: Mortality experience in a cohort exposed to amosite. *Occupational and Environmental Medicine* 55(3): 155-160.

McConnell EE. 2005 (October 27). *Personal Communication to Mary Paxton for the Committee on Asbestos: Selected Health Effects.* Available in IOM Public Access Files.

McConnell E, Kamstrup O, Musselman R, Hesterberg T, Chevalier J, Miller W, Thevenaz P. 1994a. Chronic inhalation study of size-separated rock and slag wool insulation fibers in Fischer 344/N rats. *Inhalation Toxicology* 6(6): 571-614.

McConnell E, Mast R, Hesterberg T, Chevalier J, Kotin P, Bernstein D, Thevenaz P, Glass L, Anderson R. 1994b. Chronic inhalation toxicity of a kaolin-based refactory cermaic fiber in Syrian golden hamsters. *Inhalation Toxicology* 6(6): 503-532.

McConnell EE, Axten C, Hesterberg TW, Chevalier J, Miller WC, Everitt J, Oberdorster G, Chase GR, Thevenaz P, Kotin P. 1999. Studies on the inhalation toxicology of two fiberglasses and amosite asbestos in the Syrian golden hamster: Part II. Results of chronic exposure. *Inhalation Toxicology* 11(9): 785-835.

McDonald JC, Liddell FD, Dufresne A, McDonald AD. 1993. The 1891-1920 birth cohort of Quebec chrysotile miners and millers: Mortality 1976-88. *British Journal of Industrial Medicine* 50(12): 1073-1081.

Meurman LO, Pukkala E, Hakama M. 1994. Incidence of cancer among anthophyllite asbestos miners in Finland. *Occupational and Environmental Medicine* 51(6): 421-425.

Neugut AI, Murray TI, Garbowski GC, Treat MR, Forde KA, Waye JD, Fenoglio-Preiser C. 1991. Association of asbestos exposure with colorectal adenomatous polyps and cancer. *Journal of the National Cancer Institute* 83(24): 1827-1828.

Peto J, Doll R, Hermon C, Binns W, Clayton R, Goffe T. 1985. Relationship of mortality to measures of environmental asbestos pollution in an asbestos textile factory. *Annals of Occupational Hygiene* 29(3): 305-355.

Piolatto G, Negri E, La Vecchia C, Pira E, Decarli A, Peto J. 1990. An update of cancer mortality among chrysotile asbestos miners in Balangero, northern Italy. *British Journal of Industrial Medicine* 47(12): 810-814.

Pira E, Pelucchi C, Buffoni L, Palmas A, Turbiglio M, Negri E, Piolatto PG, La Vecchia C. 2005. Cancer mortality in a cohort of asbestos textile workers. *British Journal of Cancer* 92(3): 580-586.

Puntoni R, Merlo F, Borsa L, Reggiardo G, Garrone E, Ceppi M. 2001. A historical cohort mortality study among shipyard workers in Genoa, Italy. *American Journal of Industrial Medicine* 40(4): 363-370.

Raffn E, Villadsen E, Lynge E. 1996. Colorectal cancer in asbestos cement workers in Denmark. *American Journal of Industrial Medicine* 30(3): 267-272.

Reid A, Ambrosini G, de Klerk N, Fritschi L, Musk B. 2004. Aerodigestive and gastrointestinal tract cancers and exposure to crocidolite (blue asbestos): Incidence and mortality among former crocidolite workers. *International Journal of Cancer* 111(5): 757-761.

Sanden A, Jarvholm B. 1987. Cancer morbidity in Swedish shipyard workers 1978-1983. *International Archives of Occupational and Environmental Health* 59(5): 455-462.

Seidman H, Selikoff IJ, Gelb SK. 1986. Mortality experience of amosite asbestos factory workers: Dose-response relationships 5 to 40 years after onset of short-term work exposure. *American Journal of Industrial Medicine* 10(5-6): 479-514.

Selikoff IJ, Seidman H. 1991. Asbestos-associated deaths among insulation workers in the United States and Canada, 1967-1987. *Annals of the New York Academy of Sciences* 643: 1-14.

Selikoff IJ, Hammond EC, Seidman H. 1979. Mortality experience of insulation workers in the United States and Canada, 1943-1976. *Annals of the New York Academy of Sciences* 330: 91-116.

Smailyte G, Kurtinaitis J, Andersen A. 2004. Cancer mortality and morbidity among Lithuanian asbestos-cement producing workers. *Scandinavian Journal of Work, Environment and Health* 30(1): 64-70.

Spiegelman D, Wegman DH. 1985. Occupation-related risks for colorectal cancer. *Journal of the National Cancer Institute* 75(5): 813-821.

Szeszenia-Dabrowska N, Urszula W, Szymczak W, Strzelecka A. 2002. Mortality study of workers compensated for asbestosis in Poland, 1970-1997. *International Journal of Occupational Medicine and Environmental Health* 15(3): 267-278.

Tola S, Kalliomaki PL, Pukkala E, Asp S, Korkala ML. 1988. Incidence of cancer among welders, platers, machinists, and pipe fitters in shipyards and machine shops. *British Journal of Industrial Medicine* 45(4): 209-218.

Vineis P, Ciccone G, Magnino A. 1993. Asbestos exposure, physical activity and colon cancer: A case-control study. *Tumori* 79(5): 301-303.

Wei EK, Giovannucci E, Wu K, Rosner B, Fuchs CS, Willett WC, Colditz GA. 2004. Comparison of risk factors for colon and rectal cancer. *International Journal of Cancer* 108(3): 433-442.

Woitowitz HJ, Lange HJ, Beierl L, Rathgeb M, Schmidt K, Ulm K, Giesen T, Woitowitz RH, Pache L, Rodelsperger K. 1986. Mortality rates in the Federal Republic of Germany following previous occupational exposure to asbestos dust. *International Archives of Occupational and Environmental Health* 57(3): 161-171.

12

Summary and Recommendations

SUMMARY

In addressing its charge of whether asbestos exposure plays a causal role in the occurrence of pharyngeal, laryngeal, esophageal, stomach, or colorectal cancer, the committee reviewed a broad array of evidence from observational and experimental research. Its review emphasized epidemiologic studies of cancer rates in cohorts of asbestos-exposed workers and of risk factors in sets of individuals with cancer at the selected sites in comparison to the general population. The observational evidence was systematically identified and evaluated for its consistency and strength of association. The committee also considered the biologic plausibility of causal associations of asbestos with cancers at the specified sites, recognizing that asbestos is an established cause of mesothelioma and lung cancer. The full committee reviewed the final integration of the evidence to assure uniformity of application of the causal criteria across the sites.

Of the five sites considered, the committee found the evidence to be *sufficient* to infer a causal relationship for laryngeal cancer; to be *suggestive* for pharyngeal, stomach, and colorectal cancers; and to be *inadequate* for esophageal cancer. Most of the non-epidemiologic evidence does not indicate any particular site as being the target of carcinogenic action by asbestos in humans; that evidence and the complementary epidemiologic evidence do establish with certainty that asbestos is a human carcinogen. Although correspondence of tumor sites in humans and experimental animals would constitute intuitively appealing evidence and would likely be mechanistically consistent, it should be noted, however, that empirical consideration of epidemiologic and experimental findings for known carcinogens have demonstrated that site-specificity is not necessarily the rule across species. Documentation of persistence of fibers at a target site would represent important evidence in support of biologic plausibility. Although inhaled asbestos fibers clearly pass by the tissues in question in this report, either directly or by swallowing secretions following clearance from the respiratory tract, investigations on fiber persistence in the target organs with definitive findings proved to be unfortunately sparse. Consequently, the epidemiologic data did, in large part, influence the committee's decision-making for these five sites.

The inference of causality for laryngeal cancer reflects the consistency of the evidence from a substantial number of both worker cohorts and general-population case-control studies, an indication of greater risk among more highly exposed persons, and the finding of an association with exposure in studies that addressed potential confounding by tobacco-smoking and alcohol consumption. In considering biologic plausibility, the committee noted that the epithelium of the larynx is similar to the respiratory epithelium lining the conducting airways of the lung. Inhaled fibers pass through the larynx and may deposit there; although fiber deposition and persistence in the larynx have not been studied extensively, there are reports of fibers and asbestos bodies being recovered from laryngeal tissues.

For all the sites for which the evidence was classified as *suggestive*, the case-control information was less abundant than for laryngeal cancer. For stomach and colorectal cancers, there actually were a few more informative cohorts, but fewer than half as many cohorts provided data on pharyngeal cancer as had on laryngeal cancer. The committee's review found less consistency among the findings of the individual studies for these sites and there was only limited indication of exposure-response relationships. Asbestos fibers could pass through the lumen of the pharynx, stomach, and colon and rectum, but it is uncertain how fibers might interact with the presumed target for carcinogenesis, the cells of the epithelium. Despite sporadic reports of asbestos bodies or fibers being recovered from stomach and colon tissue, information was lacking on the fiber doses received by target cells in the gastrointestinal epithelium. Relevant animal evidence was available from feeding studies, which showed the induction of colon polyps in rats but not the production of malignancy.

The evidence was most sparse for cancer of the esophagus, for which the designation was *inadequate*. There was a suggestion of an exposure-response relationship from the available cohort studies, but the summary estimate of 0.99 for any asbestos exposure was indicative of no association. Only three case-control studies were identified, and investigation of potential confounding was limited. Animal-feeding studies did not show production of esophageal cancers.

RECOMMENDATIONS

This committee was charged with reviewing evidence on a widely used material that is known to cause respiratory malignancy. Asbestos has been extensively investigated as a cause of mesothelioma and lung cancer with epidemiologic and experimental approaches. However, its potential to cause malignancy at other sites that may also be exposed to substantial numbers of asbestos fibers has not been as extensively investigated; little effort has gone into determining delivered or effective dose at these extrapulmonary sites. Much of the information reviewed by the committee came from cohort studies of workers that focused on investigating respiratory effects; information on risks of other diseases, including cancers at the site covered by this committee's charge, was reported only incidentally. Other evidence came from case-control studies directed at the causes of the cancers at the sites of interest, but these studies were not specifically designed to address asbestos exposure and their exposure assessments varied in quality.

The committee's review identified limitations of the available evidence that contributed uncertainty to its conclusions. Although the committee was not charged with developing a research agenda to address the information gaps, its review found many research needs. Research should address the relevance of physical and chemical characteristics of asbestos fibers to carcinogenicity. Studies directed at doses of fibers received by organs other than the lung are needed; mechanistic studies directed at these organs could prove to be a useful complement to ongoing work on the respiratory carcinogenicity of asbestos fibers. Studies involving animal models with high risk for cancer of the designated sites might also be useful. In addition, consideration should be given to approaches to strengthen the epidemiologic information on asbestos exposure and risk of cancers at the sites in the committee's charge. Information might be gained from further follow-up of some of the cohorts of asbestos-exposed workers; however, the committee is concerned that further study of these cohorts may no longer be possible in that most were initiated decades ago and their records may not have been maintained. Some effort might be made to determine whether key cohorts could be followed up or new studies started on potentially informative populations.

APPENDIX A

Agendas of Public Meetings Held by the Committee on Asbestos: Selected Health Effects

FIRST PUBLIC MEETING

Tuesday, July 26, 2005
Keck Building, Room 203
500 Fifth Street NW
Washington, DC

- Welcome, opening remarks, and discussion of agenda for open session
  Jonathan Samet, M.D.
  Committee Chair

- Charge to the committee
  Rose Marie Martinez
  Director, Board on Population Health and Public Health Practice

- Mineralogical properties of asbestos influencing its toxicity
  Jeffrey Post, Ph.D.
  Department of Mineral Sciences
  Smithsonian National Museum of National History
  Washington, DC

- Extra-pulmonary exposure to asbestos
  Ronald Dodson, Ph.D., F.C.C.P., F.A.H.A.
  ERI Consulting
  Tyler, Texas

- Mechanisms of fiber-induced toxicity
  Agnes Kane, Ph.D., M.D.
  Brown University
  Providence, Rhode Island

SECOND PUBLIC MEETING

Wednesday, October 5, 2005
Keck Building, Room 109
500 Fifth Street NW
Washington, DC

- Opening remarks, discussion of agenda for open session
  Jonathan Samet, M.D.
  Committee Chair

- Properties of asbestos involved in mechanisms of action leading to mesothelioma
  Brooke Mossman, Ph.D.
  University of Vermont
  Burlington, Vermont

- Molecular biology of carcinogenesis in gastrointestinal tissues (particularly of the esophagus, stomach, colon, and rectum)
  Karl Kelsey, M.D.
  Harvard School of Public Health
  Boston, Massachusetts

THIRD PUBLIC MEETING

Wednesday, November 16, 2005
NAS Building, Room 150
2101Constitution Avenue NW
Washington, DC

- Opening remarks, discussion of agenda for open session
  Jonathan Samet, M.D.
  Committee Chair

- Meta-analysis issues
  Steve Goodman
  Johns Hopkins University School of Medicine
  Baltimore, Maryland

- Synopsis concerning animal studies
  Ernest E. McConnell (response presented by Rogene Henderson)
  ToxPath, Inc
  Raleigh, North Carolina

- Dosimetry of asbestos fibers
  Frederick Miller, Ph.D.
  Fred J. Miller and Associates LLC
  Cary, North Carolina

- Observed fiber counts in tissues: respiratory versus non-respiratory
  Victor Roggli, M.D. (by teleconference)
  Durham Veterans Administration Medical Center
  Durham, North Carolina

APPENDIX B

Lineage and Design Properties of Studies on Cohorts Informative for Selected Cancers

TABLE B.1 Lineage and Design Properties of Studies on Cohorts Informative for Selected Cancers

Cohort Population (location—number, description)	Type of Exposure	Number of Workers[a]
Patients with Asbestos-Related Disease		
1. Italy— 631 women compensated for asbestosis	implied high exposure to asbestos 1. mainly chrysotile 2. mainly crocidolite	1. 276 textile workers 2. 278 asbestos cement workers
2. Finland— a. 1,376 asbestosis patients b. 4,887 patients with pleural disease		
3. Poland— a. 907 men with asbestosis b. 490 women with asbestosis		
4. US clinical trial monitoring asbestos-exposed men	men with asbestos exposure in clinical trial of lung cancer prevention	1,839 asbestos-exposed (smoking-eligible) vs 7,924 heavy smokers (not asbestos-exposed)
Mining		
5. Wittenoom Gorge, Western Australia	crocidolite	6,000 men
		6,505 men 411 women
		6,506 men
		6,493 men 415 women
		~5,700 men alive in 1980

Temporal Definition	Follow-Up	Citation[b]
alive and on asbestosis compensation roles 12/31/1979	1/1/1980-10/30/1997	**Germani et al. (1999)**
1964-1995	1967-1995	**Karjalainen et al. (1999)**
diagnosed 1970-1997	1999	**Szeszenia-Dabrowska et al. (2002)**
	prospective for 10-18 yrs (1984-2004)	**Aliyu et al. (2005)**
1943-1966		Hobbs et al. (1980)
1943-1966	1980	**Armstrong et al. (1988)**
1943-1966	1980	de Klerk et al. (1989)
1943-1966	2000	Berry et al. (2004)
1943-1966	1979-2000	**Reid et al. (2004)**

continues

TABLE B.1 Continued

Cohort Population (location—number, description)	Type of Exposure	Number of Workers[a]
6. Quebec, Canada—Asbestos and Thetford Mines	chrysotile	6,091 male miners
		11,788 men and women
		544
	chrysotile, also exposed to crocidolite	workers at factory in Asbestos, Quebec
		10,939 men 440 women
		10,939 men 440 women
		5,351 men surviving through 1976 of original 10,939 men
		10,918 men
7. Finland—Paakkila and Maljasalmi Mines	anthophyllite	1,092
	anthophyllite	1,092
	anthophyllite	736 men, 167 women
8. Balangero, Italy	chrysotile	932
	chrysotile	1,094
9. Northern Transvaal, South Africa—North West Cape Blue and Penge Mines	1. crocilodite 2. amosite	7,317 white men 1. 3,430 2. 3,212 3. 675 both
10. Libby, MT, US—NIOSH sample	tremolite-actinolite	
	tremolite-actinolite	575 men
	tremolite	1. 569 men 2. 406 men

Temporal Definition	Follow-Up	Citation[b]
employed in 1950, ≥ 5 yrs exposure	1955	Braun and Truan (1958)
born 1881-1920; with >1 mo working	11/1/1966	McDonald et al. (1971)
employees with ≥ 20 yr in 1961	1977	Nicholson et al. (1979)
born 1881-1920; with >1 mo working	1975	McDonald and Liddell (1979)
born 1881-1920; with >1 mo working	1975	McDonald et al. (1980)
born 1891-1920; with >1 mo before 1967	1975	Liddell et al. (1984)
born 1891-1920; with >1 mo working	1976-1988	**McDonald et al. (1993)**
born 1891-1920; with >1 mo working	1992	**Liddell et al. (1997)**
1/1/1936-6/30/1967, ≥ 3 mo	5/201969	Meurman et al. (1974)
1/1/1936-6/30/1967, ≥ 3 mo	9/1/1977	Meurman et al. (1979)
worked ≥ 3 mo 1/1/1936-6/30/1967; alive 1/1/1953	1953-1991	**Meurman et al. (1994)**
> 1 mo 1930-1965; alive 1/1/1946	1946-1975	Rubino et al. (1979)
1946-1987, > 1 yr	1987	**Piolatto et al. (1990)**
1945-1955	1980	**Sluis-Cremer et al. (1992)**
		Amandus et al. (1987)
pre-1970; > 1 yr	1981	**Amandus and Wheeler (1987)**
1. pre-1970; > 1 yr 2. pre-1963; > 1 yr	1. 1981 2. June 1983	Amandus et al. (1988)

continues

TABLE B.1 Continued

Cohort Population (location—number, description)	Type of Exposure	Number of Workers[a]
Insulation Manufacture / Insulators		
11. Canada/USA		1. 632 men
		1. 632 men 3. 17,800 men (including survivors of 1 and 2)
a. 632 male insulation workers before 1943 in NY/NJ		**1. 632 men** 2. 833 men 3. 17,800 men
		17,800 men
		17,800 men
b. Paterson, NJ, US—820 men producing amosite asbestos insulation for shipbuilding	amosite	**820 men**
	amosite	820 men
		17,800 men
c. 17,800 male members in 1967 of asbestos insulation unions		**17,800 men**
12. Uxbridge, UK—Cape [insulation] Boards Plant	amosite	4,820 male asbestos workers
	amosite	4,825 men
	1947-1973 amosite and small amt chrysotile; 1973 only amosite	autopsies on 48 workers
13. East London, UK—1,400 male laggers [subgroups 1 and 2 make up population 32]	crocidolite, amosite and chrysotile	1. ~3,000 male factory workers 2. ~700 female factory
		3. ~1,400 laggers (insulators)
14. Tyler, TX, US—753 white male asbestos pipe-insulation plant workers	amosite	753 white men

Temporal Definition	Follow-Up	Citation[b]
1. members < 1943	1943-1962	Selikoff et al. (1964)
1. members < 1943 3. in union 1/1/1967	1. 1943-1971 3. 1967-1971	Selikoff (1974)
1. members < 1943 2. joined 1943-1962 3. in union 1/1/1967	**1. 1943-1976** 2. hire date—1976 3. 1967-1976	**Selikoff et al. (1979)**
in union 1/1/1967	1967-1976	Selikoff et al. (1980)
in union 1/1/1967	1967-1979	Seidman et al. (1982)
1941-1945	**1985**	**Seidman et al. (1986)**
1941-1945	1988	Ribak et al. (1989)
in union 1/1/1967	1967-1986	Seidman and Selikoff (1990)
in union 1/1/1967	**1967-1986**	**Selikoff and Seidman (1991)**
1947-1979	1947-1980	**Acheson et al. (1984)**
1947-1979	1986	Gardner et al. (1988)
		Gibbs et al. (1994)
1 and **3. began 4/1/1933-3/31/1964, > 1 mo** 2. began 1936-1942 workers	1980	**Berry et al. (2000)**
worked at plant during operation (1954-1972) or during clean-up; alive in 1964	1964-1993	**Levin et al. (1998)**

continues

TABLE B.1 Continued

Cohort Population (location—number, description)	Type of Exposure	Number of Workers[a]
Asbestos Textile Workers		
15. Italy—889 male and 1,077 female textile workers		889 men, 1,077 women
16. Rochdale, Northern England	asbestos (textile) workers	chrysotile 1°, crocidolite
	asbestos textiles	chrysotile 1°, crocidolite
	asbestos workers	
	asbestos textiles	chrysotile 1°, crocidolite
	asbestos textiles	chrysotile, crocidolite
	chrysotile, crocidolite	3,222 men and 283 women
17. Charleston, SC, USA—asbestos textile workers	chrysotile	
	chrysotile	
	chrysotile	1,261 white men
	chrysotile	1,261 men
	chrysotile only	2,543 men (black and white, reason so much larger?)
	chrysotile	3,022 subjects; 1. 1,247 white men 2. 546 black men 3. 1,229 white women
	chrysotile	3,022 subjects; 1. 1,247 white men 2. 546 black men 3. 1,229 white women

Temporal Definition	Follow-Up	Citation[b]
1946-1984, ≥ 1 mo	1996	Pira et al. (2005)
113 men	> 20 yr completed 1922-1953	Doll (1955)
1. 198 men 2. 427 men and 175 women	1. > 20 yr completed 1916-1961 2. > 10 yr expo; hired > 1932	Knox et al. (1965)
113 men		Hill et al. (1966)
878: 658 men and 220 women	1916-1966, > 10 yrs	Knox et al. (1968)
1,106	1916-1972	Peto et al. (1977)
1916-1983	6/30/1983	Peto et al. (1985)
		Dement et al. (1982)
1930-1975		Dement et al. (1983a)
1940-1975, > 1 mo	1975	Dement et al. (1983b)
1940-1975	1975	Finkelstein (1984)
> 1 mo working before 1958	1977	McDonald et al. (1983)
1940-1975	1990	Brown et al. (1994)
1940-1975	1990	Dement et al. (1994)

continues

TABLE B.1 Continued

Cohort Population (location—number, description)	Type of Exposure	Number of Workers[a]
Asbestos Cement		
18. Denmark—Danish Eternit Ltd. cement factory	chrysotile, crocidolite and amosite	5,686 men
	chrysotile mostly (only < 1946), amosite, crocilodite	7,979 men 583 women
	mainly chrysotile; amosite, crocilodite	7,887 men 576 women
		7,887 men, 576 women
19. Emilia Romagna, Italy—10 cement factories	chrysotile, crocidolite	3,341
20. Casale Monferrato, Italy—asbestos cement production	crocidolite and chrysotile	2,608 men 759 women
	chrysotile, crocidolite	2,605 men 762 woman
21. Lithuainia—Daugeliai and Akmene Factories	chrysotile—almost only	1,285 men 602 women
22. Southern Sweden—asbestos cement plant	>95% chrysotile; crocidolite and amosite	1,929 men
		981 male asbestos cement workers
23. Tamworth, England, UK—TAC Construction Materials Ltd.	chrysotile—almost only	1,510 men 657 women
24. New Orleans, LA, US—workers at two asbestos cement plants	primarily chrysotile, 1. some crocidolite and amosite 2. crocidolite	1. 1,898 men at plant 1 2. 3,594 men at plant 2
	chrysotile, amosite, crocidolite	839 men

Temporal Definition	Follow-Up	Citation[b]
1943-1976	1976	Clemmensen and Hjalgrim-Jensen (1981)
ever 1928-1984; alive 1943	1943-1984	**Raffn et al. (1989)**
1928-1984	1943-1990	**Raffn et al. (1996)**
1928-1984	1943-1990	Raffn et al. (1998)
1952-1987	1989	**Giaroli et al. (1994)**
worked anytime 1950-1980	1964-4/15/1986	**Botta et al. (1991)**
worked anytime 1950-1980	1965-1993	Magnani et al. (1996)
pre-1978	2000	**Smailyte et al. (2004a)**
1907-	1985	Albin et al. (1988)
1907-1977	1986	**Albin et al. (1990)**
> 1 yr employed; 15 yrs latency	1958-1989	**Jakobsson et al. (1994)**
1941-1983	1984	**Gardner et al. (1986)**
employed before 1970; 20 yr latency	Oct 1980	**Hughes et al. (1987)**
had clinical exam in 1969 with x-ray	1983	Hughes and Weill (1991)

continues

TABLE B.1 Continued

Cohort Population (location—number, description)	Type of Exposure	Number of Workers[a]
Friction Materials		
25. Ontario, Canada—two automotive parts factories		1,314 men 343 women
26. Ferodo, UK—friction materials factory	crocidolite, chrysolite	9,113 men 4,347 women
	chrysotile; some crocidolite <1945	13,460
	crocidolite, chrysolite	9,104 men 4,346 women
	chrysotile	9,104 men 4,346 women
27. USSR	chrysotile	1. 156 2. 2,834
28. New York, US—friction products manufacture	chrysotile	1. 2,057 men 2. 268 men 54 women
Generic "Asbestos Workers"		
29. China—eight asbestos factories	chrysotile	5,893 men and women
30. Qingdao, China—asbestos plant	chrysotile	160 men 370 women
31. Federal Republic of Germany—asbestos-related workers from national register	(smoking info)	3,735 men and women 1. 665 exposure ended <1972 2. 3,070 exposure ended >1971
		616 women
		3,372 men 616 women

Temporal Definition	Follow-Up	Citation[b]
1/1/1950; > 1 yr	1985	**Finkelstein (1989a)**
1941-1979	1979	Newhouse et al. (1982)
1942-1979	1979	Berry and Newhouse (1983)
1941-1979	1986	Newhouse and Sullivan (1989)
1941-1986	1986	**Berry (1994)**
1. working in FP shop 1/1/1966 2. Yoroslavl plant, > 3yr	1. 1984 2. 1949-1988	**Kogan et al. (1993)**
1. ? 2. current employees	1. 1937-1980	**Parnes (1990)**
worked > 15 yr	1986	**Zhu and Wang (1993)**
pre-1972; > 1 yr	1994	**Pang et al. (1997)**
> 3 yrs expo before1977	1977-1982	**Woitowitz et al. (1986)**
> 3 yrs expo before 1977	1977-1988	Rosler et al. (1994)
	1977-1988?	Rosler and Woitowitz (1995)

continues

TABLE B.1 Continued

Cohort Population (location—number, description)	Type of Exposure	Number of Workers[a]
32. East London, UK—3000 male and 700 female asbestos factory workers [subgroup 3 makes up population 13]	crocidolite, small amount chrysotile, amosite after 1926	4,835 men 922 women after limit cohort to enhance tracking
	crocidolite, amosite and chrysotile	>4,000 workers 1,327 severe expo
	crocidolite, amosite and chrysotile	1. 3,232 male factory workers 2. 922 female factory workers 3. 1,368 male laggers
	crocidolite, amosite and chrysotile	1. ~3,000 male factory workers 2. 932 female factory workers 3. ~1,400 laggers
	crocidolite, amosite and chrysotile	1. ~3,000 male factory workers 2. 932 female factory workers 3. ~1,400 laggers
33. Lancashire, UK—gas mask manufacture	chrysotile and crocidolite	1,327 women
34. England and Wales, UK—national survey of asbestos workers	various types of asbestos	31,150 men traced and examined of 33,079 total
35. US—asbestos industry retirees	production or maintenance service employees for asbestos company	1,464 men
		1,348 men 65 yr old; full expo and job history
	amosite, chrysotile, crocidolite	1,348 men
	amosite, chrysotile, crocidolite	1,075 men of above who worked in US
	amosite, chrysotile, crocidolite	1,074 men

Temporal Definition	Follow-Up	Citation[b]
worked 4/1/1933-3/31/1964, > 1 mo	5/1/1965	Newhouse (1969)
began 1936-1942	1968	Newhouse et al. (1972)
worked 4/1/1933-3/31/1964, > 1 mo		Newhouse and Berry (1973)
1 and 3. began 4/1/1933-3/31/1964 2. began 1936-1942	1975	Newhouse and Berry (1979)
1 and 3. began 4/1/1933-3/31/1964 2. began 1936-1942	1980	Newhouse et al. (1985b)
1 and 3. began 4/1/1933-3/31/1964, > 1 mo **2. began 1936-1942**	1980	**Berry et al. (2000)**
1939	1951-1980	**Acheson et al. (1982)**
asbestos work first before 1969 or only after 1969 (max 12 yr latency)	1981	**Hodgson and Jones (1986)**
retired 1941-1967	1969	Enterline et al. (1972)
1941-1967	1969	Enterline et al. (1973)
1941-1967	1969	Enterline and Henderson (1973)
1941-1967	1973	Henderson and Enterline (1979)
1941-1967	1980	**Enterline et al. (1987)**

continues

TABLE B.1 Continued

Cohort Population (location—number, description)	Type of Exposure	Number of Workers[a]
Other Occupations with Substantial Asbestos Exposure		
36. Ontario, Canada—members of plumbers' and pipe fitters' union		25,285 men
37. Finland—7,775 male shipyard workers	asbestos one of many toxic exposures	12,693 men: 1,689 welders, 4,308 platers, 6,003 machinists, 693 pipe fitters (608 in shipyard)
38. Tuscany, Italy—railway carriage construction and repair	chrysotile, crocidolite	734 men
39. Genoa, Italy—ship repair, refitting, and construction	asbestos one of many toxic exposures	2,348 men
	asbestos one of many toxic exposures	2,190 men
	asbestos one of many toxic exposures	3,984 men
40. Gothenburg, Sweden—shipyard workers	shipyards sprayed mostly amosite; crocidolite used on 4 naval ships in 1950s	272 men
	shipyard insulation workers	248
	asbestos and other potenially toxic agents (metal fumes and solvents)	383 men (18 not fully IDed)
	handled chrysotile (around spraying of amosite, some crocidolite); asbestos use stopped in 1972	3,902 participated in health program 1977-1979 (self-selected for belief ever exposed to asbestos)
	chrysotile, mainly	3,893

[a]Number of subjects with information necessary for analysis (as used in this report's meta-analyses and reported in tables in Appendix D) may have been less.
[b]Full citations can be found in the reference list for Chapter 6.

Temporal Definition	Follow-Up	Citation[b]
1950-1999	1999	**Finkelstein and Verma (2004)**
1945-1960, > 1 yr	1953-1981	**Tola et al. (1988) [incidence]**
1945-1969	1970-1997	**Battista et al. (1999)**
worked any time before 1952; alive 1960	1960-1969	Puntoni et al. (1977)
worked any time 1960-1970	1960-1975	Puntoni et al. (1979)
worked any time 1960-1980	1960-1995	**Puntoni et al. (2001)**
active in union 1970	1970-1979	Sanden et al. (1984)
	1970-1994	Jarvholm and Sanden (1988)
insured worker dying 1960-1979 at 40-67 yrs of age		Sanden et al. (1985)
	1978-1983	**Sanden and Jarvholm (1987) [incidence]**
		Sanden et al. (1992)

APPENDIX C

Description of Case-Control Studies of All Selected Cancers as Related to Exposure to Asbestos

TABLE C.1 Description of Case-Control Studies of All Selected Cancers as Related to Exposure to Asbestos

Reference[a]	Population	Number of Cases[b]
Ahrens et al. 1991	Male laryngeal-cancer cases identified in one hospital in Bremen, Germany, in 1986 with histologic confirmation; male controls with nonneoplastic disease selected from same hospital and matched on age and residence	100 laryngeal
Berrino et al. 2003	Male cases of laryngeal and hypopharyngeal cancer, less than 55 yr old, diagnosed in six European centers in 1979-1982 with histologic confirmation; controls selected from census lists, electoral rolls, or population registries and matched for sex and age	215 laryngeal and 100 hypopharyngeal
Brown et al. 1988	White, male laryngeal-cancer cases, 30-79 yr old, diagnosed in 56 hospitals along Gulf Coast of Texas in 1975-1980; controls selected through Texas Department of Health mortality tapes, drivers license records, HCFA-provided Medicare records, and matched on age, vital status, ethnicity, county of residence	183 laryngeal
Burch et al. 1981	Laryngeal cancer cases diagnosed in southern Ontario in 1977-1979; neighborhood controls matched on sex, age	204 laryngeal (184 men and 20 women)

Number of Controls[b]	Relevant Exposures	Exposure Assessment	Analysis; Adjustment for Potential Confounders
100	Asbestos	In-person interview with standardized questionnaire covering lifetime occupational history with exposure checklist	Unconditional logistic regression; smoking, alcohol consumption, age
819	Asbestos	Interview with standardized questionnaire assessing jobs held at least 1 year; job titles coded; panel of industrial hygienists and occupational physicians assessed probabilities of exposure to specific agents	Unconditional logistic regression; study centre, age, tobacco-smoking, consumption of alcohol, SES, dietary variables, other agents; Boffetta et al. (2003) analyzed same study population in terms of occupation and industry
250	Asbestos	Interview (self-reports or proxy) assessing lifetime occupational and residential histories, lifestyle factors, demographic characteristics; industrial hygienist classified job titles for exposure to specific agents	Logistic regression; cigarette smoking, alcohol consumption
204	Asbestos	In-person interview with standardized questionnaire assessing lifetime occupational history and lifestyle factors; self-reported agents and occupational epidemiologist classification	Discordant pairs, RR; smoking

continues

TABLE C.1 Continued

Reference[a]	Population	Number of Cases[b]
Cocco et al. 1994	Male gastric cancer cases, 35-74 yr old, diagnosed and histologically confirmed in 1985-1987 in four areas of Italy; population controls randomly selected and matched for gender and age	640 gastric
De Stefani et al. 1998	Male laryngeal-cancer cases, 30-75 yr old, diagnosed in five hospitals in Montevideo, Uruguay, in 1993-1995; cancer controls selected from same hospitals and timeframe	112 laryngeal
Demers et al. 1994	Colon and rectum cancer cases, 40-84 yr-old white males, diagnosed in 1984-1987 through the Metropolitan Detroit Cancer Surveillance System (SEER); controls selected through RDD	261 colon and rectum
Dietz et al. 2004	Laryngeal cancer cases diagnosed at the Department of Otolaryngology, Head and Neck Surgery university hospitals of Heidelberg and Manheim and town hospitals of Ludwigshafen, Darmstadt and Heilbronn, Germany, in 1998-2000; population controls selected from local registries and matched on sex and age	257 laryngeal (236 men and 21 women)
Dumas et al. 2000	Male rectal cancer cases, 35-70 yr old, diagnosed in 19 large Montreal-area hospitals in 1979-1985 and histologically confirmed for one of 19 cancer sites; frequency-matched by approximate age, population-based controls also chosen from electoral lists, RDD	257 rectal

Number of Controls[b]	Relevant Exposures	Exposure Assessment	Analysis; Adjustment for Potential Confounders
959	Asbestos	Interview assessing work histories (job title and duration); jobs coded and JEM applied for six specific agents	Logistic regression; age, study area, residence type, migration, family gastric cancer history, quetelet index, total caloric, protein, and vitamin C intake
509 (for asbestos analysis, 352 excluding subjects with colorectal cancer)	Asbestos	In-person interview with standardized questionnaire assessing lifetime occupational histories and exposure to specific agents	Unconditional logistic regression; age, residence, education, income, tobacco-smoking and type, alcohol consumption
183	Asbestos	Telephone interview assessing lifetime work, medical, and lifestyle histories; occupations and industries coded and assigned likelihoods of asbestos exposure	Unconditional logistic regression; age, smoking
769 (702 men and 67 women)		In-person interview with standardized questionnaire assessing lifetime occupational history, tobacco and alcohol use; quantification using job-specific supplementary questionnaires validated for asbestos	Conditional logistic regression; age, sex, smoking, alcohol consumption
1,295 cancer, 533 population	Chrysotile; amphiboles	In-person interviews with specific question on details of each job subject had; analyzed and coded by team of chemists and industrial hygienists (about 300 exposures) on semi-quantitative scale	Unconditional logistic regression; age, education, respondent status, cigarette-smoking, beer consumption, BMI

continues

TABLE C.1 Continued

Reference[a]	Population	Number of Cases[b]
Ekstrom et al. 1999	Gastric cancer cases, 40-79 yr old, residing in one of five counties, born in Sweden, and diagnosed in 1989-1995, identified and histologically confirmed by participating clinicians from all hospitals in the study area; controls randomly selected from the population register	565 gastric
Elci et al. 2002	Male laryngeal-cancer cases diagnosed in Oncology Treatment Center of Social Security Agency Okmeydani Hospital in Istanbul, Turkey, in 1979-1984 with histologic confirmation; controls selected from same hospital, timeframe among cases of HD, cancers of skin (nonmelanoma), testis, bone, male breast as well as benign lesions	940 laryngeal
Fredriksson et al. 1989	Colon cancer cases, 30-75 yr old, identified through the Swedish Cancer Registry among patients diagnosed in 1980-1983; cases resident of the Umea region and alive during the study's data collection; randomly selected population controls from the National Population Register frequency-matched on age, sex	329 colon (165 men and 164 women)
Garabrant et al. 1992	English-speaking, white, male cases of colon cancer, 45-70 yr old, diagnosed in 1983-1986, and identified through the Los Angeles County Cancer Surveillance Program; neighborhood controls matched on gender and date of birth	419 colon
Gerhardsson de Verdier et al. 1992	Colorectal-cancer cases identified through local hospitals and Regional Cancer Registry in Stockholm, Sweden in 1986-1988; cases histologically confirmed and subjects limited to those born in Sweden in 1907-1946 and lived half their lives there; population controls randomly selected from Stockholm County population registry	352 colon (163 men and 189 women); 217 rectal (107 men and 110 women)

Number of Controls[b]	Relevant Exposures	Exposure Assessment	Analysis; Adjustment for Potential Confounders
1,164	Asbestos	In-person interview with professional interviewer; occupational epidemiologists to assess type of exposure and duration from self-reports of exposure and job titles	Unconditional logistic regression; age, sex
1,519	Asbestos	In-person interview with standardized questionnaire assessing lifetime occupational history, tobacco and alcohol use; industrial hygienist performed JEM exposure assignments	Unconditional logistic regression; age, smoking, alcohol consumption
658 (330 men and 328 women)	Asbestos	Mailed questionnaire assessing occupational history (job titles); telephone interviews followed if necessary; exposure to high or low grade of asbestos independently coded by two physicians and one hygienist	Mantel-Haenszel; age, sex, physical activity
419	Asbestos	In-person interview with standardized questionnaires assessing past 30 years of occupational exposures, physical activity and weight, medical history, family cancer history, and a modified Semiquantitative Food Frequency Questionnaire	Conditional logistic regression; family history of large bowel cancer, total caloric intake, carbohydrates, calcium, weight, and physical activity
512 (236 men and 276 women)	Asbestos	Questionnaire administered in person or through mail with follow-up telephone survey; exposure to list of chemicals or employment in specified occupations determined	Unconditional logistic regression; age, sex, nutritional intake markers, BMI, physical activity, family history of colorectal cancer

continues

TABLE C.1 Continued

Reference[a]	Population	Number of Cases[b]
Goldberg et al. 2001	Male cases and controls, 35-70 yr old, diagnosed in 19 large Montreal-area hospitals in 1979-1985 and histologically confirmed for one of 19 cancer sites; frequency-matched by approximate age; population-based controls also chosen from electoral lists and with RDD	497 colon
Gustavsson et al. 1998	Oral-cavity, oro- and hypopharyngeal-, laryngeal-, and esophageal-cancer cases among all Swedish men, 40-79 yr old, residing in two regions with reporting from departments of oncology and surgery in 1988-1990; controls randomly selected from population registers and matched on age, region	545 total, including: 138 pharyngeal, 157 laryngeal, 122 esophageal
Hardell 1981	Men from Umea region, 25-85 yr old, diagnosed with adenocarcinoma of colon reported to Swedish Cancer Registry 1978-1979; controls from Umea region assembled for two previous studies were used as referents	154 colon
Hillerdal 1980	Male gastrointestinal cancer cases diagnosed in Uppsala county in 1968-1972 obtained through the Swedish Cancer Registry with chest x-rays retrieved through the General Health Survey; controls selected 3:1 based on age, sex, and year of x-ray	386 total (21 esophagus, 148 stomach, 8 small intestine, 108 large intestine, and 101 rectum)
Hinds et al. 1979	White, male laryngeal cancer cases diagnosed in 3 counties of Washington through the Cancer Surveillance System in 1976-1977; neighborhood controls matched on sex, race, age	47 laryngeal
Krstev et al. 2005	Stomach cancer cases, 21-79 yr old, diagnosed at 22 hospitals and eight endoscopic centers in Warsaw, Poland, in 1994-1996; controls randomly selected from an electronic registry and matched on gender and age	443 stomach (285 men and 158 women)

Number of Controls[b]	Relevant Exposures	Exposure Assessment	Analysis; Adjustment for Potential Confounders
1,514 cancer, 533 population	Asbestos	In-person interviews with specific question on detail of each job subject had; analyzed and coded by team of chemists and industrial hygienists (about 300 exposures) on semi-quantitative scale	Unconditional logistic regression; age, respondent status, ethnicity, non-occupational factors (such as cigarette-smoking, alcohol consumption)
641	Asbestos	Interview with standardized questionnaire assessing lifestyle and environmental factors; occupational hygienist assigned exposure intensity, probability to 17 specific occupational exposures	Unconditional logistic regression; age, region, alcohol consumption, tobacco-smoking
541	Asbestos	Responses to mailed questionnaire on work history, chemical exposures, and lifestyle factors interpreted to determine ever-never status for asbestos exposure.	Mantel-Haenszel analysis stratified on age and urban vs rural residence
1,158	Asbestos	Evidence of pleural plaques on chest x-rays regarded as indirect proof of asbestos exposure	Standardized incidence ratio (observed/ expected)
47	Asbestos	In-person interview (or next-of-kin for deceased) with standardized questionnaire assessing lifetime occupational history and lifestyle factors	Matched pairs, RR
479 (313 men and 166 women)	Asbestos	In-person interview with standardized questionnaire assessed lifetime occupational history and exposure to numerous specific agents	Unconditional logistic regression; age, education, smoking, lifetime number of jobs held

continues

TABLE C.1 Continued

Reference[a]	Population	Number of Cases[b]
Luce et al. 2000	Cases of laryngeal and hypopharyngeal cancer identified from the Cancer Registry of New Caledonia in 1993-1995 among residents living there at least 5 years and 18 years old; population controls selected from electoral rolls and matched on sex and age	23 larynx (20 men and 3 women); 5 hypopharynx
Marchand et al. 2000	Male cases of laryngeal and hypopharyngeal cancer diagnosed in 15 hospitals in six cities in France in 1989-1991; hospital, cancer controls selected	315 laryngeal 206 hypopharyngeal
Merletti et al. 1991	Male oral- and oropharyngeal cancer cases, 26-92 yr old, diagnosed in Turin, Italy, in 1982-1984; controls selected randomly from resident files, stratified by age, sex	86 oral cavity or oropharyngeal (12 specifically oropharyngeal)
Muscat and Wynder 1992	White, male laryngeal cancer cases diagnosed and histologcally confirmed at eight hospitals in New York, Illinois, Michigan, and Pennsylvania in 1985-1990; hospital controls randomly selected and matched on hospital, age, and year of interview	194 laryngeal
Neugut et al. 1991	Colorectal cancer cases among males, 35-84 yr old, undergoing colonoscopy in three NYC medical centers in 1986-1988; colonoscopy controls free of invasive colon carcinomas, inflammatory bowel disease, or colon polyps	51 colorectal

Number of Controls[b]	Relevant Exposures	Exposure Assessment	Analysis; Adjustment for Potential Confounders
305 total (matched also to 228 lung cancer cases, etc.)	Pö, a whitewash containing tremolite asbestos	In-person (or next-of-kin for deceased) interview with standardized questionnaire assessed lifetime occupational and lifestyle history and residence in whitewashed houses	Unconditional logistic regression; age, ethnicity, smoking, alcohol
305	Asbestos	In-person interview with standardized questionnaire assessing lifetime occupational history, tobacco and alcohol use; JEM exposure assignments	Unconditional logistic regression; age, smoking, alcohol consumption; Goldberg et al. (1997) analyzed same study population in terms of occupation and industry, while Menvielle et al. (2004) analyzed the occupational information from an SES perspective
373	Asbestos	In-person interview with standardized questionnaire assessing lifetime occupational history; job titles coded; industrial hygienists applied JEM to determine exposures to 13 agents	Unconditional logistic regression; age, education, birthplace, tobacco-smoking, alcohol consumption
184	Asbestos	In-person interview assessed occupational history and exposure to specific agents; occupation and exposure linkage system applied to determine exposure probability and intensity	Multiple logistic regression; age, education, smoking, alcohol, quetelet index
195	Asbestos	Telephone interview or mailed questionnaire assessed self-reported exposure to asbestos with occupational history used as verification	Multiple logistic regression; age

continues

TABLE C.1 Continued

Reference[a]	Population	Number of Cases[b]
Olsen and Sabroe 1984	Laryngeal cancer cases, less than 75 yr old, diagnosed in 1980-1982 through five department of oncology in Denmark; population controls matched 4:1 through municipal registries and matched on sex, age	326 laryngeal (276 men and 50 women)
Parent et al. 1998	Male cases and controls, 35-70 yr old, diagnosed in 19 large Montreal-area hospitals in 1979-1985 and histologically confirmed for one of 19 cancer sites; frequency-matched by approximate age; population-based controls also chosen from electoral lists and with RDD	250 stomach
Parent et al. 2000	Male cases and controls, 35-70 yr old, diagnosed in 19 large Montreal-area hospitals in 1979-1985 and histologically confirmed for one of 19 cancer sites; frequency-matched by approximate age; population-based controls also chosen from electoral lists and with RDD	99 esophageal (63 squamous-cell carcinoma, 23 adenocarcinomas, and 13 uncertain morphology)
Shettigara and Morgan 1975	Male cases of laryngeal cancer diagnosed at Toronto General Hospital and resident of metropolitan Toronto in 1974; neighborhood controls matched on sex and age	43 laryngeal
Spiegelman and Wegman 1985	Cases of colon and rectal cancer and cancer controls selected from sample of Third National Cancer Survey of incident cancers in seven US metropolitan areas and two states in 1969-1971; digestive and occupationally associated cancers (respiratory, urinary, bone, skin, buccal, pharyngeal, leukemia) excluded from controls	370 colon (218 men and 152 women); 175 rectal (119 men and 56 women); 8 large intestine (6 men and 2 women)
Stell and McGill 1973	Male laryngeal cancer cases diagnosed consecutively in one Liverpool hospital; hospital controls matched on age	100 laryngeal

Number of Controls[b]	Relevant Exposures	Exposure Assessment	Analysis; Adjustment for Potential Confounders
1,134 (971 men and 163 women)	Asbestos	In-person interview with standardized questionnaire assessing lifetime occupational and lifestyle histories, exposure to specific agents	Logistic regression; age, tobacco, alcohol consumption, sex
2,289 cancer, 533 population	Chrysotile asbestos, amphibole asbestos	In-person interviews with specific question on detail of each job subject had; analyzed, coded by team of chemists and industrial hygienists (about 300 exposures) on semi-quantitative scale	Unconditional logistic regression; age, respondent status, birthplace, education, cigarette-smoking
2,299 cancer, 533 population	Asbestos	In-person interviews with specific question on detail of each job subject had; analyzed, coded by team of chemists and industrial hygienists (about 300 exposures) on semi-quantitative scale	Unconditional logistic regression; age, respondent status, birthplace, educational level, beer consumption, spirits consumption, β-carotene index, cigarette-smoking (length, pattern)
43	Asbestos	In-person interview with standardized questionnaire assessing age at first exposure and duration of exposure to asbestos and other agents	Discordant pairs
1,861 total (626 men and 1,245 women)	Asbestos	Interviews conducted on primary, secondary occupations, industries, duration; exposure assignment according to NIOSH National Occupational Hazard Survey protocol	Logistic regression; age, race, marital status, region, income group, educational level, body mass, nutritional scores
100	Asbestos	In-person interview with questionnaire assessing occupational history	Chi-square

continues

TABLE C.1 Continued

Reference[a]	Population	Number of Cases[b]
Vineis et al. 1993	Colon cancer cases diagnosed in 1990-1991 at the Main Hospital of Torino, Italy; controls selected from a 10% sample of patients with nontraumatic conditions in 1989-1990	131 colon (74 men and 57 women)
Wortley et al. 1992	Laryngeal cancer cases, 20-74 yr old, identified through the Hutchinson Cancer Research Center (SEER participant) in Seattle of western Washington residents in 1983-1987; controls selected through RDD and matched on age and sex	235 laryngeal
Zagraniski et al. 1986	White, male cases of laryngeal cancer diagnosed in two New Haven hospitals in 1975-1980; white, male general surgery controls	87 laryngeal
Zheng et al. 1992a	Oral- and pharyngeal-cancer cases, 20-75 yr old, identified through population-based cancer registry as newly diagnosed in 1988-1990; controls randomly selected from Shanghai Resident Registry, matched on age, sex	204 oral or pharyngeal (115 men and 89 women)
Zheng et al. 1992b	Laryngeal cancer cases, 20-75 yr old, identified through population-based cancer registry as newly diagnosed in 1988-1990; controls randomly selected from Shanghai Resident Registry, matched on age, sex	201 laryngeal (177 men and 24 women)

NOTE: BMI = body mass index; HCFA = Health Care Financing Administration; HD = Hodgkin's disease; JEM = job exposure matrix; NIOSH = National Institute for Occupational Safety and Health; OR = odds ratio; RDD = random-digit dialing; SES = socio-economic status.

[a]Full citations can be found in the reference list for Chapter 6.

[b]Number of cases and controls with information necessary for analysis (as used in this report's meta-analyses and reported in tables in Appendix E) may have been less.

Number of Controls[b]	Relevant Exposures	Exposure Assessment	Analysis; Adjustment for Potential Confounders
463 (254 men and 209 women)	Jobs with potential exposure to asbestos	Self-reported job titles coded and selected as exposed for: stone cutter, mechanic or pipes and boilers, pipefitter, steamfitter, boilermaker, mechanic at heating company, and pipe installer	Mantel-Haenszel OR; age
547	Asbestos	In-person interview with standardized questionnaire assessing lifetime occupational history; industrial hygienists performed JEM exposure assignments	Multiple logistic regression; smoking, drinking, age, education
153	Asbestos work	In-person interview with standardized questionnaire assessing lifetime occupational history and lifestyle factors	Condition logistic regression; tobacco, alcohol consumption
414 (269 men and 145 women)	Asbestos	In-person interview with standardized questionnaire assessing lifestyle factors and occupational exposures	Chi-squared test
414 (269 men and 145 women)	Asbestos	In-person interview with standardized questionnaire assessing lifestyle factors	Unconditional logistic regression; age, smoking, education

APPENDIX D

Cohort Results Tables

TABLE D.1 Pharyngeal Cancer and Exposure to Asbestos—Cohort Studies

Reference*	Study Population	Exposed Cases	Estimated RR (95% CI)
Mining			
Reid et al. 2004	5,685 male crocidolite mining and milling workers in western Australia (incidence 1980-2000—pharynx)	**16**	**1.88 (1.15-3.07)**
Piolatto et al. 1990	1,058 male chrysotile miners in northern Italy (oropharynx)	6	**2.31 (0.85-5.02)**[a]
	Duration of exposure (years)		
	< 10	5	4.55 (1.47-10.61)[a]
	10-20	1	2.00 (0.05-11.14)[a]
	> 20	0	0.0 (0.0-4.10)[a]
Sluis-Cremer et al. 1992	7,317 male amosite and crocidolite miners in South Africa (lip, oral cavity, pharynx)	10	**2.14 (1.03-3.94)**
	Amosite subcohort	1	0.42 (0.0-1.97)
	Crocidolite subcohort	5	2.94 (1.16-6.18)
Insulation Manufacture/Insulators (laggers)			
Berry et al. 2000	1,400 male asbestos factory workers in east London, UK (pharynx, buccal cavity) (laggers)	0	**0.0 (0.0-8.79)**[a]

continues

TABLE D.1 Pharyngeal Continued

Reference*	Study Population	Exposed Cases	Estimated RR (95% CI)
Selikoff and Seidman 1991	17,800 male members of asbestos insulation unions in Canada and US in 1967 (oropharynx)	**48**	**2.18 (1.62-2.91)**[a]
Levin et al. 1998	783 white male asbestos pipe insulation factory in Tyler, TX (pharynx, buccal cavity)	**1**	**1.07 (0.03-5.95)**
Asbestos Textile Workers			
Pira et al. 2005	1,966 textile employees in Italy (oral, pharynx)	**7**	**2.26 (0.90-4.65)**
	Duration of employment (years)		
	< 1	4	3.89 (1.06-9.96)[a]
	1 to < 5	2	2.52 (0.30-9.10)[a]
	5 to < 10	0	0
	10+	**1**	**1.33 (0.03-7.41)**[a]
	Time since first employment (years)		
	< 15	3	3.36 (0.69-9.83)[a]
	15 to < 25	4	3.63 (0.99-9.30)[a]
	25 to < 35	0	0
	35+	0	0
	Time since last exposure (years)		
	Ongoing to < 3	1	1.86 (0.05-10.38)[a]
	3 to < 15	2	1.79 (0.22-6.46)[a]
	15 to < 25	4	4.72 (1.29-12.08)[a]
	25 to < 35	0	0
	35+	0	0
	Age at first exposure (years)		
	< 25	0	0
	25 to < 35	2	2.57 (0.31-9.27)[a]
	35+	5	2.62 (0.85-6.12)[a]
	Sex		
	889 men	7	2.54 (1.0-5.23)[a]
	1,077 women	0	0
Asbestos Cement			
Raffn et al. 1989	7,996 male asbestos-cement industry workers in Denmark (buccal cavity, pharynx) (incidence)	**13**	**0.79 (0.42-1.35)**
Giaroli et al. 1994	3,341 male asbestos-cement workers in Italy (mouth, pharynx)	0	0 (0-1.37)[b]

TABLE D.1 Pharyngeal Continued

Reference*	Study Population	Exposed Cases	Estimated RR (95% CI)
Hughes et al. 1987	5,492 male asbestos-cement manufacturing plant employees in New Orleans, LA (buccal, pharynx)		
	Plants combined (20 year lag)	**11**	**0.90 (0.45-1.61)[a]**
	Plant 1	5	1.13 (0.37-2.64)[a]
	Plant 2	6	0.77 (0.28-1.67)[a]
Parnes 1990	2,057 male brake-lining and disk-manufacturing workers in Albany, NY (buccal cavity, pharynx)	**3**	**1.83 (0.37-5.19)[a]**
Generic "Asbestos Workers"			
Berry et al. 2000	Asbestos factory workers in east London, UK (buccal cavity, pharynx)		
	3,000 men	**5**	**2.17 (0.70-5.07)[a]**
	Low/mod < 2 years	1	1.59 (0.04-8.84)[a]
	Low/mod > 2 years	1	2.04 (0.05-11.37)[a]
	Severe < 2 years	2	2.94 (0.36-10.62)[a]
	Severe > 2 years	1	2.00 (0.05-11.14)[a]
	700 women	0	0.00 (0.00-7.10)[a]
Enterline et al. 1987	1,074 white male production and maintenance workers at US asbestos company (buccal cavity, pharynx)	**5**	**1.39 (0.45-3.24)[a]**
Other Occupations with Substantial Asbestos Exposure			
Battista et al. 1999	734 male railway carriage construction and repair workers in Italy (mouth, pharynx)	**3**	**2.65 (0.72-6.86)[b]**
Puntoni et al. 2001	3,984 male shipyard workers in Genoa, Italy (oropharynx)	**16**	**0.97 (0.56-1.58)**

NOTE: CI = Confidence interval; RR = relative risk. Figures are for mortality unless otherwise indicated. Data points included in meta-analyses are bolded.

* Full citations can be found in the reference list for Chapter 6.

[a]95% CIs calculated with standard methods from observed and expected numbers presented in original paper.

[b]90% CIs reported.

TABLE D.2 Laryngeal Cancer and Exposure to Asbestos—Cohort Studies

Reference*	Study Population	Exposed Cases	Estimated RR (95% CI)
Patients with Asbestos-Related Disease			
Germani et al. 1999	631 women compensated for asbestosis in Italy	**1**	**8.09 (0.21-45.08)**
	Textile industry (n = 276)	0	0.0 (0.0-60.10)[a]
	Asbestos cement industry (n = 278)	1	16.09 (0.42-89.66)
Karjalainen et al. 1999	Asbestos-related disease patients in Finland (incidence)		
	Men		
	1,287 with asbestosis	**5**	**4.2 (1.4-9.8)**
	4,708 with benign pleural disease	**1**	**0.5 (0.0-2.7)**
	Women		
	89 with asbestosis	0	0 (0.0-340.0)
	179 with benign pleural disease	0	0 (0.0-460.0)
Szesznia-Dabrowska et al. 2002	902 male workers compensated for asbestosis in Poland	**1**	**0.43 (0.01-2.40)**[a]
Mining			
Armstrong et al. 1988	6,505 male crocidolite miners and millers in Western Australia (mortality to 1980)	**2**	**0.68 (0.17-2.74)**
Reid et al. 2004	5,685 male crocidolite mining and milling workers in western Australia (incidence 1980-2000)	**19**	**1.82 (1.16-2.85)**
Liddell et al. 1997	8,923 male chrysotile miners and millers in Quebec (mortality 1950-1992)	**36**	**1.11 (0.79-1.55)**[a]
	Cumulative exposure to age 55 (million particles per cubic foot-yrs) among 7,728 living to age 55	30	1.04 (0.70-1.48)[a]
	< 300	24	1.03 (0.66-1.53)[a]
	< 3	7	1.45 (0.58-2.99)[a]
	3 to < 10	6	1.71 (0.63-3.72)[a]
	10 to < 30	2	0.51 (0.06-1.84)[a]
	30 to < 60	1	0.34 (0.01-1.89)[a]
	60 to < 100	3	1.11 (0.23-3.24)[a]
	100 to < 200	2	0.59 (0.07-2.13)[a]
	200 to < 300	3	1.45 (0.30-4.24)[a]

TABLE D.2 Laryngeal Continued

Reference*	Study Population	Exposed Cases	Estimated RR (95% CI)
	> 300	6	**1.08 (0.40-2.35)**[a]
	300 to < 400	4	3.12 (0.85-7.99)[a]
	400 to < 1000	2	0.64 (0.08-2.31)[a]
	1000+	0	0.00 (0.00-3.24)[a]
Meurman et al. 1994	Anthophyllite asbestos miners in Finland (incidence)		
	736 men (3+ months of exposed time)	4	**1.75 (0.48-4.47)**
	Moderate exposure	1	1.33 (0.03-7.40)
	Heavy exposure	3	**1.95 (0.40-5.69)**
	5+ years of exposed time	2	3.03 (0.37-10.9)
	Moderate exposure	0	0 (0.00-36.2)
	Heavy exposure	2	**3.60 (0.44-13.0)**
	167 women (3+ months of exposed time)	0	0 (0.00-123.0)
Piolatto et al. 1990	1,058 male chrysotile miners in northern Italy	8	**2.67 (1.15-5.25)**[a]
	Duration of exposure (years)		
	< 10	3	2.31 (0.48-6.75)[a]
	10-20	0	0 (0.00-6.15)[a]
	> 20	5	**4.55 (1.47-10.61)**[a]
	Age at first exposure (years)		
	< 30	5	3.57 (1.16-8.34)[a]
	30+	3	1.88 (0.39-5.48)[a]
	Time since first exposure (years)		
	< 20	2	4.00 (0.48-14.44)[a]
	20-30	2	2.50 (0.30-9.02)[a]
	≥ 30	4	2.35 (0.64-6.02)[a]
	Time since last exposure (years)		
	Ongoing	2	4.00 (0.48-14.44)[a]
	≤ 10	3	4.29 (0.88-12.53)[a]
	> 10	3	1.67 (0.34-4.87)[a]
	Cumulative dust exposure (fiber-years)		
	< 100	1	1.43 (0.04-7.96)[a]
	100-400	2	2.22 (0.27-8.02)[a]
	> 400	5	**3.85 (1.25-8.98)**[a]
Sluis-Cremer et al. 1992	7,317 male amosite and crocidolite miners in South Africa	5	**1.86 (0.60-4.34)**
	Amosite subcohort	2	1.44 (0.25-4.52)
	Crocidolite subcohort	3	3.09 (0.84-7.98)

continues

TABLE D.2 Laryngeal Continued

Reference*	Study Population	Exposed Cases	Estimated RR (95% CI)
Insulation Manufacture/Insulators (laggers)			
Selikoff and Seidman 1991	17,800 male members of asbestos insulation unions in Canada and US in 1967	18	1.70 (1.01-2.69)[a]
Berry et al. 2000	1,400 male asbestos factory workers in east London, UK (laggers)	0	0.00 (0.0-15.38)[a]
Levin et al. 1998	753 white male workers in asbestos pipe insulation factory in Tyler, TX	1	2.21 (0.06-12.29)
Asbestos Textile Workers			
Pira et al. 2005	1,966 textile employees in Italy	7	2.38 (0.95-4.90)
	Duration of employment (years)		
	< 1	1	1.05 (0.03-5.87)[a]
	1 to < 5	3	3.98 (0.82-11.63)[a]
	5 to < 10	2	3.90 (0.47-14.09)[a]
	10+	1	1.38 (0.03-7.67)[a]
	Time since first employment (years)		
	< 15	1	1.06 (0.03-5.92)[a]
	15 to < 25	1	0.98 (0.02-5.46)[a]
	25 to < 35	5	7.32 (2.37-17.09)[a]
	35+	0	0
	Time since last exposure (years)		
	Ongoing to < 3	0	0
	3 to < 15	3	2.71 (0.56-7.93)[a]
	15 to < 25	2	2.67 (0.32-9.62)[a]
	25 to < 35	2	4.99 (0.60-18.00)[a]
	35+	0	0
	Age at first exposure (years)		
	< 25	1	3.84 (0.10-21.38)[a]
	25 to < 35	1	1.57 (0.04-8.76)[a]
	35+	5	2.44 (0.79-5.71)[a]
	Sex		
	889 men	7	2.46 (0.99-5.06)[a]
	1,077 women	0	0
Peto et al. 1985	Asbestos textile factory workers in Rochdale, UK		
	283 women	0	0.0 (0.00-61.50)[b]
	3,211 men	4	1.55 (0.42-3.97)[b]
	< 10 years in scheduled areas		
	Time since first employment		
	< 20 years	0	0.0 (0.00-4.24)[b]
	20+ years	4	3.70 (1.01-9.48)[b]

TABLE D.2 Laryngeal Continued

Reference*	Study Population	Exposed Cases	Estimated RR (95% CI)
	10+ years in scheduled areas		
	Time since first employment		
	< 20 years	0	0.0 (0.00-19.42)[b]
	20+ years	0	0.0 (0.00-8.20)[b]
Dement et al. 1994	3,022 asbestos textile plant workers in South Carolina	4	**1.55 (0.53-3.55)**
	White males	3	2.31 (0.63-5.96)
	White females	0	0.0 (0.00-12.72)[b]
	Black males	1	1.02 (0.05-4.84)
Asbestos Cement			
Raffn et al. 1989	7,996 male asbestos-cement industry workers in Denmark (incidence)	14	**1.66 (0.91-2.78)**
	Duration of employment, 15 years latency		
	< 5 years	2	0.81 (0.09-2.94)
	≥ 5 years	6	**2.27 (0.83-4.95)**
	First employment 1928-40, 15 years latency	5	**5.50 (1.77-12.82)**
Giaroli et al. 1994	3,341 male asbestos-cement workers in Italy	2	**0.82 (0.15-2.59)**
Botta et al. 1991	Asbestos-cement workers in Italy		
	2,608 men	5	**0.70 (0.23-1.64)**
	759 women	0	**0.0 (0.00-369.0)[b]**
Smailyte et al. 2004	1,285 male asbestos-cement producers in Lithuania (incidence)	7	**1.4 (0.7-2.9)**
	Duration of employment (years)		
	< 1	0	0.0 (0.0-4.1)[b]
	1-4	3	1.6 (0.5-4.8)
	5-9	2	3.0 (0.8-12.5)
	≥ 10	2	1.3 (0.4-5.7)
	25+ years since first exposure	3	1.4 (0.29-4.09)[a]
Gardner et al. 1986	2,090 chrysotile asbestos cement products workers in England	1	0.91 (0.02-5.06)[b]
Hughes et al. 1987	5,492 male asbestos-cement manufacturing plant employees in New Orleans, LA		
	Plants combined (20 year lag)	3	**0.56 (0.11-1.62)[a]**
	Plant 1	2	1.00 (0.12-3.61)[a]
	Plant 2	1	0.30 (0.01-1.64)[a]

continues

TABLE D.2 Laryngeal Continued

Reference*	Study Population	Exposed Cases	Estimated RR (95% CI)
Friction Materials			
Finkelstein 1989	1,314 male workers in automotive parts factory in Ontario	3	8.54 (1.76-24.97)[a]
	Duration of employment (years)		
	1 to < 20	0	0.00 (0.00-36.27)[a]
	≥ 20	3	11.90 (2.46-34.79)[a]
Berry 1994	9,104 male friction materials factory workers in the UK	6	0.64 (0.23-1.39)
Parnes et al. 1990	2,057 male brake-lining and disk-manufacturing workers in Albany, NY	3	4.03 (0.80-11.39)[a]
	Duration of employment (years)		
	0-4	2	6.64 (0.76-22.70)[a]
	5+	1	2.24 (0.06-12.41)[a]
Generic "Asbestos Workers"			
Berry et al. 2000	Asbestos factory workers in east London, UK		
	3,000 men	3	2.05 (0.42-6.01)[a]
	Low/mod	0	0.00 (0.00-5.27)[a]
	Severe < 2 years	2	4.65 (0.56-16.79)[a]
	Severe > 2 years	1	3.03 (0.08-16.88)[a]
	700 women	0	0.00 (0.00-26.36)[a]
Enterline et al. 1987	1,074 white male production and maintenance workers at US asbestos company	2	1.14 (0.14-4.13)[a]
Other Occupations with Substantial Asbestos Exposure			
Finkelstein and Verma 2004	25,285 male pipe-trade workers in Ontario		
	20+ years since start of membership (latency)	14	1.32 (0.72-2.21)
Tola et al. 1988	7,775 male shipyard workers in Finland (incidence)	24	1.20 (0.77-1.79)
Battista et al. 1999	734 male railway carriage construction and repair workers in Italy	5	2.40 (0.95-5.05)[c]
Puntoni et al. 2001	3,984 male shipyard workers in Genoa, Italy	32	1.64 (1.12-2.32)
	Time since first exposure (years)		
	0-19	5	1.36 (0.44-3.17)[a]
	20-29	4	0.93 (0.25-2.38)[a]
	30-39	6	1.58 (0.58-3.44)[a]
	≥ 40	17	2.20 (1.28-3.52)[a]

TABLE D.2 Laryngeal Continued

Reference*	Study Population	Exposed Cases	Estimated RR (95% CI)
	Duration of exposure (years)		
	0-14	6	1.14 (0.42-2.48)[a]
	15-24	8	1.59 (0.69-3.13)[a]
	≥ 25	**18**	**1.96 (1.16-3.10)**[a]
	Age at hire (years)		
	0-24	15	2.36 (1.32-3.89)[a]
	25-34	9	1.89 (0.87-3.59)[a]
	≥ 35	8	0.96 (0.41-1.89)[a]
	Period of hire ≤ 1940	22	2.36 (1.48-3.57)[a]
	Insulation workers	**3**	**8.52 (1.76-24.91)**[a]

NOTE: CI = Confidence interval; RR = relative risk. Figures are for mortality unless otherwise indicated. Data points included in meta-analyses are bolded.

* Full citations can be found in the reference list for Chapter 6.

[a]95% CIs calculated with standard methods from observed and expected numbers presented in original paper.

[b]SMR and 95% CIs calculated with standard methods from observed and expected numbers presented in original paper.

[c]90% CIs reported.

TABLE D.3 Esophageal Cancer and Exposure to Asbestos—Cohort Studies

Reference*	Study Population	Exposed Cases	Estimated RR (95% CI)
Patients with Asbestos-Related Disease			
Karjalainen et al. 1999	Asbestos-related disease patients in Finland (incidence)		
	Men		
	1,287 with asbestosis	1	1.0 (0.0-5.5)
	4,708 with benign pleural disease	1	0.5 (0.0-2.7)
	Women		
	89 with asbestosis	1	10.5 (0.3-58.2)
	179 with benign pleural disease	0	0.0 (0.0-92.6)
Szesznia-Dabrowska et al. 2002	902 male workers compensated for asbestosis in Poland	1	0.65 (0.01-2.40)[a]
Mining			
Armstrong et al. 1988	6,505 male crocidolite miners and millers in Western Australia (mortality to 1980)	3	0.72 (0.23-2.22)
Reid et al. 2004	5,685 male crocidolite mining and milling workers in western Australia		
	Incidence	10	1.11 (0.60-2.07)
	Mortality	8	0.89 (0.44-1.78)
McDonald et al. 1993	5,335 chrysotile miners and millers in Quebec (1976-1988)	10	0.73 (0.35-1.34)[a]
Meurman et al. 1994	Anthophyllite asbestos miners in Finland (incidence)		
	736 men (3+ months of exposed time)	3	1.99 (0.41-5.81)
	Moderate exposure	1	1.70 (0.04-9.44)
	Heavy exposure	2	2.18 (0.26-7.88)
	5+ years of exposed time	2	5.00 (0.61-18.1)
	Moderate exposure	0	0 (0.00-61.0)
	Heavy exposure	2	5.92 (0.72-21.4)
	167 women (3+ months of exposed time)	1	2.86 (0.07-15.9)
	Moderate exposure	1	8.68 (0.22-48.4)
	Heavy exposure	0	0 (0.00-16.1)
Insulation Manufacture/Insulators (laggers)			
Selikoff and Seidman 1991	17,800 male members of asbestos insulation unions in Canada and US in 1967	30	1.68 (1.13-2.40)[a]
Seidman et al. 1986	820 men producing amosite asbestos insulation in Paterson, NJ, US	1	0.49 (0.01-2.70)[b]

TABLE D.3 Esophageal Continues

Reference*	Study Population	Exposed Cases	Estimated RR (95% CI)
Selikoff et al. 1979	632 male insulation workers in New York and New Jersey, US before 1943	1	0.71 (0.02-3.98)[b]
	<35 years	0	0.0 (0.00-9.04)[a]
	35 + years	1	1.00 (0.03-5.57)[b]
Acheson et al. 1984	4,820 male insulation board factory workers in Uxbridge, UK	2	1.00 (0.12-3.61)[a]
Berry et al. 2000	1,400 male asbestos factory workers in east London, UK (laggers)	0	0.0 (0.00-4.79)[b]
Levin et al. 1998	753 white male workers in asbestos pipe insulation factory in Tyler, TX	2	2.32 (0.28-8.39)
Asbestos Textile Workers			
Peto et al. 1985	Asbestos textile factory workers in Rochdale, UK		
	283 women	0	0.0 (0.00-11.53)[b]
	3,211 men	11	1.67 (0.83-2.99)[b]
	< 10 years in scheduled areas		
	Time since first employment		
	< 20 years	2	1.11 (0.13-4.01)[b]
	20+ years	6	1.92 (0.70-4.17)[b]
	10+ years in scheduled areas		
	Time since first employment		
	< 20 years	0	0.0 (0.00-9.71)[b]
	20+ years	3	2.36 (0.49-6.91)[b]
Asbestos Cement			
Albin et al. 1990	Asbestos cement workers in southern Sweden (esophagus, stomach, duodenum—too broad for meta-analysis)	23	1.0 (0.5-2.0)
	≥ 40 fiber-years/ml	na	1.7 (0.2-3.3)
Gardner et al. 1986	2,090 chrysotile asbestos cement products workers in England	1	0.29 (0.01-1.59)[b]
Hughes et al. 1987	5,492 male employees at two asbestos-cement manufacturing plants in New Orleans, LA (20 year lag)	12	0.93 (0.48-1.62)[a]
	Duration of exposure (20 year lag)		
	≤ 1 year	7	0.88 (0.35-1.80)[a]
	> 1 year - 5 years	3	1.25 (0.26-3.65)[a]
	> 5 years - 15 years	0	0.0 (0.00-4.61)[a]
	> 15 years	2	1.11 (0.13-4.01)[a]

continues

TABLE D.3 Esophageal Continues

Reference*	Study Population	Exposed Cases	Estimated RR (95% CI)
Generic "Asbestos Workers"			
Woitowitz et al. 1986	Asbestos-exposed workers in Germany (esophagus/stomach—too broad for meta)		
	3,070 workers with exposure after 1972	13	1.82 (0.97-3.12)[a]
	665 workers with exposure complete by 1972	2	1.42 (0.17-5.13)[a]
Berry et al. 2000	Asbestos factory workers in east London, UK		
	3,000 men	7	**1.70 (0.68-3.50)**[b]
	Low/mod < 2 years	2	1.80 (0.22-6.50)[b]
	Low/mod > 2 years	2	2.27 (0.28-8.20)[b]
	Severe < 2 years	2	1.59 (0.19-5.73)[b]
	Severe > 2 years	1	**1.15 (0.0-6.40)**[b]
	700 women	5	**5.62 (1.82-13.11)**[b]
	Low/mod	1	6.25 (0.16-34.81)[b]
	Severe < 2 years	2	3.92 (0.47-14.16)[b]
	Severe > 2 years	2	**9.09 (1.10-32.82)**[b]
Hodgson and Jones 1986	31,150 male asbestos workers in England and Wales, UK	6	**0.64 (0.23-1.39)**[a]
	Cumulative exposure (years)		
	< 10	0	0.00 (0.00-2.64)[a]
	10-20	2	0.65 (0.08-2.33)[a]
	≥ 20	4	**0.80 (0.22-2.05)**[a]
Enterline et al. 1987	1,074 white male production and maintenance workers at US asbestos company	4	**1.36 (0.37-3.47)**[a]
Other Occupations with Substantial Asbestos Exposure			
Finkelstein and Verma 2004	25,285 male pipe-trade workers in Ontario		
	20+ years since start of membership (latency)	30	**1.27 (0.86-1.81)**
Puntoni et al. 2001	3,984 male shipyard workers in Genoa, Italy	11	0.77 (0.38-1.38)

NOTE: CI = Confidence interval; na = not available; RR = relative risk. Figures are for mortality unless otherwise indicated. Data points included in meta-analyses are bolded.

* Full citations can be found in the reference list for Chapter 6.

[a]95% CIs calculated with standard methods from observed and expected numbers presented in original paper.

[b]SMR and 95% CIs calculated with standard methods from observed and expected numbers presented in original paper.

TABLE D.4 Stomach Cancer and Exposure to Asbestos—Cohort Studies

Reference*	Study Population	Exposed Cases	Estimated RR (95% CI)
Patients with Asbestos-Related Disease			
Germani et al. 1999	631 women compensated for asbestosis in Italy	**2**	**0.45 (0.05-1.61)**
	Textile industry (n = 276)	2	1.09 (0.13-3.93)
	Asbestos cement industry (n = 278)	0	0.0 (0.0-1.41)[a]
Karjalainen et al. 1999	Asbestos-related disease patients in Finland (incidence)		
	Men		
	1,287 with asbestosis	**4**	**0.7 (0.2-1.9)**
	4,708 with benign pleural disease	**11**	**1.3 (0.6-2.3)**
	Women		
	89 with asbestosis	**1**	**2.2 (0.1-12.1)**
	179 with benign pleural disease	**0**	**0.0 (0.0-17.4)**
Szesznia-Dabrowska et al. 2002	902 male workers compensated for asbestosis in Poland	**5**	**0.70 (0.23-1.63)**
Mining			
Armstrong et al. 1988	6,505 male crocidolite miners and millers in Western Australia (mortality to 1980)	**17**	**1.16 (0.72-1.87)**
de Klerk et al. 1989	Nested analysis of 17 cases vs 343 controls among Western Australian miners		
	5+ years of employment	**0**	**0.0 (0.0-6.4)**
	50+ average f/ml at worksites	**1**	**0.4 (0.0-4.2)**
Reid et al. 2004	5,685 male crocidolite mining and milling workers in western Australia		
	Incidence (1980-2000)	27	1.31 (0.82-1.75)
	Mortality	**21**	**1.39 (0.91-2.14)**
Liddell et al. 1997	8,923 male chrysotile miners and millers in Quebec (mortality 1950-1992)	**183**	**1.24 (1.07-1.44)**[a]
	Cumulative exposure to age 55 (million particles per cubic foot—yrs) among 7,728 living to age 55	158	1.26 (1.07-1.48)[a]
	< 300	118	1.16 (0.96-1.39)[a]
	< 3	32	1.41 (0.98-2.01)[a]
	3 to < 10	22	1.38 (0.87-2.09)[a]
	10 to < 30	15	0.89 (0.50-1.47)[a]
	30 to < 60	13	1.07 (0.57-1.83)[a]
	60 to < 100	13	1.16 (0.62-1.98)[a]
	100 to < 200	16	1.15 (0.66-1.87)[a]
	200 to < 300	7	0.80 (0.32-1.65)[a]

continues

TABLE D.4 Stomach Continued

Reference*	Study Population	Exposed Cases	Estimated RR (95% CI)
	> 300	40	**1.69 (1.22-2.32)**
	300 to < 400	7	1.29 (0.52-2.66)[a]
	400 to < 1000	16	1.21 (0.69-1.96)[a]
	1000+	17	3.21 (1.87-5.14)[a]
Meurman et al. 1994	Anthophyllite asbestos miners in Finland (incidence)		
	736 men (3+ months of exposed time)	13	**1.42 (0.76-2.43)**
	Moderate exposure	6	1.71 (0.63-3.72)
	Heavy exposure	7	**1.24 (0.50-2.56)**
	5+ years of exposed time	3	1.26 (0.26-3.68)
	Moderate exposure	1	2.86 (0.07-15.9)
	Heavy exposure	2	**0.99 (0.12-3.56)**
	167 women (3+ months of exposed time)	1	0.67 (0.02-3.71)
	Moderate exposure	1	1.89 (0.05-10.5)
	Heavy exposure	0	0.00 (0.00-3.81)
Piolatto et al. 1990	1,058 male chrysotile miners in northern Italy	12	**0.94 (0.49-1.65)[a]**
	Duration of exposure (years)		
	< 10	4	0.69 (0.19-1.77)[a]
	10-20	5	1.79 (0.58-4.17)[a]
	> 20	3	**0.75 (0.15-2.19)[a]**
Amandus et al. 1987	575 male tremolite-exposed vermiculite miners in Libby, MT	2	**1.24 (0.15-4.49)**
Insulation Manufacture/Insulators (laggers)			
Selikoff and Seidman 1991	17,800 male members of asbestos insulation unions in Canada and US in 1967	38	1.29 (0.92-1.78)[a]
Seidman et al. 1986	820 men producing amosite asbestos insulation in Paterson, NJ, US	11	1.90 (0.95-3.40)[a]
Selikoff et al. 1979	632 male insulation workers in New York and New Jersey, US before 1943	19	**3.52 (2.12-5.49)[b]**
	Duration of exposure (years)		
	< 20	0	0.00 (0.00-36.9)[b]
	20-35	6	4.00 (1.47-8.71)[b]
	> 35	13	3.42 (1.82-5.85)[b]
Acheson et al. 1984	4,820 male insulation board factory workers in Uxbridge, UK	7	0.94 (0.38-1.94)[a]
Berry et al. 2000	1,400 male asbestos factory workers in east London, UK (laggers)	2	0.77 (0.09-2.78)[a]

TABLE D.4 Stomach Continued

Reference*	Study Population	Exposed Cases	Estimated RR (95% CI)
Levin et al. 1998	753 white male workers in asbestos pipe insulation factory in Tyler, TX	0	0.0 (0.00-3.35)[a]
Asbestos Textile Workers			
Pira et al. 2005	1,966 textile employees in Italy	**15**	**1.20 (0.67-1.98)**
	Duration of employment (years)		
	< 1	5	1.42 (0.46-3.31)[a]
	1 to < 5	2	0.63 (0.08-2.27)[a]
	5 to < 10	6	2.64 (0.97-5.75)[a]
	10+	2	0.57 (0.07-2.06)[a]
	Time since first employment (years)		
	< 15	5	1.37 (0.44-3.20)[a]
	15 to < 25	6	1.48 (0.54-3.22)[a]
	25 to < 35	3	1.00 (0.21-2.92)[a]
	35+	1	0.57 (0.01-3.17)[a]
	Time since last exposure (years)		
	Ongoing to < 3	2	0.87 (0.11-3.14)[a]
	3 to < 15	6	1.29 (0.47-2.81)[a]
	15 to < 25	4	1.21 (0.33-3.10)[a]
	25 to < 35	2	1.20 (0.15-4.33)[a]
	35+	1	1.90 (0.05-10.58)[a]
	Age at first exposure (years)		
	< 25	2	1.31 (0.16-4.73)[a]
	25 to < 35	1	0.38 (0.01-2.12)[a]
	35+	12	1.45 (0.75-2.53)[a]
	Sex		
	889 men	11	1.16 (0.58-2.08)[a]
	1,077 women	4	1.34 (0.37-3.43)[a]
Peto et al. 1985	Asbestos textile factory workers in Rochdale, UK		
	283 women	2	1.85 (0.22-6.69)[a]
	3,211 men	**29**	**1.00 (0.67-1.44)**[b]
	< 10 years in scheduled areas		
	Time since first employment		
	< 20 years	9	0.89 (0.41-1.69)[b]
	20+ years	9	0.77 (0.35-1.46)[b]
	10+ years in scheduled areas		
	Time since first employment		
	< 20 years	2	0.92 (0.11-3.31)[b]
	20+ years	9	**1.80 (0.82-3.42)**[b]

continues

TABLE D.4 **Stomach** Continued

Reference*	Study Population	Exposed Cases	Estimated RR (95% CI)
Dement et al. 1994	3,022 asbestos textile plant workers in South Carolina	9	0.90 (0.47-1.56)
	White males	3	0.77 (0.21-2.00)
	White females	0	0.00 (0.00-1.55)[b]
	Black males	6	1.60 (0.69-3.15)
Asbestos Cement			
Raffn et al. 1989	7,996 male asbestos-cement industry workers in Denmark (incidence)	43	1.43 (1.03-1.93)
	Duration of employment, 15 years latency		
	< 5 years	13	1.77 (0.94-3.02)
	≥ 5 years	15	1.27 (0.70-2.07)
	First employment 1928-40, 15 years latency	8	1.69 (0.73-3.33)
Botta et al. 1991	Asbestos-cement workers in Italy		
	2,608 men	17	0.81 (0.47-1.30)
	759 women	4	1.36 (0.37-3.48)
Smailyte et al. 2004	Asbestos-cement producers in Lithuania (incidence)		
	602 women	4	1.2 (0.4-3.2)
	1,285 men	14	0.9 (0.5-1.5)
	Duration of employment (years)		
	< 1	1	0.4 (0.1-2.6)
	1-4	8	1.4 (0.7-2.8)
	5-9	2	0.8 (0.2-3.3)
	≥ 10	3	0.6 (0.2-1.9)
	25+ years since first exposure	4	0.6
Albin et al. 1990	Asbestos cement workers in southern Sweden (esophagus, stomach, duodenum—grouping too broad for inclusion in meta-analysis)	23	1.0 (0.5-2.0)
	≥ 40 fiber-years/ml	na	1.7 (0.2-3.3)
Gardner et al. 1986	2,090 chrysotile asbestos cement products workers in England	15	1.09 (0.61-1.81)[b]
Hughes et al. 1987	5,492 male asbestos-cement manufacturing plant employees in New Orleans, LA (20 year lag)	22	1.13 (0.71-1.71)[a]
	Duration of exposure (20 year lag)		
	≤ 1 year	14	1.20
	> 1 year-5 years	5	1.35
	> 5 years-15 years	2	1.54
	> 15 years	1	0.37

TABLE D.4 Stomach Continued

Reference*	Study Population	Exposed Cases	Estimated RR (95% CI)
Friction Materials			
Kogan et al. 1993	2,834 friction product workers in Yaroslavl, Russia	**14**	**0.58 (0.32-0.98)[a]**
	Males	3	0.45 (0.09-1.33)[a]
	Females	11	0.70 (0.35-1.25)[a]
Generic "Asbestos Workers"			
Zhu and Wang 1993	5,893 chrysotile factory workers in China	**28**	**2.40 (1.60-3.47)[a]**
Pang et al. 1997	Chrysotile asbestos plant workers in China	5	4.40 (1.43-10.27)[b]
	160 men	5	7.87 (2.55-18.38)[b]
	370 women	0	0.00 (0.00-7.37)[b]
Woitowitz et al. 1986	Asbestos-exposed workers in Germany (esophagus/stomach—too broad for meta)		
	3,070 workers with exposure after 1972	13	1.82 (0.97-3.12)[a]
	665 workers with exposure complete by 1972	2	1.42 (0.17-5.13)[a]
Berry et al. 2000	Asbestos factory workers in east London, UK		
	3,000 men	**21**	**1.24 (0.77-1.89)[a]**
	Low/mod < 2 years	4	0.89 (0.24-2.29)[a]
	Low/mod > 2 years	3	0.82 (0.17-2.39)[a]
	Severe < 2 years	9	1.82 (0.83-3.44)[a]
	Severe > 2 years	5	1.30 (0.42-3.03)[a]
	700 women	5	1.42 (0.46-3.32)[a]
	Low/mod	1	1.50 (0.04-8.31)[a]
	Severe < 2 years	1	0.51 (0.01-2.84)[a]
	Severe > 2 years	3	3.41 (0.70-9.97)[a]
Acheson et al. 1982	1,327 women in gas-mask manufacture in Lancashire, UK	**9**	**1.20 (0.55-2.28)[a]**
Hodgson and Jones 1986	31,150 male asbestos workers in England and Wales, UK	**27**	**1.00 (0.66-1.46)[a]**
	Cumulative exposure (years)		
	< 10	6	1.50 (0.55-3.27)[a]
	10-20	10	1.16 (0.56-2.14)[a]
	≥ 20	11	0.77 (0.38-1.38)[a]
Enterline et al. 1987	1,074 white male production and maintenance workers at US asbestos company	**20**	**1.80 (1.10-2.78)[a]**

continues

TABLE D.4 Stomach Continued

Reference*	Study Population	Exposed Cases	Estimated RR (95% CI)
Other Occupations with Substantial Asbestos Exposure			
Finkelstein and Verma 2004	25,285 male pipe-trade workers in Ontario		
	20+ years since start of membership (latency)	**21**	**0.67 (0.41-1.02)**
Tola et al. 1988	7,775 male shipyard workers in Finland (incidence)	**63**	**0.80 (0.61-1.02)**
Battista et al. 1999	734 male railway carriage construction and repair workers in Italy	**13**	**1.31 (0.77-2.08)**[c]
Puntoni et al. 2001	3,984 male shipyard workers in Genoa, Italy	**67**	**1.14 (0.89-1.45)**
Sanden et al. 1987	3,787 male shipyard workers in Sweden (incidence)	**3**	**0.88 (0.18-2.58)**[b]
	20 year latency	3	1.07 (0.22-3.13)[b]
	Heavy exposure	1	0.77 (0.02-4.28)[b]

NOTE: CI = Confidence interval; na = not available; RR = relative risk. Figures are for mortality unless otherwise indicated. Data points included in meta-analyses are bolded.

* Full citations can be found in the reference list for Chapter 6.

[a]95% CIs calculated with standard methods from observed and expected numbers presented in original paper.

[b]SMR and 95% CIs calculated with standard methods from observed and expected numbers presented in original paper.

[c]90% CIs reported.

TABLE D.5 Colorectal[a] Cancer and Exposure to Asbestos—Cohort Studies

Reference*	Study Population	Exposed Cases	Estimated RR (95% CI)
Patients with Asbestos-Related Disease			
Germani et al. 1999	631 women compensated for asbestosis in Italy (large and small intestine, plus rectum)	11	2.18 (1.09-3.90)
	Colon and sigma	8	2.38 (1.03-3.90)
	Textile industry (n = 276)	5	3.67 (1.20-8.60)
	Asbestos cement industry (n = 278)	2	1.16 (0.14-4.21)
	Rectum	1	0.62 (0.02-3.45)
	Textile industry (n = 276)	0	0.0
	Asbestos cement industry (n = 278)	0	0.0
Karjalainen et al. 1999	Asbestos-related disease patients in Finland (incidence)		
	Men—colorectal	23	1.1 (0.7-1.7)[c]
	Colon	11	1.0 (0.5-1.9)[c]
	1,287 with asbestosis	3	0.9 (0.2-2.5)
	4,708 with benign pleural disease	8	1.1 (0.5-2.1)
	Rectum	12	1.2 (0.6-2.2)[c]
	1,287 with asbestosis	4	1.3 (0.3-3.2)
	4,708 with benign pleural disease	8	1.2 (0.5-2.4)
	Women—colon only	3	4.2(0.9-12.3)[c]
	89 with asbestosis	2	4.6 (0.6-16.5)
	179 with benign pleural disease	1	3.4 (0.1-1.91)
Szesznia-Dabrowska et al. 2002	Workers compensated for asbestosis in Poland		
	902 men—colorectal	3	0.66 (0.14-1.92)[c]
	Colon	1	0.51 (0.01-2.84)[b]
	Rectum, anus	2	0.77 (0.09-2.78)
	489 women—colorectal	3	1.38(0.29-4.04)[c]
	Colon	2	1.99 (0.24-7.19)
	Rectum, anus	1	0.86 (0.02-4.79)[b]
Aliyu et al. 2005	3,897 male participants in the Beta-Carotene and Retinol Efficacy Trial (colorectal)	85	2.0 (1.6-2.5)
	1,847 with pleural abnormality: positive	51	1.40 (0.88-2.23)
	24 with radiographic profusion: 3/2 to 3/+	1	1.38 (0.18-10.6)
	156 with >40 years in high-risk trade	3	0.49 (0.12-2.00)
	707 with >41 years since first exposure	29	1.20 (0.48-3.04)

continues

TABLE D.5 Colorectal[a] Continued

Reference*	Study Population	Exposed Cases	Estimated RR (95% CI)
Mining			
Armstrong et al. 1988	6,505 male crocidolite miners and millers in Western Australia (mortality to 1980)	**14**	**0.70 (0.41-1.18)**
Reid et al. 2004	5,685 male crocidolite mining and milling workers in western Australia		
	Incidence (1979-2000)	88	1.05 (0.85-1.29)
	Mortality	**49**	**1.31 (0.99-1.74)**
McDonald et al. 1993	5,335 chrysotile miners and millers in Quebec (1976-1988)	**73**	**0.82 (0.65-1.04)[b]**
Meurman et al. 1994	Anthophyllite asbestos miners in Finland with more than 3 months exposure (incidence)		
	736 men—colorectal	**3**	**0.55 (0.11-1.60)**
	Moderate exposure	2	1.06 (0.13-3.82)
	Heavy exposure	**1**	**0.28 (0.01-1.56)**
	5+ years of exposed time (212 men)	2	1.27 (0.15-4.60)
	Moderate exposure	1	3.85 (0.10-21.4)
	Heavy exposure	**1**	**0.76 (0.02-4.25)**
	167 women—colorectal	4	2.61 (0.71-6.69)[c]
	Colon	3	3.45 (0.71-10.1)
	Moderate exposure	1	3.14 (0.08-17.4)[b]
	Heavy exposure	2	3.66 (0.44-13.2)
	Rectum	1	1.52 (0.04-8.44)
	Moderate exposure	0	0.00 (0.00-15.2)
	Heavy exposure	1	2.39 (0.06-13.3)
Piolatto et al. 1990	1,058 male chrysotile miners in northern Italy (intestinal)	**6**	**0.91 (0.33-1.98)[b]**
	Duration of exposure (years)		
	< 10	3	1.03 (0.21-3.02)[b]
	10-20	0	0.00 (0.00-2.84)[b]
	> 20	**3**	**1.30 (0.27-3.81)[b]**

TABLE D.5 Colorectal[a] Continued

Reference*	Study Population	Exposed Cases	Estimated RR (95% CI)
Insulation Manufacture/Insulators (laggers)			
Selikoff and Seidman 1991	17,800 male members of asbestos insulation unions in Canada and US in 1967	**121**	**1.37 (1.14-1.64)**[b]
Seidman et al. 1986	820 men producing amosite asbestos insulation in Paterson, NJ, US	**22**	**1.85 (1.16-2.80)**[b]
Selikoff et al. 1979	632 male insulation workers in New York and New Jersey, US before 1943	**23**	**2.77 (1.76-4.16)**[c]
	Duration of exposure (years)		
	< 20	0	0.00 (0.00-18.45)[c]
	20-35	7	3.68 (1.48-7.59)[c]
	> 35	**16**	**2.58 (1.48-4.19)**[c]
Acheson et al. 1984	4,820 male insulation board factory workers in Uxbridge, UK	10	1.31 (0.63-2.42)[b]
	Colon	6	**1.37 (0.50-2.98)**[b]
	Rectum	4	**1.24 (0.34-3.17)**[b]
Berry et al. 2000	1,400 male asbestos factory workers in east London, UK (laggers)	8	2.86 (1.23-5.63)[b]
	Colon	**7**	**4.32 (1.73-8.90)**[b]
	Rectum	**1**	**0.85 (0.02-4.72)**[b]
Levin et al. 1998	753 white male workers in asbestos pipe insulation factory in Tyler, TX	6	1.67 (0.61-3.63)[b]
	Colon	6	**2.07 (0.76-4.51)**
	Rectum	0	**0.0 (0.00-5.27)**[b]
Asbestos Textile Workers			
Pira et al. 2005	1,966 textile employees in Italy	**16**	**1.45 (0.83-2.35)**
	Duration of employment (years)		
	< 1	7	2.23 (0.89-4.59)[b]
	1 to < 5	1	0.35 (0.01-1.95)[b]
	5 to < 10	3	1.46 (0.30-4.28)[b]
	10+	5	**1.67 (0.54-3.89)**[b]
	Time since first employment (years)		
	< 15	2	0.86 (0.10-3.10)[b]
	15 to < 25	2	0.55 (0.07-1.98)[b]
	25 to < 35	7	2.24 (0.89-4.58)[b]
	35+	5	2.64 (0.32-9.54)[b]

continues

TABLE D.5 Colorectal[a] Continued

Reference*	Study Population	Exposed Cases	Estimated RR (95% CI)
	Time since last exposure (years)		
	During to < 3	0	0.00 (0.0-2.69)[b]
	3 to < 15	5	1.34 (0.43-3.13)[b]
	15 to < 25	6	1.83 (0.67-3.98)[b]
	25 to < 35	3	1.52 (0.31-4.45)[b]
	35+	2	2.91 (0.35-10.51)[b]
	Age at first exposure (years)		
	< 25	3	1.63 (0.34-4.77)[b]
	25 to < 35	2	0.75 (0.09-2.71)[b]
	35+	11	1.68 (0.84-3.01)[b]
	Sex		
	889 men	10	1.39 (0.67-2.56)[b]
	1,077 women	6	1.56 (0.57-3.40)[b]
Peto et al. 1985	Asbestos textile factory workers in Rochdale, UK		
	283 women	4	1.98 (0.54-5.07)[b]
	3,211 men	20	0.75 (0.46-1.16)[c]
	< 10 years in scheduled areas		
	< 20 years since first employment	5	0.60 (0.19-1.40)[c]
	20+ years since first employment	8	0.68 (0.29-1.33)[c]
	10+ years in scheduled areas		
	< 20 years since first employment	2	1.18 (0.14-4.25)[c]
	20+ years since first employment	5	1.03 (0.33-2.40)[c]
Asbestos Cement			
Raffn et al. 1996	7,887 male asbestos-cement industry workers in Denmark (incidence)	102	1.22 (0.99-1.48)
	Years since first employment		
	0-14	23	1.02 (0.65-1.53)
	> 15	79	1.29 (1.02-1.61)
	first employed 1928-1950	39	1.47 (1.05-2.01)
Botta et al. 1991	Asbestos-cement workers in Italy		
	2,608 men	11	0.65 (0.33-1.17)
	759 women	7	1.80 (0.72-3.70)

TABLE D.5 Colorectal[a] Continued

Reference*	Study Population	Exposed Cases	Estimated RR (95% CI)
Smailyte et al. 2004a	Asbestos-cement producers in Lithuania (incidence)		
	602 women	3	0.8 (0.1-1.8)
	1,285 men	17	**1.6 (1.0-2.6)**
	Duration of employment (years)		
	< 1	4	2.2 (0.8-5.7)
	1-4	2	0.5 (0.2-2.1)
	5-9	3	1.8 (0.6-5.6)
	≥ 10	8	**2.4 (1.2-4.7)**
	25+ years since first exposure	7	**1.6 (0.6-3.3)** [b]
Albin et al. 1990	1,465 male asbestos-cement workers in southern Sweden (mortality 1927-1986)	26	1.5 (0.7-3.0)
	≥ 40 fiber-years/ml	na	3.4 (1.2-9.5)
Jakobsson et al. 1994	981 male industrial workers in Sweden (asbestos cement) (incidence 1958-1989)	**26**	**1.47 (0.96-2.15)**[b]
	Right colon	12	2.38 (1.23-4.16)
	Left colon	1	0.22 (0.00-1.18)
	Rectum	13	1.65 (0.88-2.83)
Gardner et al. 1986	2,090 chrysotile asbestos cement products workers in England	**11**	**0.71 (0.36-1.28)**[c]
	Colon	6	0.65 (0.24-1.42)[c]
	Rectum	5	0.81 (0.26-1.88)[c]
Hughes et al. 1987	5,492 male asbestos-cement manufacturing plant employees in New Orleans, LA		
	Plants combined (20 year lag)	21	0.90 (0.56-1.38)[b]
	Plant 1	10	1.20 (0.58-2.21)[b]
	Plant 2	11	0.73 (0.36-1.31)[b]
	Duration of exposure (20 year lag)		
	≤ 1 year	11	0.79 (0.39-1.41)[b]
	> 1 year - 5 years	5	1.11 (0.36-2.59)[b]
	> 5 years - 15 years	1	0.67 (0.02-3.74)[b]
	> 15 years	4	**1.21 (0.33-3.09)**[b]
Generic "Asbestos Workers"			
Woitowitz et al. 1986	Asbestos-exposed workers in Germany		
	3,070 workers with exposure after 1972	5	**0.79 (0.26-1.84)**[b]
	665 workers with exposure complete by 1972	3	**2.15 (0.44-6.29)**[b]

continues

TABLE D.5 Colorectal[a] Continued

Reference*	Study Population	Exposed Cases	Estimated RR (95% CI)
Berry et al. 2000	Asbestos factory workers in east London, UK		
	3,000 men	**22**	**1.36 (0.85-2.06)[c]**
	Colon		
	Low/mod < 2 years	3	1.21 (0.25-3.54)[c]
	Low/mod > 2 years	3	1.49 (0.31-4.36)[c]
	Severe < 2 years	3	1.11 (0.23-3.25)[c]
	Severe > 2 years	**8**	**4.06 (1.75-8.00)[c]**
	Rectum		
	Low/mod < 2 years	2	1.06 (0.13-3.82)[c]
	Low/mod > 2 years	0	0.00 (0.00-2.38)[c]
	Severe < 2 years	3	1.46 (0.30-4.28)[c]
	Severe > 2 years	**0**	**0.00 (0.00-2.41)[c]**
	700 women	**7**	**1.19 (0.48-2.44)[c]**
	Colon		
	Low/mod	0	0.00 (0.00-5.13)[c]
	Severe < 2 years	2	0.87 (0.11-3.15)[c]
	Severe > 2 years	**1**	**1.00 (0.03-5.57)[c]**
	Rectum		
	Low/mod	0	0.00 (0.00-10.85)[c]
	Severe < 2 years	4	3.70 (1.01-9.48)[c]
	Severe > 2 years	**0**	**0.00 (0.00-7.85)[c]**
Hodgson and Jones 1986	31,150 male asbestos workers in England and Wales, UK	**16**	**0.54 (0.31-0.88)[c]**
	Colon—cumulative exposure (years)	6	0.36 (0.13-0.78)[b]
	< 10	1	0.40 (0.01-2.23)[b]
	10-20	2	0.36 (0.04-1.31)[b]
	≥ 20	**3**	**0.54 (0.11-1.57)[c]**
	Rectum—cumulative exposure (years)	10	0.77 (0.37-1.43)[b]
	< 10	1	0.52 (0.01-2.93)[b]
	10-20	2	0.47 (0.06-1.72)[b]
	≥ 20	**7**	**1.03 (0.41-2.12)[b]**
Enterline et al. 1987	1,074 white male production and maintenance workers at US asbestos company	**23**	**1.15 (0.73-1.73)[b]**
	Colon	14	0.98 (0.54-1.65)[b]
	Rectum	9	1.59 (0.73-3.02)[b]

TABLE D.5 Colorectal[a] Continued

Reference*	Study Population	Exposed Cases	Estimated RR (95% CI)
Other Occupations with Substantial Asbestos Exposure			
Finkelstein and Verma 2004	25,285 male pipe-trade workers in Ontario 20+ years since start of membership (latency)	**96**	**1.16 (0.94-1.42)**
Tola et al. 1988	7,775 male shipyard workers in Finland (incidence)	**35**	**0.79 (0.55-1.10)**
Battista et al. 1999	734 male railway carriage construction and repair workers in Italy	**6**	**0.93 (0.41-1.84)[d]**
Puntoni et al. 2001	3,984 male shipyard workers in Genoa, Italy	**59**	**1.00 (0.76-1.29)**
Sanden et al. 1987	3,787 male shipyard workers in Sweden (incidence)	3	0.38 (0.08-1.1)
	Rectum	**3**	**0.45 (0.09-1.33)[c]**
	Heavy or very heavy exposure	**2**	**0.65 (0.08-2.33)[c]**
	Colon	0	0.00 (0.00-3.00)[c]

NOTE: CI = Confidence interval; na = not available; RR = relative risk. Figures are for mortality unless otherwise indicated. Data points included in meta-analyses are bolded.

* Full citations can be found in the reference list for Chapter 6.

[a]Statistics from original paper presented here; when RRs were calculated for colon and rectum separately, combined RRs for colorectal cancer were derived for use in meta-analysis.

[b]95% CIs calculated with standard methods from observed and expected numbers presented in original paper.

[c]SMR and 95% CIs calculated with standard methods from observed and expected numbers presented in original paper.

[d]90% CIs reported.

APPENDIX E

Case-Control Results Tables

TABLE E.1 Pharyngeal Cancer and Exposure to Asbestos—Case-Control Studies

Reference*	Study Population	Exposed Cases	Estimated RR (95% CI)
Berrino et al. 2003	100 male cases of hypopharyngeal cancer from six centers in Southern Europe, < 55 years old (adjusted for smoking and alcohol consumption)		
	Possible	na	1.8 (0.9-3.9)
	Probable	na	1.8 (0.6-5.0)
	(More detailed findings from combined analysis with 215 cases of laryngeal cancer on Table E.2)		
Luce et al. 2000	5 hypopharyngeal cancer cases among residents of New Caledonia		
	Whitewash from tremolite asbestos	1	0.64 (0.01-6.68)
Marchand et al. 2000	206 hypopharyngeal cancer cases among male residents of six cities in France (adjusted for smoking and alcohol consumption)		
	Any exposure	161	1.80 (1.08-2.99)
	Low cumulative exposure	52	1.92 (1.03-3.57)
	Intermediate	52	1.40 (0.74-2.63)
	High	57	2.14 (1.14-4.01)

continues

TABLE E.1 Pharyngeal Continued

Reference*	Study Population	Exposed Cases	Estimated RR (95% CI)
Gustavsson et al. 1998	138 pharyngeal cancer cases among male residents of two regions in Sweden (adjusted for smoking and alcohol consumption)		
	Asbestos (low)	24	1.01 (0.57-1.80)
	Asbestos (high)	22	1.08 (0.62-1.91)
Zheng et al. 1992b	115 male oral or pharyngeal cancer cases among residents of Shanghai, China		
	Asbestos, occupational exposure	**16**	**1.81 (0.91-3.60)**[a]
Merletti et al. 1991	86 oral cavity or oropharynx (n = 12) cancer cases among male residents of Turin, Italy (adjusted for smoking and alcohol consumption)		
	Any exposure	**45**	**1.1 (na)**
	Probable or definite	3	0.4 (na)

NOTES: CI = Confidence interval; na = not available; RR = relative risk. Data points included in meta-analyses are bolded.

* Full citations can be found in the reference list for Chapter 6.

[a]OR and 95% CI calculated with standard methods from observed numbers of exposed cases and controls in original paper.

TABLE E.2 Laryngeal Cancer and Exposure to Asbestos—Case-Control Studies

Reference*	Study Population	Exposed Cases	Estimated RR (95% CI)
Berrino et al. 2003	213 male cases of endolaryngeal cancer from six centers in Southern Europe, < 55 years old		
	Possible	na	1.7 (1.0-3.0)
	Probable	**na**	**1.8 (0.8-4.0)**
	Combined analysis with 100 hypopharyngeal cancer cases		
	Asbestos (JEM-derived agent), any exposure	215	1.6 (1.0-2.5)
	10+ years duration and 20+ years lag	121	1.4 (0.8-2.4)
	Likelihood of exposure		
	Possible	175	1.7 (1.1-2.8)
	Probable	40	1.9 (0.9-3.8)
	Duration of exposure		
	< 10 years	na	1.3 (0.6-2.7)
	10-19 years	na	1.4 (0.7-2.7)
	≥ 20 years	na	1.7 (0.9-3.0)
			p-trend > 0.05
	Tertiles of weighted exposure		
	1	na	1.4 (0.8-2.3)
	2	na	1.9 (1.2-3.2)
	3	na	1.6 (1.0-2.6)
			p-trend = 0.037
Dietz et al. 2003	257 laryngeal cancer cases among residents of Rhein-Neckar region, Germany		
	Asbestos	59	1.3 (0.8-2.1)
Elci et al. 2002	940 laryngeal cancer cases among male residents of Istanbul, Turkey (smoking-adjusted)		
	Asbestos (JEM-derived agent)	150	1.0 (0.8-1.3)
	Glottis	28	0.8 (0.5-1.2)
	Supraglottis	71	1.0 (0.8-1.4)
	Other laryngeal	51	1.2 (0.9-1.7)
	Intensity of exposure		
	Low	45	0.9 (0.6-1.3)
	Medium	93	1.2 (0.9-1.6)
	High	12	0.6 (0.3-1.1)
	Probability of exposure		
	Low	121	1.2 (0.9-1.5)
	Medium	20	0.6 (0.4-1.1)
	High	9	0.7 (0.3-1.5)

continues

TABLE E.2 Laryngeal Continued

Reference*	Study Population	Exposed Cases	Estimated RR (95% CI)
Luce et al. 2000	20 laryngeal cancer cases among male residents of New Caledonia (all smokers)		
	Whitewash from tremolite asbestos	3	**0.72 (0.22-2.30)**
	Melanesians	2	0.71 (0.14-3.63)
	Non-Melanesians	1	0.60 (0.07-5.22)
Marchand et al. 2000	296 laryngeal cancer cases among male residents of six cities in France (smoking-adjusted)		
	Any exposure	**216**	**1.24 (0.83-1.90)**
	Low cumulative exposure	67	1.10 (0.66-1.82)
	Intermediate	72	1.20 (0.73-1.99)
	High	77	**1.47 (0.87-2.46)**
	Supraglottic, any exposure	56	1.12 (0.61-2.05)
	Low cumulative exposure	15	0.84 (0.38-1.84)
	Intermediate	22	1.31 (0.62-2.76)
	High	19	1.27 (0.58-2.78)
	Glottic and subglottic, any exposure	75	1.15 (0.68-1.95)
	Low cumulative exposure	27	1.19 (0.62-2.27)
	Intermediate	21	0.90 (0.45-1.78)
	High	27	1.44 (0.73-2.83)
	Epilarynx, any exposure	77	1.77 (0.94-3.30)
	Low cumulative exposure	22	1.45 (0.67-3.13)
	Intermediate	25	1.69 (0.79-3.64)
	High	30	2.22 (1.05-4.71)
De Stefani et al. 1998	112 laryngeal cancer cases among male residents of Montevideo, Uruguay (smoking-adjusted)		
	Asbestos (self-reported agent)	23	**1.8 (0.9-3.2)**
	1-20 years	4	0.9 (0.3-2.7)
	20+ years	**19**	**2.4 (1.2-4.8)**
	Supraglottic	na	2.3 (0.9-5.7)
	Glottic	na	2.9 (0.8-10.5)
Gustavsson et al. 1998	157 laryngeal cancer cases among male residents of two regions in Sweden		
	Asbestos (low)	28	1.21 (0.73-2.02)
	Asbestos (high)	**34**	**1.69 (1.05-2.74)**
	Quartile I	13	1.16 (1.02-1.32)
	Quartile II	15	1.35 (1.04-1.74)
	Quartile III	16	1.56 (1.06-2.30)
	Quartile IV	**18**	**1.82 (1.08-3.04)**
			p-trend = 0.02

TABLE E.2 Laryngeal Continued

Reference*	Study Population	Exposed Cases	Estimated RR (95% CI)
Muscat and Wynder 1992	186 laryngeal cancer cases among white, male residents of New York, Illinois, Michigan, and Pennsylvania, US		
	Asbestos, any exposure	66	1.1 (0.7-1.9)
	Glottis	40	1.3 (0.7-2.7)
	Supraglottis	26	1.1 (0.5-2.6)
Wortley et al. 1992	235 laryngeal cancer cases among residents of western Washington state, US		
	Asbestos—peak		
	None	145	1.0
	Low	3	1.2 (0.6-7.1)
	Medium	57	1.3 (0.8-2.0)
	High	30	1.1 (0.6-1.9)
	Asbestos—duration		
	< 1 year	151	1.0
	1-9	50	1.0 (0.5-2.1)
	≥ 10	34	1.2 (0.6-2.3)
	Asbestos—exposure scores		
	< 5	173	1.0
	5-19	25	1.1 (0.6-2.1)
	≥ 20	37	1.4 (0.7-2.5)
Zheng et al. 1992a	201 laryngeal cancer cases among residents of Shanghai, China (smoking-adjusted)		
	Asbestos, occupational exposure	26	2.0 (1.0-4.3)
Ahrens et al. 1991	85 laryngeal cancer cases among male residents of Bremen, Germany (smoking-adjusted)		
	Asbestos	na	1.1 (0.5-2.4)
Brown et al. 1988	180 laryngeal cancer cases among male residents along Gulf Coast of Texas (smoking-adjusted)		
	Asbestos	88	1.5 (1.0-2.2)
	< 5 years	20	1.3 (0.7-2.6)
	5-14	24	2.2 (1.1-4.3)
	≥ 15	40	1.4 (0.8-2.4)
	unknown	4	
Zagraniski et al. 1986	92 laryngeal cancer cases among white, male residents of New Haven, CT (smoking-adjusted)		
	Asbestos workers (ever held occupation)	11	1.1 (0.4-2.9)

continues

TABLE E.2 Laryngeal Continued

Reference	Study Population	Exposed Cases	Estimated RR (95% CI)
Olsen and Sabroe 1984	276 male laryngeal cancer cases among residents of Denmark (smoking-adjusted)		
	Asbestos	**17**	**1.8 (1.0-3.4)**
Burch et al. 1981	184 laryngeal cancer cases among male residents of southern Ontario, Canada (smoking-adjusted)		
	Self-reported asbestos exposure	36	1.6 ($p = 0.069$)
	Occupational hygienist classified exposure	**14**	**2.3 ($p = 0.052$)**
Hinds et al. 1979	47 laryngeal cancer cases among male residents of three counties in WA; self-reported asbestos exposure		
	All subtypes	**25**	**1.75 ($p = 0.21$)**
	Glottis	na	1.29 ($p = 0.63$)
	Supraglottis	na	4.00 ($p = 0.22$)
Shettigara and Morgan 1975	43 laryngeal cancer cases among male hospital patients in Toronto, Canada		
	Asbestos	**10**	**∞ (0 exposed controls)**
Stell and McGill 1973	100 laryngeal cancer cases among male hospital patients in Liverpool, UK		
	Asbestos	**31**	**14.53 (4.27-49.43)**[a]

NOTES: CI = Confidence interval; na = not available; RR = relative risk. Data points included in meta-analyses are bolded.

* Full citations can be found in the reference list for Chapter 6.

[a]OR and 95% CI calculated with standard methods from observed numbers of exposed cases and controls in original paper.

TABLE E.3 Esophageal Cancer and Exposure to Asbestos—Case-Control Studies

Reference*	Study Population	Exposed Cases	Estimated RR (95% CI)
Parent et al. 2000	99 esophageal cancer cases among male residents of Montreal, Canada; IH-derived agent: chrysotile asbestos (smoking-adjusted)		
	All subtypes		
	Any exposure	21	1.4 (0.8-2.4)
	Nonsubstantial	19	1.4 (0.8-2.5)
	Substantial	2	1.3 (0.3-6.2)
	63 squamous-cell carcinomas		
	Any exposure	17	2.0 (1.1-3.8)
	Nonsubstantial	16	2.1 (1.1-4.0)
	Substantial	1	1.1 (0.1-9.7)
Gustavsson et al. 1998	122 esophageal cancer cases among male residents of two regions in Sweden; IH-derived agent (smoking-adjusted)		
	Asbestos (low)	22	1.21 (0.67-2.17)
	Asbestos (high)	21	1.00 (0.54-1.82)
Hillerdal 1980	Gastrointestinal carcinoma cases among male residents of Uppsala county, Sweden (exposure = pleural plaques)		
	21 esophageal	1	2.86 (0.07-15.91)[a]

NOTES: CI = Confidence interval; na = not available; RR = relative risk. Data points included in meta-analyses are bolded.

* Full citations can be found in the reference list for Chapter 6.

[a]OR and 95% CI calculated with standard methods from observed and expected numbers presented in original paper.

TABLE E.4 Stomach Cancer and Exposure to Asbestos—Case-Control Studies

Reference*	Study Population	Exposed Cases	Estimated RR (95% CI)
Krstev et al. 2005	443 stomach cases among residents of Warsaw, Poland		
	285 males, ever exposed	**42**	**1.5 (0.9-2.4)**
	1-9 years	19	1.2 (0.6-2.3)
	≥ 10 years	**23**	**1.9 (0.9-3.8)**
	158 females, ever exposed	1	0.3 (0.03-3.0)
	1-9 years	1	0.4 (0.0-6.0)
	≥ 10 years	**0**	**—**
Ekstrom et al. 1999	**565 gastric cancer cases among residents of Sweden**	**155**	**1.11 (0.87-1.42)**
Parent et al. 1998	250 male gastric cancer cases among residents of Montreal, Canada		
	Chrysotile asbestos		
	Nonsubstantial	43	1.2 (0.8-1.7)
	Substantial	**4**	**0.7 (0.2-1.8)**
	Amphibole asbestos		
	Nonsubstantial	10	0.6 (0.3-1.2)
	Substantial	**3**	**1.9 (0.6-6.9)**
Cocco et al. 1994	640 gastric cancer cases among male residents of Italy		
	Ever exposed	**239**	**0.7 (0.5-1.1)**
	21+ years	**na**	**1.4 (0.6-3.0)**
Hillerdal 1980	Gastrointestinal carcinoma cases among male residents of Uppsala county, Sweden (exposure = pleural plaques)		
	148 stomach	**6**	**2.40 (0.88-5.22)[a]**

NOTES: CI = Confidence interval; na = not available; RR = relative risk. Data points included in meta-analyses are bolded.

* Full citations can be found in the reference list for Chapter 6.

[a]95% CI calculated with standard methods from observed and expected numbers presented in original paper.

TABLE E.5 Colorectal Cancer and Exposure to Asbestos—Case-Control Studies

Reference*	Study Population	Exposed Cases	Estimated RR (95% CI)
Goldberg et al. 2001	497 colon cancer cases among male residents of Montreal, Canada; industrial-hygiene-derived agent		
	Adjusted for age and non-occupational factors		
	Nonsubstantial	60	0.9 (0.6-1.3)
	Substantial	18	2.1 (1.1-4.0)
	Further adjusted for occupational factors		
	Nonsubstantial	60	0.9 (0.6-1.3)
	Substantial	18	1.8 (0.9-3.6)
	Frequency		
	1-5%	21	0.9 (0.5-1.6)
	6-30%	49	1.1 (0.7-1.5)
	> 30%	8	1.5 (0.6-3.7)
	Concentration		
	Low	40	0.9 (0.6-1.4)
	Medium	32	1.2 (0.8-1.8)
	High	6	1.4 (0.4-4.3)
	Duration (10-year increment)	78	1.1 (0.9-1.2)
Dumas et al. 2000	257 rectal cancer cases among male residents of Montreal, Canada		
	Chrysotile, any	30	0.7 (0.5-1.0)
	Substantial	3	0.5 (0.2-1.6)
	Amphiboles, any	11	0.7 (0.3-1.2)
	Substantial	2	1.5 (0.3-7.6)
Demers et al. 1994	261 colorectal cancer cases among white males residents of southeast Michigan	15	0.5 (0.3-1.0)
	Duration (years)		
	< 20	9	0.6 (0.3-1.5)
	20+	6	0.4 (0.1-1.2)
	Latency (years)		
	< 40	5	0.4 (0.1-1.3)
	40+	10	0.6 (0.2-1.4)
Vineis et al. 1993	74 colon cancer cases among male residents of industrialized northern Italy (job titles)		
	Jobs with putative asbestos exposure	4	4.8 (1.05-21.5)
Garabrant et al. 1992	419 male colon cancer cases among residents of Los Angeles County, CA		
	Never exposed	353	1.00

continues

TABLE E.5 Colorectal Continued

Reference*	Study Population	Exposed Cases	Estimated RR (95% CI)
	No latency		
	Any exposure	**66**	**0.99 (0.66-1.50)**
	Asbestos on hands and clothes		
	Did not get on hands or clothes	17	2.32 (0.87-6.23)
	Got on hands or clothes	49	0.82 (0.52-1.30)
	Use of mask		
	Did not wear mask	55	0.95 (0.61-1.46)
	Wore mask	11	1.43 (0.49-4.17)
	Frequency of exposure		
	< 5 times/week	18	1.00 (0.50-2.00)
	≥ 5 times/week	**31**	**0.79 (0.43-1.46)**
	Brief, intense exposure	17	1.48 (0.64-3.38)
	Ordinal trend		$p = 0.70$
	Duration of exposure (years)		
	< 5	24	0.98 (0.53-1.84)
	5-14	20	1.47 (0.67-3.22)
	≥ 15	22	0.76 (0.39-1.49)
	Continuous trend		$p = 0.61$
	Ordinal trend		$p = 0.81$
	Time since first exposure (years)		
	< 1-14	10	1.66 (0.54-5.10)
	15-29	21	1.37 (0.65-2.91)
	≥ 30	35	0.77 (0.45-1.31)
	Continuous trend		$p = 0.61$
	Ordinal trend		$p = 0.66$
	Cumulative exposure index		
	1-30	41	1.26 (0.74-2.15)
	31-60	11	0.80 (0.34-1.88)
	≥ 61	**14**	**0.65 (0.28-1.51)**
	Continuous trend		$p = 0.22$
	Ordinal trend		$p = 0.46$
	15-year latency		
	Exposed, latency > 15 years	56	0.93 (0.60-1.44)
	Asbestos on hands and clothes		
	Did not get on hands or clothes	12	1.75 (0.62-4.94)
	Got on hands or clothes	44	0.83 (0.51-1.33)
	Use of mask		
	Did not wear mask	46	0.86 (0.55-1.37)
	Wore mask	10	1.95 (0.55-6.90)
	Frequency of exposure		
	< 5 times/week	14	0.83 (0.39-1.76)
	≥ 5 times/week	30	0.93 (0.49-1.77)
	Brief, intense exposure	12	1.14 (0.46-2.87)
	Ordinal trend		$p = 0.78$

TABLE E.5 Colorectal Continued

Reference	Study Population	Exposed Cases	Estimated RR (95% CI)
	Duration of exposure (years)		
	< 5	19	0.74 (0.37-1.47)
	5-14	21	1.60 (0.75-3.44)
	≥ 15	16	0.69 (0.30-1.55)
	Continuous trend		$p = 0.58$
	Ordinal trend		$p = 0.79$
	Cumulative exposure index		
	1-30	36	1.07 (0.63-1.81)
	31-60	10	0.94 (0.33-2.65)
	≥ 61	10	0.55 (0.21-1.47)
	Continuous trend		$p = 0.33$
	Ordinal trend		$p = 0.40$
Gerhardson de Verdier et al. 1992	Colon and rectal cancer cases among male residents of Stockholm, Sweden; self-reported agents		
	163 colon cancers	**22**	**1.9 (0.9-4.2)**
	Right colon	16	2.6 (1.2-5.9)
	Left colon	3	0.5 (0.1-1.9)
	107 rectal cancers	**17**	**1.9 (0.8-4.6)**
	Colorectal cancer: latency (years)		
	1-19	5	1.4 (0.3-9.9)
	20+	34	2.0 (1.0-3.9)
	1-29	12	1.6 (0.5-5.0)
	30+	27	2.0 (1.0-4.4)
	1-39	22	1.4 (0.7-3.0)
	40+	17	3.2 (1.1-11.5)
Neuget et al. 1991	51 colorectal cancer cases among males undergoing colonoscopy in 3 NYC medical centers		
	Asbestos exposure	10	**1.8 (0.8-5.6)**
	Significant exposure	3	**4.3 (0.8-23.5)**
Fredriksson et al. 1989	329 colon cancer cases among residents of Umea, Sweden		
	Asbestos, low grade	na	1.2 (0.6-2.4)
	Asbestos, high grade	**na**	**2.1 (0.8-5.8)**
Spiegelman and Wegman 1985	Colorectal cancer cases in seven US metropolitan areas and two states; JEM-derived agent		
	Males: 343 colorectal cancer	**na**	**1.28 ($p = 0.17$)**
	224 colon cancer only	na	1.22 ($p = 0.33$)
	Females: 208 colorectal cancer	**na**	**1.08 ($p = 0.65$)**
	171 colon cancer only	na	1.09 ($p = 0.64$)

continues

TABLE E.5 Colorectal Continued

Reference*	Study Population	Exposed Cases	Estimated RR (95% CI)
Hardell 1981	153 colon cancer cases among male residents of Umea, Sweden		
	Asbestos, any	**16**	**1.9 (1.0-3.6)**
Hillerdal 1980	Gastrointestinal carcinoma cases among male residents of Uppsala county, Sweden (exposure = pleural plaques)		
	108 colon	**3**	**1.67 (0.34-4.87)**[a]
	101 rectal	**3**	**1.76 (0.36-5.16)**[a]

NOTES: CI = Confidence interval; na = not available; RR = relative risk. Data points included in meta-analyses are bolded.

* Full citations can be found in the reference list for Chapter 6.

[a]OR and 95% CI calculated with standard methods from observed and expected numbers presented in original paper.

APPENDIX F

Initial Analyses of Available Data Concerning Cancers of Colon and/or Rectum and Asbestos Exposure

After culling all the data available concerning either colon or rectal cancers and exposure to asbestos from the cohort and case-control studies, the committee conducted preliminary analyses to determine whether conclusions should or could be derived separately for the colon and for the rectum. As presented by the original researchers, there were three sets of findings that grouped themselves:

A. findings on just the colon,
B. findings on just the rectum, and
C. findings on colon and rectum combined.

The summary tables and plots on the following pages are the result of the initial analyses of these three datasets; unfortunately the graphic quality of these preliminary runs was poor.

For almost all the cohort studies reporting on either of these two sites individually, if data on one were given, the corresponding information on the other was also present. Furthermore, because most of the cohort studies presented the expected number of cancers at a site as well as the number observed, the statistics for the combined sites could accurately be recalculated. Since adjustment for confounders had generally not been performed for the cohort studies, this approach posed no compromise on the refinement of the analysis.

For the (fewer) case-control studies (all of which had analyses involving some adjustment for confounders), when the results were not presented in combined form, only one of the two sites had been studied. The committee was, therefore, not in a position to derive statistics for the combined statistics where they were not already available.

Colon cancer is more prevalent than rectal cancer, representing more than 70% of the cases when the two sites are combined. Therefore, colon cancer can be considered to dominate the calculations. The risk factors for cancers at these two segments of the intestinal tract are not well enough understood to be distinguished.

Having scanned the plots for evidence of systematic differences between the results for colon and rectal cancers and discussed the options for deriving a valid and useful conclusions, the committee agreed to conduct its meta-analyses of the epidemiologic data on colon and rectal cancers on datasets with the sites combined and to draw a single conclusion about causality for the combined sites (as stated in the Fairness in Asbestos Injury Resolution, or FAIR, legislation and the committee's charge).

A. Results for colon cancer and asbestos exposure

COLON

Study Type	Plot	Comparison	Strata*	No. of Studies	99% CI for summary RR	Between study SD
CA-CO	1	Any v none	All	9	(0.94, 1.77)	.14
	2		EQ = 1,2	4	(0.87, 1.55)	.00
			EQ = 3	5	(0.91, 3.88)	0.19
	3		EQ = 1,2 Adjusted			
			EQ = 1,2 Unadjusted			
	4a	High v none	EQ = 1,2 Use highest reported RR	3	(0.58, 3.00)	.32
	4b		EQ = 1,2 Use lowest reported RR	3	(0.45, 2.94)	.25
Cohort	1	Any v none	All	16	(0.91, 2.06)	.42
	2		EQ = 1,2	7	(.61, 2.09)	.51
			EQ = 3	9	(1.14, 2.70)	.00
	3	High v none	EQ = 1,2	4	(0.60, 4.83)	.59

* Not enough studies to report subgroups of adjusted RR.

1. Results from cohort studies

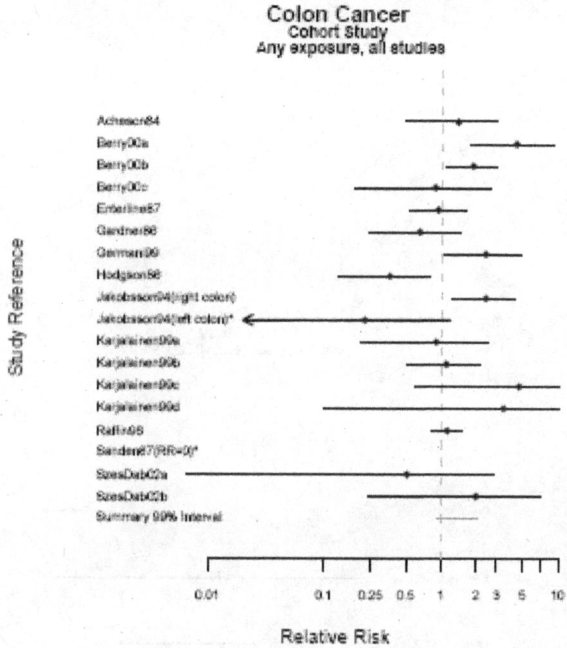

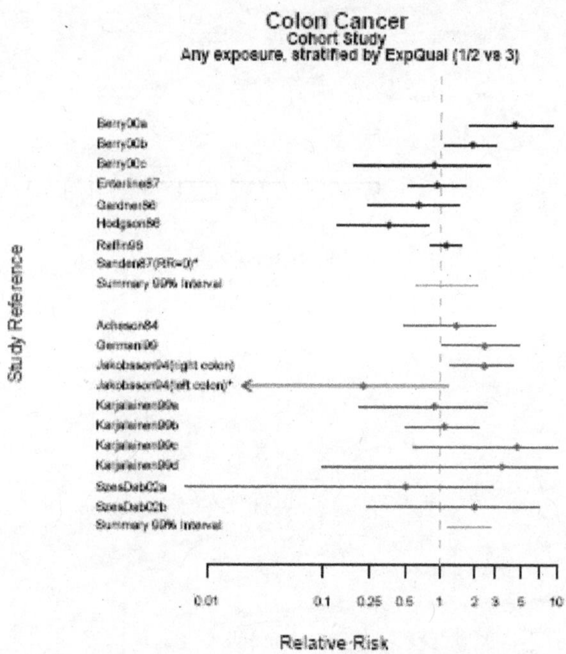

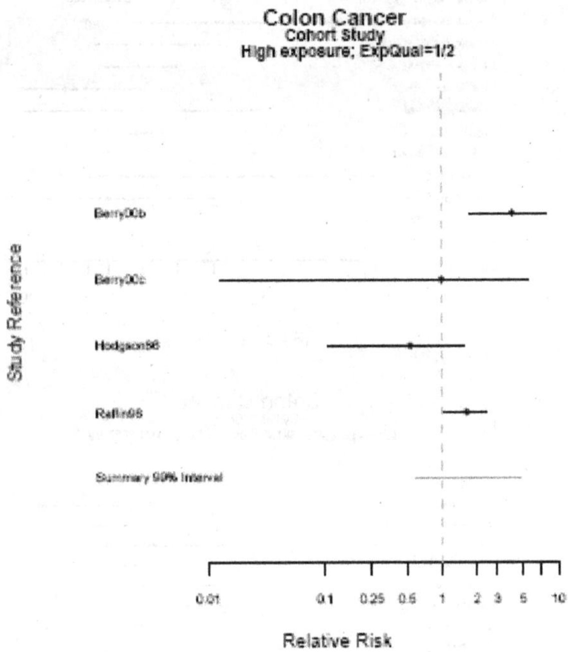
Colon Cancer
Cohort Study
High exposure; ExpQual=1/2
Study Reference
Berry00b
Berry00c
Hodgson98
Raffn98
Summary 99% Interval
0.01
0.1
0.25
0.5
1
2
3
5
10
Relative Risk

2. Results from case-control studies

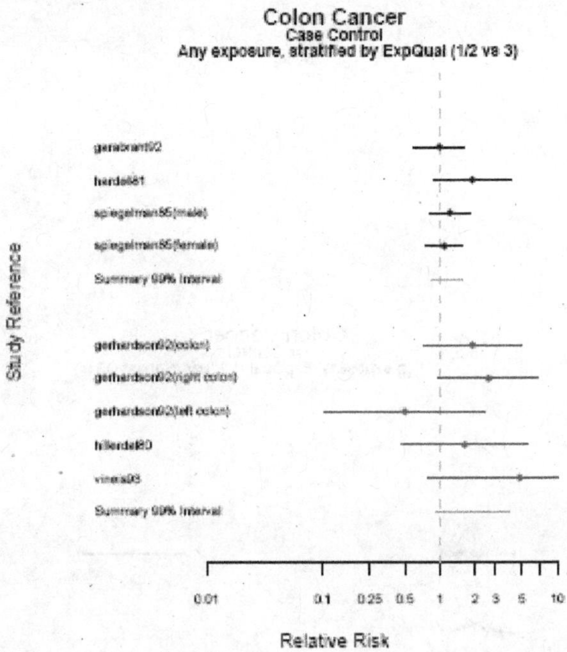

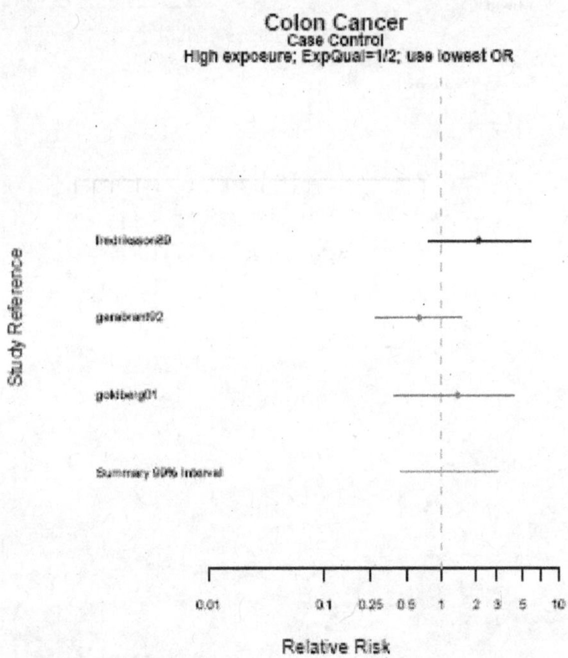

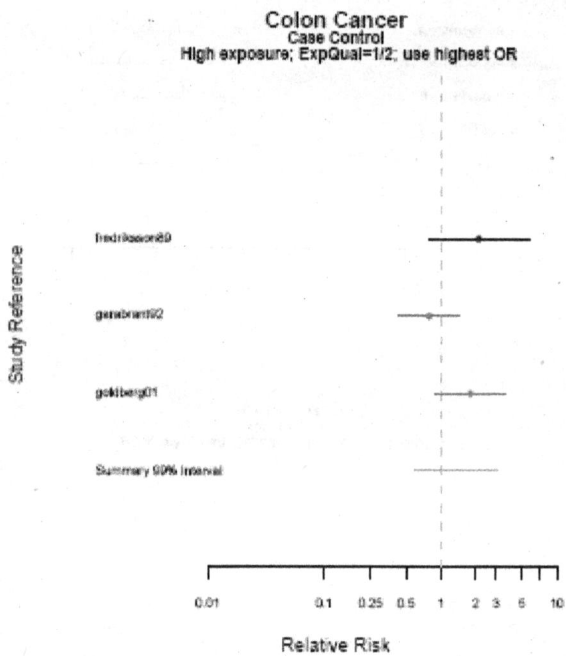
Colon Cancer
Case Control
High exposure; ExpQual=1/2; use highest OR
Study Reference
goldberg01
Summary 90% Interval
0.01
0.1
0.25
0.5
1
2
3
5
10
Relative Risk

B. Results for rectal cancer and asbestos exposure

RECTAL

Study Type	Plot	Comparison	Strata*	No. of Studies	99% CI for summary RR	Between study SD
CA-CO	1	Any v none	All	4	(0.50, 1.67)	0.29
	2		EQ = 1,2	2	(0.44, 1.10)	.00
			EQ = 3	2	(0.65, 5.13)	.00
	3		EQ = 1,2 Adjusted			
			EQ = 1,2 Unadjusted			
	4	High v none	EQ = 1,2	2	(0.17, 3.10)	.00
Cohort	1	Any v none	All	15	(0.97, 1.60)	.00
	2		EQ = 1,2	8	(0.91, 1.62)	.00
			EQ = 3	7	(0.81, 2.21)	.00
	3	High v none	EQ = 1,2	3	(0.67, 2.01)	.33

* Not enough studies to report subgroups of adjusted RR.

1. Results from cohort studies

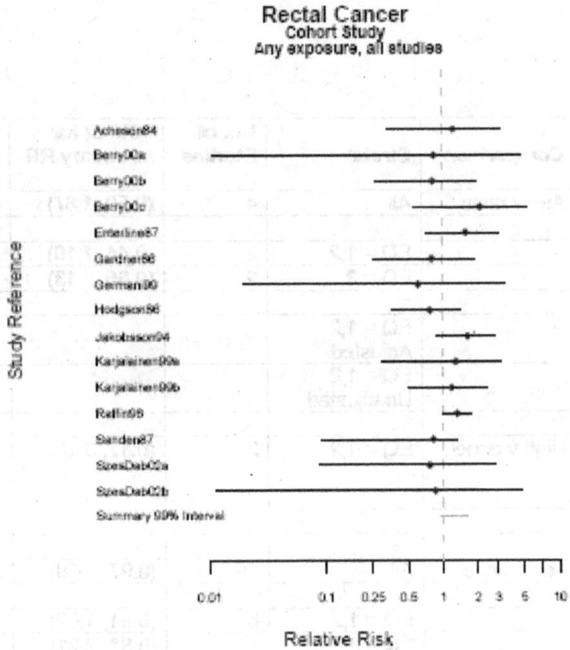

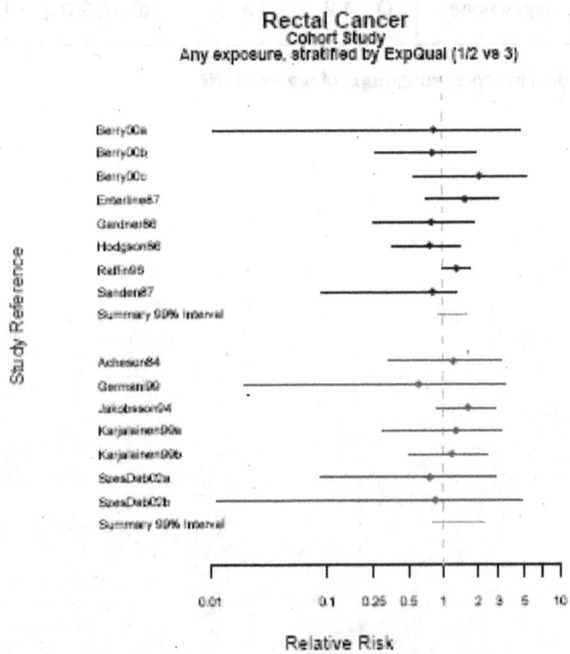

2. Results from case-control studies

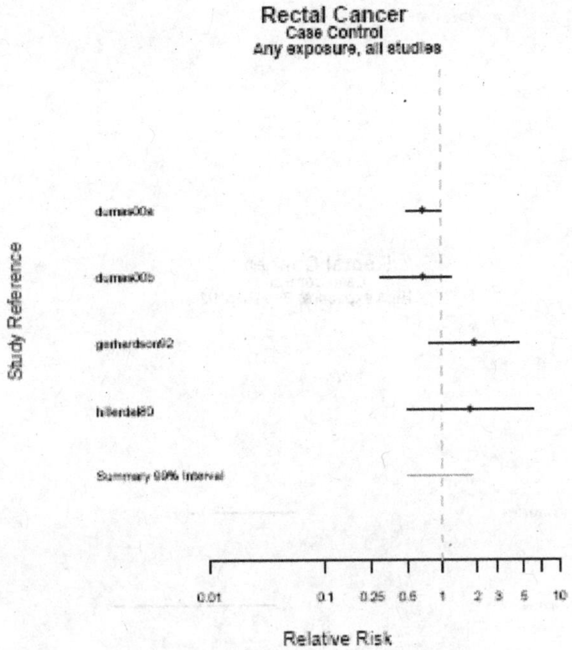

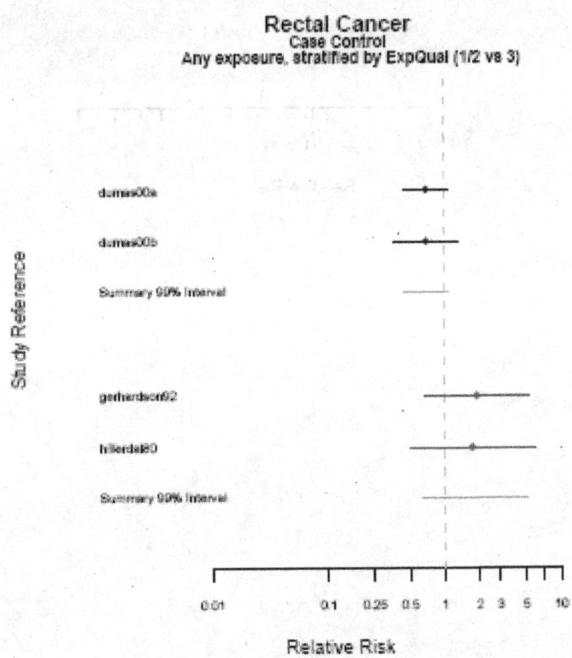

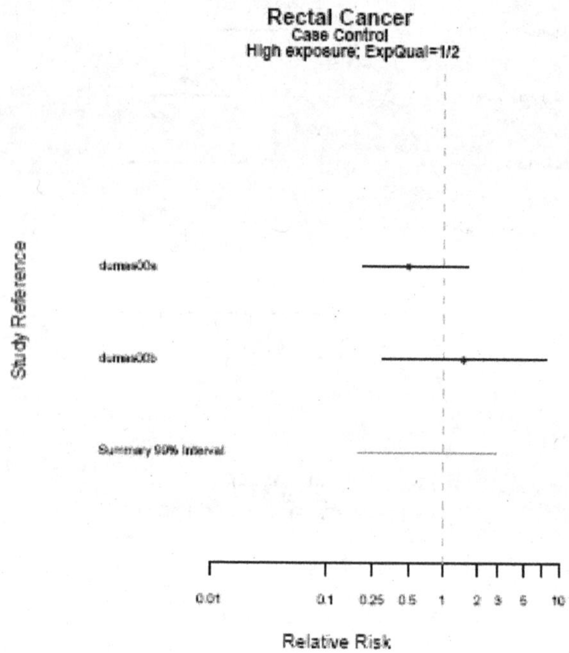
Rectal Cancer
Case Control
High exposure; ExpQual=1/2
Study Reference
dumas00a
dumas00b
Summary 99% Interval
0.01
0.1
0.25
0.5
1
2
3
5
10
Relative Risk

C. Results for colon or rectal cancer and asbestos exposure

COLORECTAL

Study Type	Plot	Comparison	Strata*	No. of Studies	99% CI for summary RR	Between study SD
CA-CO	1	Any v none	All	4	(0.69, 1.66)	.21
	2		EQ = 1,2	3	(0.63, 1.67)	.24
			EQ = 3	1		
	3		EQ = 1,2 Adjusted			
			EQ = 1,2 Unadjusted			
	4	High v none	EQ = 1,2	2	(0.18, 1.44)	.00
Cohort	1	Any v none	All	25	(0.96, 1.44)	.30
	2		EQ = 1,2	18	(.95, 1.56)	.51
			EQ = 3	7	(.69, 1.60)	.29
	3	High v none	EQ = 1,2 Use highest reported RR	9	(1.31, 2.53)	.00
			EQ = 1,2 Use lowest reported RR	9	(0.91, 2.70)	.33

* Not enough studies to report subgroups of adjusted RR.

1. Results from cohort studies

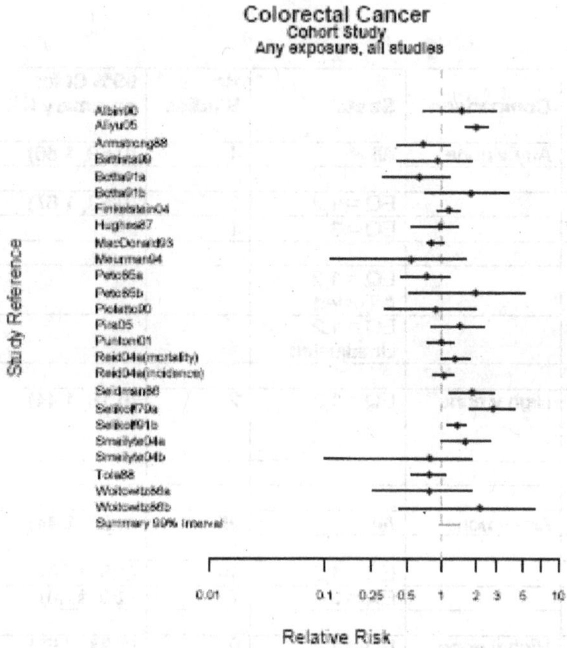

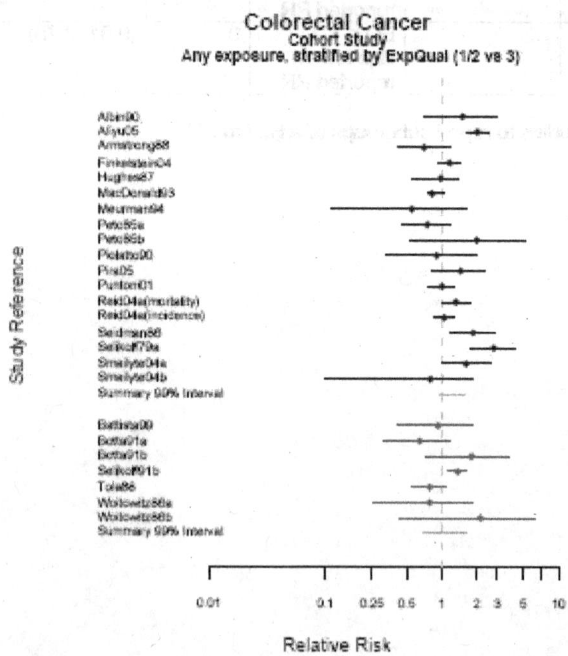

2. Results from case-control studies

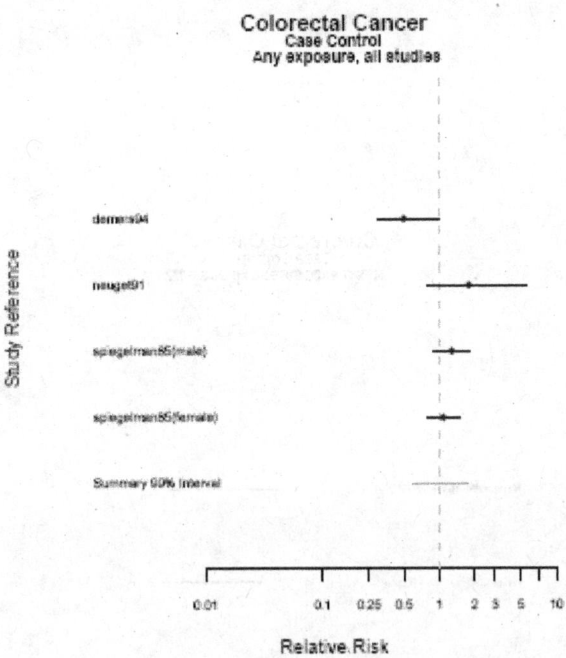

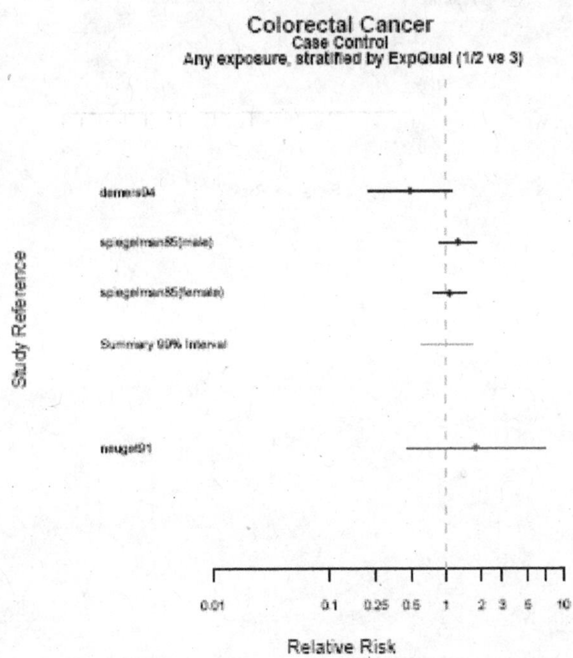

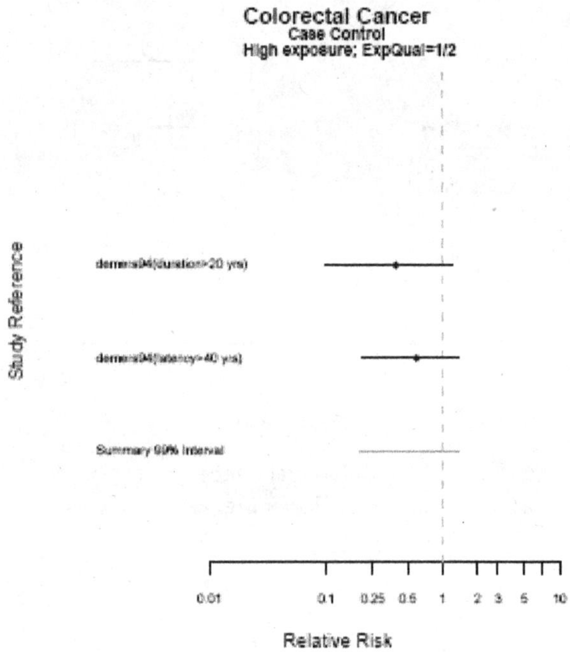
Colorectal Cancer
Case Control
High exposure; ExpQual=1/2
Study Reference
demers94(duration>20 yrs)
demers94(latency>40 yrs)
Summary 99% Interval
0.01
0.1
0.25
0.5
1
2
3
5
10
Relative Risk

APPENDIX G

Committee on Asbestos: Selected Health Effects

Jonathan M. Samet, M.D., M.S. (*Chair, IOM Member*), is professor and chairman of the Department of Epidemiology at the Johns Hopkins Bloomberg School of Public Health. He earned his M.D. from the University of Rochester School of Medicine and Dentistry and an M.S. in epidemiology from the Harvard School of Public Health. He is board-certified in internal medicine and the subspecialty of pulmonary disease. He was formerly professor and chief of the Pulmonary and Critical Care Division in the Department of Medicine at the University of New Mexico School of Medicine. He is past-president of the Society for Epidemiologic Research and the American College of Epidemiology. He has served on the US Environmental Protection Agency Science Advisory Board. He is an editor of *Epidemiology*. Dr. Samet was awarded the Surgeon General's Medallion in 1990. He has served in numerous National Academies committees, and chaired the National Research Council Committee on Health Risks of Exposure to Radon (BEIR VI) and the Committee on Research Priorities for Airborne Particulate Matter. He is also the chair of the Research Council's Board on Environmental Studies and Toxicology. He was elected to the Institute of Medicine (IOM) in 1997.

Lonnie R. Bristow, M.D., M.A.C.P. (*IOM Member*), was president of the American Medical Association (AMA), after earlier serving as vice chair and chair of the AMA's Board of Trustees. He is a board-certified internist and has practiced medicine for more than 30 years. Dr. Bristow's research interests and expertise are eclectic, and over the decades his writings have included papers on medical ethics, socialized medicine as practiced in Great

Britain and Canada, health-care financing in the United States, professional-liability insurance problems, sickle-cell anemia, and coronary-care unit use. Dr. Bristow recently retired from private practice, but continues his other activities as a professional consultant. In addition, he is a reviewer for the *Journal of the American Medical Association.* He was chair of IOM's Committee on the Quality of Health Care in America, which wrote the widely read reports *To Err Is Human* and *Crossing the Quality Chasm* in 1999 and 2001, respectively. Dr. Bristow was elected to IOM in 1978.

Harvey Checkoway, M.P.H., Ph.D., is professor in the Departments of Environmental and Health Sciences and of Epidemiology at the University of Washington School of Public Health and Community Medicine. He received his M.P.H. from Yale University and his doctorate in epidemiology from the University of North Carolina, Chapel Hill. His research and teaching are in occupational and environmental determinants of chronic diseases. Research projects for which Dr. Checkoway has been principal investigator include epidemiologic studies of cancer mortality in nuclear workers, cancer mortality in phosphate-industry workers, silicosis and lung cancer in silica-exposed diatomaceous-earth industry workers, lung cancer among chromate-exposed aerospace workers, reproductive hazards among lead-smelter workers, and environmental and genetic risk factors for Parkinson's disease.

Paul Demers, M.Sc., Ph.D., is associate professor at the University of British Columbia School of Occupational and Environmental Hygiene. He obtained his doctorate in epidemiology from the University of Washington. His research interests include occupational cancer, occupational respiratory disease, and occupational risk factors for sinonasal cancer. His current research projects concern cancer among sawmill workers exposed to wood dust and fungicides, occupational noise exposure, and the risk of injuries and heart disease among sawmill workers.

Ellen Eisen, M.S., Sc.D., is adjunct professor in the Department of Environmental Health at the Harvard School of Public Health and professor of epidemiology in the Department of Work Environment at the University of Massachusetts, Lowell. She received an M.S. in biostatistics, an Sc.D. in biostatistics and occupational health from the Harvard School of Public Health, and an M.S. in operations research and statistics from Massachusetts Institute of Technology. Dr. Eisen is interested in a variety of methodologic issues in occupational epidemiology, particularly new statistical methods to improve analysis of exposure-response data. She did early work toward standardizing measurement of pulmonary function for field studies. She has served on several National Academies committees.

George W. Guthrie, M.A., Ph.D., received his M.A. and doctorate in minerology-crystallography from Johns Hopkins University. He is a scientist at Los Alamos National Laboratory with the Geology and Geochemistry Group. His research interests include the health effects of minerals and concrete. Dr. Guthrie is interested in the mineralogic mechanisms that cause disease and is working to identify potential mineralogic properties important in disease, including mineral-catalyzed oxidation-reduction, cation exchange, and surface structure.

Rogene Henderson, Ph.D., D.A.B.T., is deputy director of the National Environmental Respiratory Center and senior biochemist and toxicologist at the Lovelace Respiratory Research Institute. Dr. Henderson also holds appointments as clinical professor of pharmacy at the University of New Mexico, Albuquerque, and as adjunct professor in the Departments of Veterinary Microbiology, Pathology, and Public Health at the School of Veterinary Medicine, Purdue University. She obtained her doctorate in chemistry from the University of Texas, was a Fulbright Scholar in physical chemistry at Ludwig Maximillians Universitaet in Munich, Germany, and is a Diplomate of the American Board of Toxicology. She has chaired the National Research Council (NRC) Subcommittee on Toxicological Hazard and Risk Assessment, Subcommittee on Pulmonary Toxicology, and standing Committee on Toxicology for six years, and she is currently a member of the Board on Environmental Studies and Toxicology. She has served as a member of the advisory council of the National Institute of Environmental Health Sciences (NIEHS) and the U.S. Environmental Protection Agency's (EPA) Science Advisory Board, Environmental Health Committee. Dr. Henderson has received numerous appointments on scientific advisory committees, including her current appointment as a member of the Health Effects Institute Research Committee. Dr. Henderson has done extensive research in the areas of lung biochemistry, the pharmacokinetics of inhaled toxins and their metabolites, and biological markers of exposure.

Joseph W. Hogan, M.S., Sc.D., is associate professor in the Bisostatistics Section and Center for Statistical Sciences Department of Community Medicine at Brown University. He received a master's degree in statistics from the University of Southern California and a doctorate in biostatistics from Harvard School of Public Health. His research interests include development of statistical methods for analyzing longitudinal data, for handling missing data, and for causal inference.

Agnes B. Kane, M.D., Ph.D., is professor and chair of the Department of Pathology and Laboratory Medicine at Brown University. She earned her M.D. and Ph.D. in experimental pathology at Temple University School of

Medicine and is board-certified in anatomic pathology. Her research has focused on mechanisms of fiber-induced toxicity, particularly on how asbestos produces mesotheliomas, using genetically engineered murine models, laser microdissection, and cDNA microarrays.

Fadlo R. Khuri, M.D., is professor in the Departments of Hematology, Oncology, Medicine, Pharmacology, and Otolaryngology at the Emory University School of Medicine. He is also associate director of clinical and translational research, chief medical officer, and director of the Aerodigestive Tract Cancer Program at the Winship Cancer Institute at Emory University. He received his M.D. from Columbia University and is board-certified in internal medicine, hematology, and medical oncology. Dr. Khuri's research focuses on molecular therapeutic and prognostic approaches to tobacco-related cancers. He has been involved in the development of novel agents for aerodigestive tract cancers and has conducted some early phase I and II studies. The goal of his research is to identify specific pathways for better molecular, prognostic, and chemopreventive approaches.

Roberta B. Ness, M.D., M.P.H., is professor and chair of the Department of Epidemiology at the University of Pittsburgh Graduate School of Public Health and director of the school's Epidemiology of Women's Health Program, the first university program of its kind in the United States. She received an M.D. from Cornell University and an M.P.H. from Columbia University. In her current position, she oversees a comprehensive effort to improve women's health through graduate-student education and research.

Michael J. Thun, M.D., M.S., is vice president of epidemiology and surveillance research at the American Cancer Society. He is also clinical professor of hematology and oncology at the Winship Cancer Institute at Emory University. He earned his M.D. from the University of Pennsylvania and his M.S. in epidemiology from the Harvard School of Public Health. Dr. Thun has a wide variety of research interests, including cancer-related aspects of smoking, aspirin and prostaglandins, alcohol abuse, heavy-metal toxicity (particularly cadmium, uranium, lead, and mercury), and occupational renal disease.

Assistants with Graphical Data

Li Su, Ph.D. candidate, Brown University
Yunxia Sui, Ph.D. candidate, Brown University

Staff

Rose Marie Martinez, Sc.D., is the director of the IOM Board on Population Health and Public Health Practices. Before joining IOM, she was senior health researcher at Mathematica Policy Research, where she studied the effects of health-system change on the public-health infrastructure, access to care for vulnerable populations, managed care, and the health-care workforce. Dr. Martinez is former assistant director of health financing and policy with the US General Accounting Office, for which she directed evaluations and policy analysis on national and public-health issues. Dr. Martinez received her doctorate from the Johns Hopkins School of Hygiene and Public Health.

Mary Burr Paxton, Ph.D., is a senior program officer in the IOM Board on Population Health and Public Health Practices. Before joining IOM, she worked as a consultant on the regulation of toxic substances and managed the conduct and analysis of several epidemiology studies on veterans' health. She received a master's of science in biostatistics from the Johns Hopkins School of Hygiene and Public Health and a doctorate in genetics from the George Washington University. She is a diplomate of the American Board of Toxicology. Dr. Paxton has worked on several National Academies reports, including *Issues in Risk Assessment, Environmental Neurotoxicology, Gulf War and Health: Insecticides and Solvents*, and *Gulf War and Health: Fuels, Combustion Products, and Propellants.*

Michael Schneider, M.P.H., is a senior program associate in the IOM Board on Population Health and Public Health Practices. He received his Masters in Public Health and an undergraduate degree in molecular and cellular biology from the University of Arizona. Michael has been with the IOM for over 5 years and has worked on several reports in the *Gulf War and Health* series.

Tia S. Carter, B.S., is a senior program assistant on the IOM Board on Population Health and Public Health Practices. She is working on a master's in health-care administration at the University of Maryland University College. She received her undergraduate degree in community health from the University of Maryland, College Park. Before coming to IOM, she worked at the Greater Washington Urban League in the Division of Aging and Health Services as the health promotions coordinator, where she was responsible for health-promotion and disease-prevention education services and activities among the elderly. *Asbestos: Selected Cancers* is Tia's first report with IOM.

